Atlas of Surgical Techniques in Trauma

Atlas of Surgical Techniques in Trauma

Edited by

Demetrios Demetriades MD PhD FACS

Professor of Surgery at the University of Southern California, and Director of Trauma, Emergency Surgery and Surgical Critical Care at the Los Angeles County and University of Southern California Medical Center, Los Angeles, California, USA

Kenji Inaba MD MSc FACS FRCSC

Associate Professor of Surgery and Emergency Medicine and Program Director for the Surgical Critical Care Fellowship and Surgery Residency at the University of Southern California, Los Angeles, California, USA

George Velmahos MD PhD FACS

John F. Burke Professor of Surgery at Harvard Medical School, and Chief of Trauma, Emergency Surgery and Surgical Critical Care at Massachusetts General Hospital, Boston, Massachusetts, USA

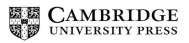

CAMBRIDGE
UNIVERSITY PRESS

CAMBRIDGE
UNIVERSITY PRESS

University Printing House, Cambridge CB2 8BS, United Kingdom

Cambridge University Press is part of the University of Cambridge.
It furthers the University's mission by disseminating knowledge in
the pursuit of education, learning and research at the highest
international levels of excellence.

www.cambridge.org
Information on this title: www.cambridge.org/9781107044593

© Cambridge University Press 2015

First published 2015

Printed in the United Kingdom by Bell and Bain Ltd

*A catalog record for this publication is available from the British
Library*

Library of Congress Cataloging in Publication data
Atlas of surgical techniques in trauma / edited by Demetrios
Demetriades, Kenji Inaba, George Velmahos.
      p. ; cm.
Includes index.
ISBN 978-1-107-04459-3 (Hardback)
I. Demetriades, Demetrios, 1951– , editor.   II. Inaba, Kenji, editor.
III. Velmahos, George C., editor.
[DNLM: 1. Wounds and Injuries–surgery–Atlases.   WO 517]
RD93
617.044–dc23   2014023642

ISBN 978-1-107-04459-3 Hardback

To my parents, my wife Elizabeth, my daughters Alexis and
Stefanie, and my son Nicky.
D. Demetriades

To my parents, wife Susie and son Koji, thank you for all of your support.
K. Inaba

To those who inspired me and those who allowed me to become a trauma
surgeon: my teachers and my parents.
G. Velmahos

Contents

List of contributors   ix
Preface   xi
Acknowledgments   xii
Introduction – Kenneth L. Mattox   xiii

Section 1 – Operating Room General Conduct

1. **Trauma operating room**   1
    Kenji Inaba and Lisa L. Schlitzkus

Section 2 – Resuscitative Procedures in the Emergency Room

2. **Cricothyrotomy**   5
    Peep Talving and Rondi Gelbard

3. **Thoracostomy tube insertion**   12
    Demetrios Demetriades and Lisa L. Schlitzkus

4. **Emergency room resuscitative thoracotomy**   18
    Demetrios Demetriades and Scott Zakaluzny

Section 3 – Head

5. **Insertion of intracranial pressure monitoring catheter**   29
    Howard Belzberg and Matthew D. Tadlock

6. **Evacuation of acute epidural and subdural hematomas**   35
    Gabriel Zada and Kazuhide Matsushima

Section 4 – Neck

7. **Neck operations for trauma: general principles**   47
    Emilie Joos and Kenji Inaba

8. **Carotid artery and internal jugular vein injuries**   53
    Edward Kwon, Daniel J. Grabo, and George Velmahos

9. **Subclavian vessels**   69
    Demetrios Demetriades and Jennifer Smith

10. **Axillary vessels**   83
    Demetrios Demetriades and Emilie Joos

11. **Vertebral artery injuries**   88
    Demetrios Demetriades and Nicholas Nash

12. **Trachea and larynx**   94
    Elizabeth R. Benjamin and Kenji Inaba

13. **Cervical esophagus**   101
    Elizabeth R. Benjamin and Kenji Inaba

Section 5 – Chest

14. **General principles of chest trauma operations**   107
    Demetrios Demetriades and Rondi Gelbard

15. **Cardiac injuries**   115
    Demetrios Demetriades and Scott Zakaluzny

16. **Thoracic vessels**   126
    Demetrios Demetriades and Stephen Varga

17. **Lung injuries**   140
    Demetrios Demetriades and Jennifer Smith

18. **Thoracic esophagus**   150
    Daniel Oh and Jennifer Smith

19. **Diaphragm injury**   162
    Lydia Lam and Matthew D. Tadlock

Section 6 – Abdomen

20. **General principles of abdominal operations for trauma**   165
    Heidi L. Frankel and Lisa L. Schlitzkus

21. **Damage control surgery**   172
    Mark Kaplan and Demetrios Demetriades

22. **Gastrointestinal tract**   180
    Kenji Inaba and Lisa L. Schlitzkus

23. **Duodenum**   189
Edward Kwon and Demetrios Demetriades

24. **Liver injuries**   198
Kenji Inaba and Kelly Vogt

25. **Splenic injuries**   209
Demetrios Demetriades and Matthew D. Tadlock

26. **Pancreas**   219
Demetrios Demetriades, Emilie Joos, and George Velmahos

27. **Urological trauma**   228
Charles Best and Stephen Varga

28. **Abdominal aorta and visceral branches**   240
Pedro G. Teixeira and Vincent L. Rowe

29. **Iliac injuries**   257
Demetrios Demetriades and Kelly Vogt

30. **Inferior vena cava**   262
Lydia Lam and Matthew D. Tadlock

Section 7 – Pelvis

31. **Surgical control of pelvic fracture hemorrhage**   273
Peep Talving and Matthew D. Tadlock

Section 8 – Upper Extremities

32. **Brachial artery injury**   281
Peep Talving and Elizabeth R. Benjamin

33. **Upper extremity fasciotomies**   288
Jennifer Smith and Mark W. Bowyer

34. **Upper extremity amputations**   294
Peep Talving and Scott Zakaluzny

Section 9 – Lower Extremities

35. **Femoral artery injuries**   303
George Velmahos and Rondi Gelbard

36. **Popliteal artery**   307
Peep Talving and Nicholas Nash

37. **Lower extremity amputations**   314
Peep Talving, Stephen Varga, and Jackson Lee

38. **Lower extremity fasciotomies**   323
Peep Talving, Elizabeth R. Benjamin, and
Daniel J. Grabo

Section 10 – Orthopedic Damage Control

39. **Orthopedic damage control**   337
Eric Pagenkopf, Daniel J. Grabo, and Peter Hammer

Index   345

Contributors

Howard Belzberg
Professor of Surgery, Division of Trauma,
Emergency Surgery and Surgical Critical Care,
University of Southern California, Los Angeles, CA, USA

Elizabeth R. Benjamin
Assistant Professor of Clinical Surgery, Division of Trauma,
Emergency Surgery and Surgical Critical Care,
University of Southern California, Los Angeles, CA, USA

Charles Best
Assistant Professor of Clinical Urology and Surgery and Chief
of Service, Department of Urology, Los Angeles County and
University of Southern California Medical Center,
Los Angeles, CA, USA

Mark W. Bowyer
Chief, Division of Trauma and Combat Surgery and Ben
Eisman Professor of Surgery, The Norman M. Rich
Department of Surgery, Uniformed Services University,
Bethesda, MD; Colonel (retired), United States Air Force, USA

Demetrios Demetriades
Professor of Surgery, University of Southern California;
Director of Trauma, Emergency Surgery and Surgical Critical
Care, Los Angeles County and University of Southern
California Medical Center, Los Angeles, CA, USA

Heidi L. Frankel
Professor of Surgery, Division of Trauma,
Emergency Surgery and Surgical Critical Care,
University of Southern California, Los Angeles, CA, USA

Rondi Gelbard
Clinical Instructor in Surgery, Division of Trauma,
Emergency Surgery and Surgical Critical Care,
University of Southern California, Los Angeles, CA, USA

Daniel J. Grabo
Assistant Professor of Clinical Surgery, Division of Trauma,
Emergency Surgery and Surgical Critical Care,
University of Southern California, Los Angeles, CA;
Lieutenant Commander, United States Navy, USA

Peter Hammer
Assistant Professor of Clinical Surgery,
Division of Trauma, Emergency Surgery and
Surgical Critical Care, University of Southern California,
Los Angeles, CA; Commander, Medical Corps, United States
Navy, USA

Kenji Inaba
Associate Professor, Surgery and Emergency Medicine and
Program Director, Surgical Critical Care Fellowship and
Surgery Residency, University of Southern California,
Los Angeles, CA, USA

Emilie Joos
Clinical Instructor, Division of Trauma, Emergency Surgery
and Surgical Critical Care, University of Southern California,
Los Angeles, CA, USA

Mark Kaplan
Professor of Surgery, Director of Trauma and Surgical
Critical Care and Director of Acute Care Surgery,
Albert Einstein Medical Center, Philadelphia, PA, USA

Edward Kwon
Assistant Professor of Clinical Surgery, Division of Trauma,
Emergency Surgery and Surgical Critical Care,
University of Southern California, Los Angeles, CA, USA

Lydia Lam
Assistant Professor of Surgery, Division of Trauma,
Emergency Surgery and Surgical Critical Care,
University of Southern California, Los Angeles, CA, USA

Jackson Lee
Associate Professor of Clinical Medicine,
Department of Orthopedics, Keck School of Medicine,
Los Angeles, CA, USA

Kazuhide Matsushima
Surgical Critical Care Fellow, Division of Trauma,
Emergency Surgery and Surgical Critical Care,
University of Southern California, Los Angeles,
CA, USA

Nicholas Nash
Clinical Instructor, Division of Trauma,
Emergency Surgery and Surgical Critical Care,
University of Southern California, Los Angeles, CA, USA

Daniel Oh
Assistant Professor of Surgery, Department of Thoracic
Surgery, University of Southern California,
Los Angeles, CA, USA

Eric Pagenkopf
Assistant Professor in Orthopedics and Director,
Navy Trauma Training Center, Los Angeles County and
University of Southern California Medical Center,
Los Angeles, CA; Captain (Retired), United States Navy, USA

Vincent L. Rowe
Professor of Surgery, Division of Vascular Surgery,
University of Southern California, Los Angeles, CA, USA

Lisa L. Schlitzkus
Surgical Critical Care Fellow, Division of Trauma,
Emergency Surgery and Surgical Critical Care,
University of Southern California, Los Angeles, CA, USA

Jennifer Smith
Assistant Professor of Surgery, Division of Trauma,
Emergency Surgery and Surgical Critical Care,
University of Southern California, Los Angeles, CA, USA

Matthew D. Tadlock
Clinical Instructor in Surgery, Division of Trauma, Emergency
Surgery and Surgical Critical Care, University of Southern
California, Los Angeles, CA; Lieutenant Commander, Medical
Corps, United States Navy, USA

Peep Talving
Assistant Professor of Surgery, Division of Trauma,
Emergency Surgery and Surgical Critical Care,
University of Southern California, Los Angeles, CA, USA

Pedro G. Teixeira
Surgical Critical Care Fellow, Division of Trauma,
Emergency Surgery and Surgical Critical Care,
University of Southern California, Los Angeles, CA, USA

Stephen Varga
Clinical Instructor, Division of Trauma,
Emergency Surgery and Surgical Critical Care,
University of Southern California, Los Angeles, CA;
Major, United States Air Force, USA

George Velmahos
John F. Burke Professor of Surgery, Harvard Medical School;
Chief of Trauma, Emergency Surgery and Surgical Critical
Care, Massachusetts General Hospital, Boston,
Massachusetts, USA

Kelly Vogt
Clinical Instructor in Surgery, Division of Trauma,
Emergency Surgery and Surgical Critical Care,
University of Southern California, Los Angeles, CA, USA

Gabriel Zada
Assistant Professor of Clinical Neurosurgery,
University of Southern California, Los Angeles, CA, USA

Scott Zakaluzny
Clinical Instructor in Surgery, Division of Trauma,
Emergency Surgery and Surgical Critical Care,
University of Southern California, Los Angeles, CA, USA

Preface

The aim of this *Atlas of Surgical Techniques in Trauma* is to provide a valuable companion in the operating room to the surgeons who provide care to the injured. It is designed to be a rapid, highly visual summary of the critical anatomy, procedural sequencing, and pitfalls associated with these procedures, ideal for trainees as well as for those in practice, as a rapid review of both common and uncommonly performed procedures prior to proceeding to the operating room.

The atlas is organized into chapters and sections according to anatomical areas. It includes more than 630 high-quality photographs and illustrations and is written in a reader-friendly format, which includes practical surgical anatomy, general principles, exposure, definitive management, and technical tips and pitfalls. It guides the surgeon, step by step, through the entire procedure, from incision to closure.

What makes this atlas unique is the use of images obtained from fresh, perfused, and ventilated human cadavers. Many hundreds of hours were spent in the USC Fresh Tissue Dissection Lab for this project. The critical aspects of each surgical exposure and procedure are clearly demonstrated in these high-fidelity models, allowing the reader to rapidly understand the technical key points, which are often difficult to convey using words alone. The extensive real-world clinical experience of the editors and senior authors in managing complex injuries at large trauma centers, combined with these high-quality operative photos and technical illustrations make this atlas an important tool in the armamentarium of the practicing surgeon.

Demetrios Demetriades, Kenji Inaba, and George Velmahos

Acknowledgments

The editors and authors greatly acknowledge the major contributions of Alexis Demetriades, Scientific Illustrator; Michael Minneti and Andrew Cervantes for coordinating and helping with the anatomical dissections and photos in the Fresh Tissue Dissection Lab.

Introduction

A contemporary focused *Atlas* of surgical techniques in trauma has been a much needed adjunct to the didactic textbooks, conferences and symposia, and other instructional material available in the field of acute care surgery and trauma. Although adjunctive descriptors have been part of many monographs and formal textbooks on the subject of trauma techniques, this unique atlas will significantly aid all who care for injured patients.

This book is *Unique* in a number of aspects. It is a work product of a single group of physicians who are, or have been in the past, in the faculty of a single institution with a singular approach to most operative techniques in this field. The surgeons in this institution, Los Angeles County & Southern California Medical Center in Los Angeles, also have integrated their educational material using human cadaver material in a standardized and innovative approach. The cadaver anatomic material is correlated in a standardized manner, facilitating an appreciation of the dynamics of exposure, control, and management. Anatomic drawings benefit the detailed learner during course instruction as well as the surgeon seeking rapid review at the time of an urgent operation. Once the reader recognizes the standardized approach to teaching, progressing through any chapter or subject in the atlas is quick and easy. This atlas material is also very amenable to small portable electronic devices, allowing a ready source for anatomy correlations, exposure recommendations, and reconstruction details – anywhere and at any time.

This *Atlas* is *Not* simply a collection of drawings. It is an Atlas textbook of techniques. It is a philosophy of surgical approaches – "a recipe." It is the type of book that would/ should have been shared with the learner by his/her mentor very early on. It is like bedtime reading – to be enthusiastically rendered to an enthusiastic recipient. It is the type of standardized material that is easily remembered and recalled because of its unique presentation.

Finally, any user of this atlas must grant me some moments of historic reflection and confession. Although I spent much of my medical school days trying to impress by taking detailed lecture notes, subscribing to and "fake reading" the *New England Journal of Medicine*, buying the recommended detailed long textbooks on the subject *de jour*, and trying to remain awake in my usual seat in the third row of the lecture room, my medical school and residency life suddenly became productively alive when I discovered the *Surgical Technique* atlases in the library. I avidly consumed these books. They were always huge and could not easily be carried around, but I managed to do just that. Becoming a surgical resident, I purchased and still own the ("big names") popular surgical technique atlases of the day (1967–1971). As the big names stopped producing new atlases with their wonderful artwork, they became historic memories on the shelves of my office. For decades, I could find no quality renewals or replacements. Now, with this well-organized, standardized, focused **Atlas of Surgical Techniques in Trauma,** those experiences no longer will be mere memories. Thank you, Demetrios and your wonderful team of artists, pathologists, and surgeons for this beautiful and innovative atlas and for the incredible learning experience it will give all caring for injured patients.

Kenneth L. Mattox, MD, FACS
Distinguished Service Professor Baylor College of Medicine
Chief of Staff/Chief of Surgery
Ben Taub General Hospital
Houston

Chapter

1

Trauma operating room

Kenji Inaba and Lisa L. Schlitzkus

Operating room

- A large operating room (OR) situated near the emergency department, elevators, and ICU should be designated as the Trauma OR to facilitate the logistics of patient flow and minimize transport. The room should be securable for high profile patients.
- A contingency plan for multiple simultaneous operations should be in place with the operating rooms in sufficient proximity to allow nursing and anesthesia cross-coverage and facilitate supervision of the surgical teams. Direct lines of communication between the OR and the resuscitation area, ICU,

other ORs, blood bank, and laboratory should be in place.
- All rooms should have ample overhead lighting as well as access to portable headlamps.
- Multiple monitors to display imaging, vital signs, and laboratory data such as thromboelastometry should be in place.
- Hybrid operating and interventional radiology suites are ideal. Both the surgical and radiology teams should be familiar with operating in the hybrid room.
- A dedicated family waiting room should be identified, and all family should be directed to this area for the postoperative discussion.

Atlas of Surgical Techniques in Trauma, ed. Demetrios Demetriades, Kenji Inaba, and George Velmahos. Published by Cambridge University Press. © Cambridge University Press 2015.

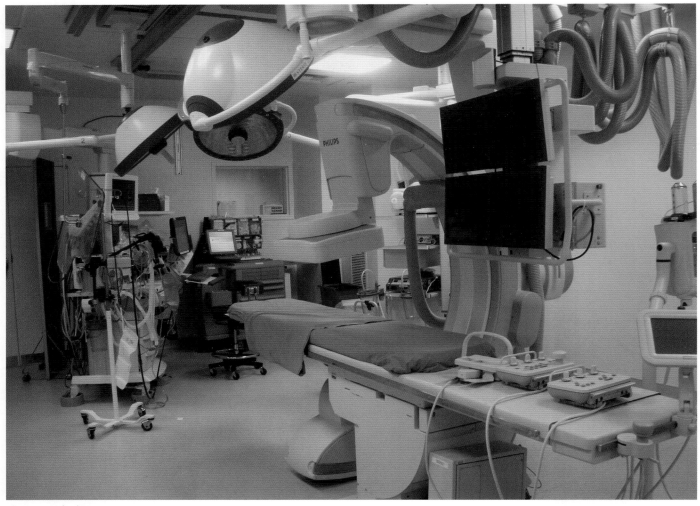

Fig. 1.1. Hybrid operating room setup.

Setup and equipment

- Nursing staff should be regularly in-serviced about the trauma room setup, supplies, and common practices such as massive transfusion to minimize problems due to service line cross-coverage.
- While all attempts should be made to count instruments and ensure a correct final count, this may be postponed in life-threatening or damage control situations. Radio-frequency ID device embedded laparotomy sponges are a useful adjunct to these emergency situations.

The following should be readily available:
- instrument trays including laparotomy, sternotomy with pneumatic sternal saw, thoracotomy, emergency airway, amputation, and peripheral vascular
- a wide selection of vascular shunts, catheters, vascular conduits, chest tubes, drains, staplers, local hemostatic agents, advanced thermal cutting devices, and temporary abdominal closure supplies

- standard suture tree including sternal closure wires, vascular sutures, and liver sutures
- adult and pediatric code cart
- high volume suction canister and device
- tourniquets
- endotracheal tube occluders
- rigid sigmoidoscope, bronchoscope, gastroscope
- portable fluoroscopy and personnel shielding devices should be immediately available for use in the OR
- an electrothermal bipolar vessel sealing system device (LigaSure device) is desirable.

Warming

- Due to the large surface area exposed, trauma patients are susceptible to hypothermia.
- The room should not be cold.
- Forced air blankets should be used.
- Warmed intravenous fluids should be available at all times.
- All irrigation fluids should be warmed.

Blood

- A type and screen should be sent immediately to the laboratory upon patient arrival to the emergency department.
- Emergency release products (uncross-matched O− or O+ packed red blood cells as well as thawed AB or low titer A plasma) should be readily available in the emergency department and in the operating room.
- A rapid transfusion device should be available.

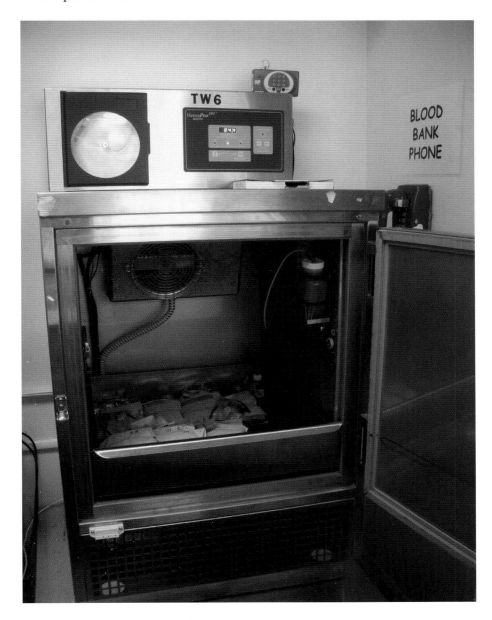

Fig. 1.2. Emergency release blood products stored in a refrigerator in the emergency department or operating room available for immediate use. Can contain uncrossed matched O+ or O− packed red blood cells and AB or low titer A plasma.

Chapter

2

Cricothyrotomy

Peep Talving and Rondi Gelbard

Surgical anatomy

- The cricothyroid membrane lies between the cricoid and thyroid cartilage and is bordered laterally by the cricothyroid muscles. In adults it is about 1 cm in height and about 2–3 cm wide, including the area covered by the two cricothyroid muscles. The actual membrane between the two muscles is approximately 1 cm wide.
- The cricoid cartilage is the only complete ring in the trachea. It serves as a stent supporting the airway and is an important attachment point for muscles and ligaments.

- The vocal cords are attached to the internal anterior surface of the thyroid cartilage, about 1 cm from the upper border of the cricothyroid membrane.
- Localizing the cricothyroid membrane rapidly can be critical in managing the difficult airway. If soft tissue trauma or obesity prevents clear identification of the thyroid and cricoid cartilage, with the neck in neutral position, place the tip of the small finger of the extended hand in the suprasternal notch. The tip of the index finger will touch the cricothyroid membrane in the midline.

(a)

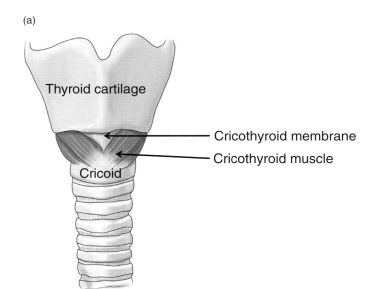

(b)

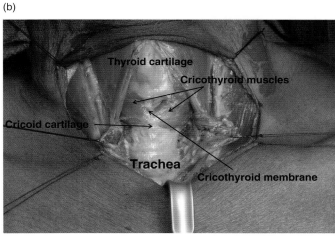

Fig. 2.1(a), (b). Anatomy of the cricothyroid space. The cricothyroid space includes the inferior border of the thyroid cartilage and the superior rim of the cricoid arch that are connected by the cricothyroid membrane, and are partially covered by the cricothyroid muscles.

Atlas of Surgical Techniques in Trauma, ed. Demetrios Demetriades, Kenji Inaba, and George Velmahos. Published by Cambridge University Press. © Cambridge University Press 2015.

(a)

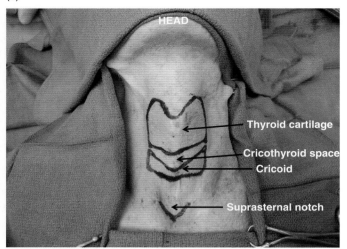

Fig. 2.2(a). Surface anatomy of the cricothyroid space. The cricothyroid space includes the inferior border of the thyroid cartilage and the superior rim of the cricoid arch. In adults the cricothyroid membrane is about 1 cm in height and about 2–3 cm wide.

(b)

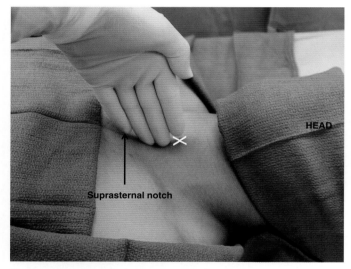

Fig. 2.2(b). Photograph demonstrating the four-finger technique for identifying the cricothyroid membrane. With the palm extended, the tip of the small finger is placed in the suprasternal notch. The tip of the index finger touches the cricothyroid membrane in the midline (x).

General principles

- Cricothyrotomy is indicated in patients requiring emergent airway management who cannot be intubated by the oral or nasal route, and cannot be oxygenated with alternative rescue techniques such as the Laryngeal mask airway, or Combitube. Severe maxillofacial trauma, or edema of the glottis are common conditions requiring cricothyrotomy.
- Cricothyrotomy is relatively contraindicated in patients under 8 years of age, because of the small size of the cricothyroid membrane and propensity to develop post-procedure stenosis. In these pediatric patients, needle jet

insufflation should be considered. For patients with suspected tracheal transection, this procedure should also be avoided.

- There is no evidence to support routine conversion of a cricothyrotomy to a formal tracheostomy.

Special instruments

- The open cricothyrotomy instrument set should include endotracheal and tracheostomy tubes (size 6 French), scalpel, tracheal hook, Senn retractors, Kelly clamp, Metzenbaum scissors, and forceps.
- Suction with an endoluminal suction catheter attachment.
- Alternatively, commercially available percutaneous cricothyrotomy sets can also be used.
- End-tidal CO_2 detector should be available.
- Adequate lighting.

(a)

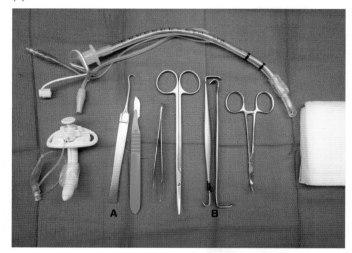

Fig. 2.3(a). Open cricothyrotomy instrument set should include endotracheal and tracheostomy tubes, scalpel, tracheal hook (A), Senn retractors (B), Kelly clamp, Metzenbaum scissors, and forceps.

(b)

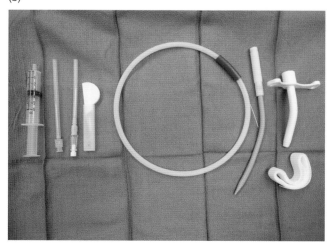

Fig. 2.3(b). Commercial percutaneous cricothyrotomy set.

Patient positioning

- Supine, with the neck in neutral position if the cervical spine has not been cleared. If cleared, the neck should be extended to facilitate this procedure.

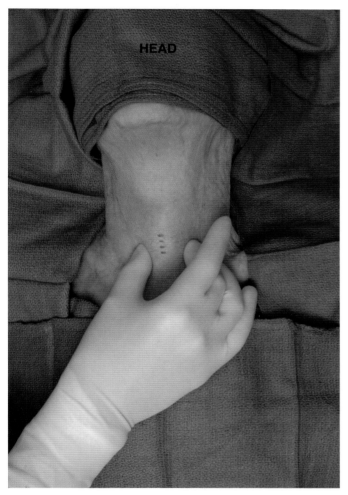

Fig. 2.4. The neck is in neutral or slightly extended position. The trachea is immobilized between the thumb and middle finger of the non-dominant hand to prevent lateral movement of the trachea during the procedure. The index finger may be used to palpate the cricothyroid space.

Technique
Percutaneous cricothyrotomy

- Begin with a 5 mm long vertical skin incision. In patients with a short and thick neck it may be difficult to palpate the cricothyroid membrane. The "four-fingers technique" as described above can help identify the cricothyroid space. This will localize the area where the initial skin incision should be made. Once the skin incision is made, re-examine the anatomy. Once the skin is breached, the underlying structures will become easier to localize. The skin incision must be sufficiently large to allow entry of the tube. Insufficient incision length is a common pitfall.
- Stabilize the thyroid cartilage between the thumb and the middle finger of the non-dominant hand to facilitate palpation of the anatomical landmarks and immobilize the airway during the procedure.
- With the dominant hand, insert the needle into the cricothyroid membrane directed caudally at a 45° angle. If time is available, the needle can be attached to a syringe that is filled with normal saline to visualize entry into the airway.
- As the needle is advanced, apply negative pressure to the syringe.
- Advance the needle until it traverses the membrane and enters the trachea, signaled by a distinct pop and aspiration of air. If saline was placed in the syringe, bubbles will be seen.
- Remove the needle and syringe, leaving the catheter in place. Advance the guide wire through the catheter. The catheter can then be removed.
- Place the dilator into the airway catheter, and insert both the dilator and catheter together over the guidewire, ensuring that guidewire is not advancing with the cannula/ dilator complex.
- Remove both the dilator and the guidewire once the airway tube is secured in the trachea.
- Secure the tube in place.

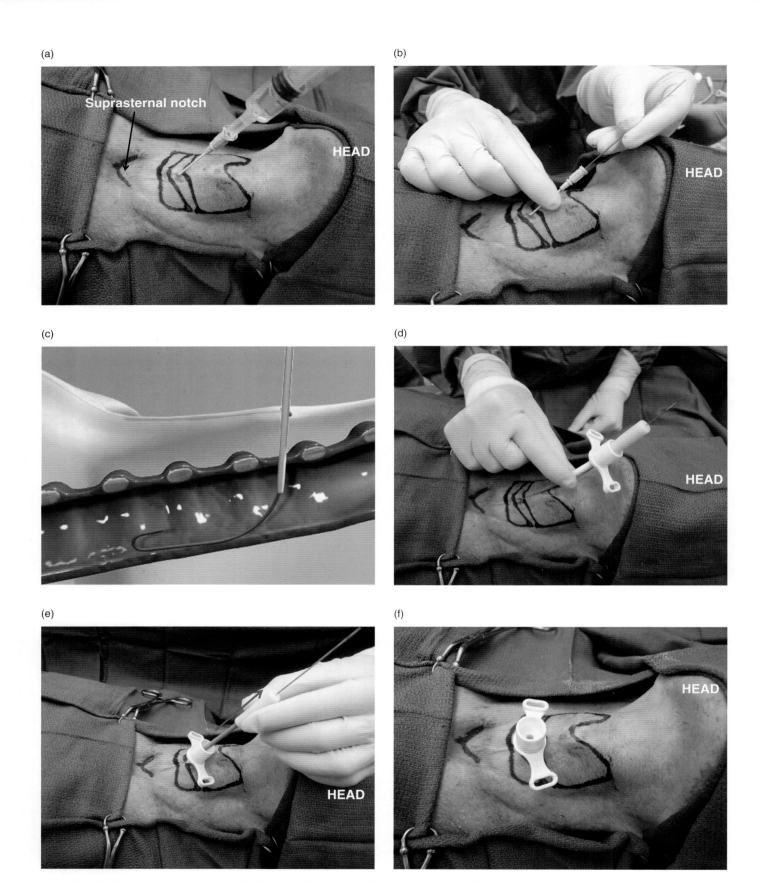

Fig. 2.5(a)–(f). Technique of percutaneous cricothyrotomy. The finder needle attached to a saline-filled syringe is inserted into the cricothyroid membrane, directed caudally at a 45° angle to avoid puncturing the posterior wall of the trachea. The needle and syringe are removed, leaving the small catheter in place. The guidewire is advanced through the catheter, and the catheter is removed once the guidewire is in place (b) and (c). The assembled dilator and airway catheter are inserted together, over the guidewire, into the trachea (d); the guidewire and dilator are removed once the airway tube has been secured (e); airway cannula in place (f).

Open cricothyrotomy

- With the non-dominant hand, stabilize the thyroid cartilage between the thumb and index finger.
- With the dominant hand, make a 3 cm midline vertical incision over the cricothyroid membrane. A transverse incision is an acceptable option, but a vertical incision is preferred because there is a decreased risk of bleeding from the anterior jugular veins and the incision is more versatile as it can easily be extended.
- Utilize the thumb and index finger of the non-dominant hand that is stabilizing the cartilage to retract the skin,

exposing the cricothyroid membrane. Senn retractors can be utilized for exposure if an assistant is available.

- Make a horizontal stab incision through the cricothyroid membrane.
- If practical, perform the incision in the lower half of the cricothyroid membrane, along the superior border of the cricoid cartilage, in order to avoid injuring the cricothyroid artery which courses through the superior half of the cricothyroid membrane.
- Insert the tracheal hook at the superior end of the cricothyroid incision and retract the thyroid cartilage cephalad.

(a)

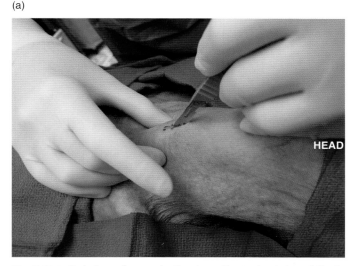

Fig. 2.6(a). Technique of open cricothyrotomy. The trachea is immobilized with the non-dominant hand. A 3-cm midline vertical skin incision is performed over the cricothyroid membrane.

(b)

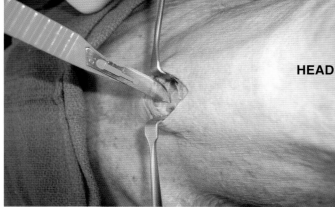

Fig. 2.6(b). A horizontal incision is made through the cricothyroid membrane to enter the trachea. This incision should be made in the lower half of the cricothyroid membrane, along the superior border of the cricoid cartilage, in order to avoid injuring the cricothyroid artery.

(c)

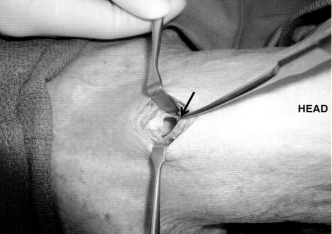

(d)

Fig. 2.6(c), (d). Following entry into the trachea, a tracheal hook is placed at the edge of the thyroid cartilage (arrow), and firm retraction is applied upward and toward the head (c). Alternatively, the tracheal hook may be placed inferiorly, on the cricoid ring with traction toward the patient's chest (d). The skin incision is retracted laterally, with Senn retractors.

- With the dominant hand, insert the cricothyrotomy tube into the trachea.
- Having the obturator in place will aid in this process. Once seated in the airway, the obturator is removed and the inner cannula can be inserted.
- Inflate the balloon with 5–10 mL of air, and confirm placement with observation of chest rise, auscultation, and assessment of end-tidal CO_2.
- Secure the tube in place and clear the airway of blood and secretions by suctioning through the cricothyrotomy tube.

(e)

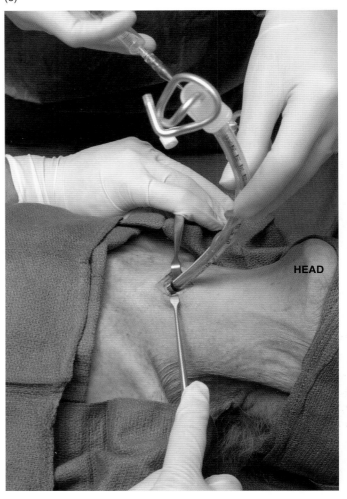

(f)

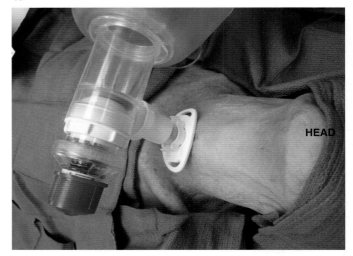

Fig. 2.6(e), (f). Insertion of the airway cannula in a caudal direction. Airway access is obtained, and appropriate location of the airway cannula is ensured with end-tidal CO_2.

Tips and pitfalls

- A cricothyrotomy may be a difficult procedure in patients with a short and thick neck.
- In obese patients, it is often difficult to palpate the cricothyroid space. In these cases, the cricothyroid membrane is usually located four finger breadths above the suprasternal notch (the "four fingers" trick). Once the skin incision is made, the underlying structures become easier to palpate.
- Reduce the risk of bleeding from the anterior jugular veins by performing a vertical skin incision.
- If the skin incision is too low, the thyroid isthmus is in the way and its division may cause bleeding.
- An insufficient skin incision is often the primary obstruction to smooth insertion of the tube into the airway.
- Incorrect placement of the tube into the subcutaneous tissues can be mitigated by immobilization of the thyroid cartilage with a tracheal hook and direct visualization of tube entry into the airway.
- The thyrohyoid space may be mistaken for the cricothyroid space and the tube is inserted too high. In order to avoid this complication, both the thyroid cartilage and cricoid ring should be clearly identified.
- Posterior tracheal wall perforation is a serious complication. Avoid pushing any instruments or the tube in the anteroposterior direction. Instead, follow the direction of the trachea.
- Cricothyrotomy can be utilized in adults for prolonged airway access with a low incidence of subglottic stenosis. The authors do not advocate routine conversion of a cricothyrotomy to a tracheostomy.
- In pediatric patients consider using needle jet insufflation rather than cricothyrotomy.

Chapter

3

Thoracostomy tube insertion

Demetrios Demetriades and Lisa L. Schlitzkus

General principles

- Strict antiseptic precautions and personal protective equipment should be used during the procedure. A single dose of prophylactic antibiotics with Cefazolin should be administered before the procedure. There is no need for further prophylaxis.
- Chest tubes can be inserted with an open or percutaneous dilational technique.
- The site of insertion is the same for open or percutaneous insertion and for hemothorax or pneumothorax at the fourth or fifth intercostal space, at or above the level of the nipple in males.
- Autotransfusion should be considered in all cases with large hemothoraces.

Positioning

The patient should be placed in the supine position with the arm abducted at 90 degrees and elbow fully extended or flexed at 90 degrees cephalad. Adduction and internal rotation of the arm is a suboptimal position and should not be used.

Site of tube insertion

- Fourth or fifth intercostal space, mid axillary line. The external landmark is at, or slightly above, the nipple level in males and at the inframammary fold in females. Insertion at this site is optimal due to the relatively thin chest wall and distance from the diaphragm, which during expiration can easily reach the sixth intercostal space.

(a)

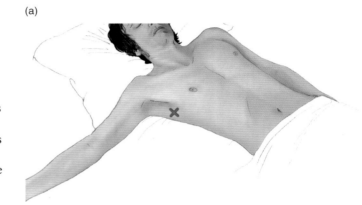

(b)

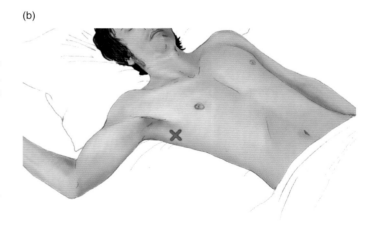

Fig. 3.1 (a)–(c). The patient should be placed in the supine position with the arm abducted at 90 degrees and elbow fully extended (a) or flexed cephalad at 90 degrees. The insertion site should be in the fourth or fifth intercostal space at the mid axillary line, at or slightly above the nipple level (b). Adduction and internal rotation of the arm is a suboptimal position and should not be used (c).

(c)

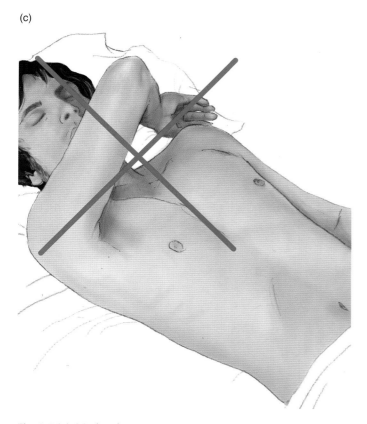

Fig. 3.1 (a)–(c). (*cont.*)

Open technique

- Usual thoracostomy tube sizes for adults are 28–32 Fr; there is no advantage to using larger tubes. For pediatric cases, refer to the Broselow tape.
- After local anesthetic is injected in the skin, soft tissue, and along the periosteum, a 1.5–2.0 cm incision is made through the skin and subcutaneous fat. The greater the soft tissue thickness, the longer the skin incision should be. An inadequate incision can compromise safe and accurate placement in the obese patient.
- A Kelly forceps is used to enter the pleural cavity. Dissection should be kept close to the upper edge of the rib to avoid injury to the intercostal vessels. The Kelly forceps is inserted into the pleural cavity in a controlled manner to avoid injury to the intrathoracic organs.
- There is no need for subcutaneous tunneling as it is painful and does not reduce the risk of empyema or air leak.
- A finger should be inserted into the pleural cavity, and swept 360 degrees to evaluate for adhesions and avoid intrapulmonary placement of the tube.
- The tube is grasped with a clamp through its distal fenestration. The distal end of the tube is clamped to avoid uncontrolled drainage of blood. The tube is firmly inserted into the pleural cavity. As soon as it enters the cavity, the clamp is released and withdrawn, while the tube is advanced in a twisting fashion towards the apex and posteriorly. Make sure that all of the tube fenestrations are in the pleural cavity. In an adult patient the tube should be inserted to 8–10 cm. Alternatively, the tube can be inserted without a clamp into the pleural cavity alongside the index finger of the non-dominant hand, which is then used to guide the tube posteriorly towards the apex. If the tube does not slide in smoothly, the tip may be caught in a fissure or by lung parenchyma. The tube should be withdrawn and re-inserted to prevent injury to the lung or other mediastinal structures.

- When the tube is in place, it should be rotated 360 degrees to prevent inappropriate kinking. If the tube does not rotate freely, it should be pulled back slightly and rotated again.

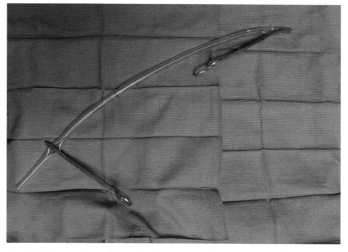

Fig. 3.2. Preparation of the chest tube: the tube is grasped with a clamp through its distal fenestration. The distal end of the tube (left) is clamped to avoid splashing of blood.

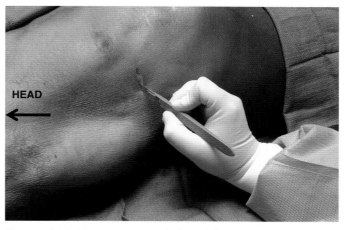

Fig. 3.3. A 1.5–2.0 cm incision is made through the skin and subcutaneous fat, in the fourth or fifth intercostal space at the mid axillary line.

(a)

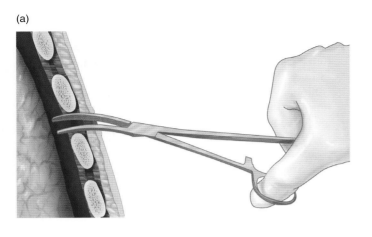

(b)

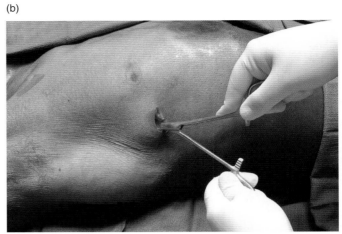

Fig. 3.4(a),(b). Kelly forceps are used to enter the pleural cavity just over the top of the rib. Spreading of the subcutaneous fat and tissue occurs as the Kelly clamp is withdrawn from the pleural cavity.

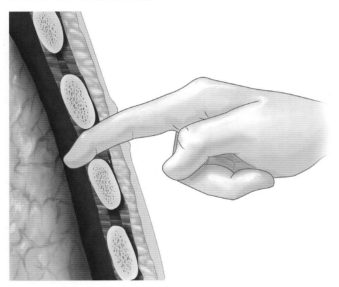

Fig. 3.5. Digital exploration of the pleural cavity to rule out adhesions.

(a)

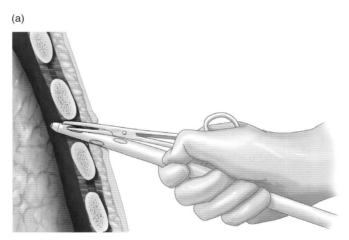

Fig. 3.6(a),(b). The tube is grasped with a Kelly clamp through its distal fenestration and is firmly forced into the pleural cavity.

(c)

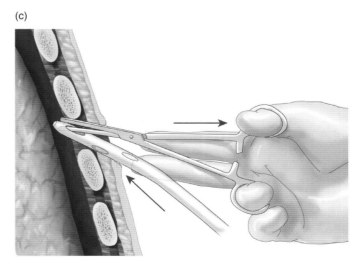

Fig. 3.6(c). When the tip of the tube enters the cavity, the clamp is released and withdrawn, while the tube is advanced in a twisting fashion towards the apex and posteriorly.

(b)

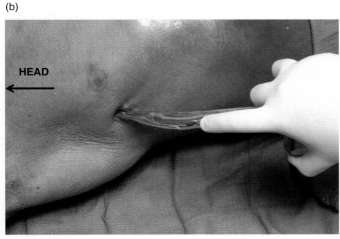

HEAD

Fig. 3.6(a),(b). (cont.)

(d)

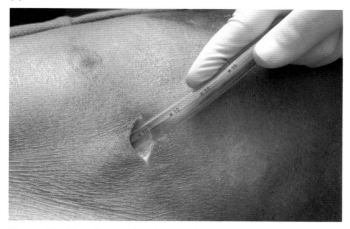

Fig. 3.6(d). Chest drain in place (in normal-weight adults, no more than 8–10 cm of the drain should be inserted into the chest).

- Connect tube to an underwater chest drainage collection system and apply wall suction at −20 cm H_2O.
- Secure tube with 0 silk. Encourage the patient to cough while sitting up, lying on their back and sides in order to promote blood drainage and lung re-expansion.
- If the incision at the insertion site is too long, it should be closed around the tube with interrupted sutures. A horizontal mattress suture may be placed around the tube and left untied to be used for wound closure at the time of tube removal. The tube is further secured to the thoracic wall with adhesive tape.

Percutaneous technique

- Less painful than the open technique.
- After infiltrating the area with local anesthetic, an introducer needle attached to a syringe with sterile saline is inserted into the chest cavity. Insert close to the upper border of the rib to avoid injury to the intercostal vessels, which are located at the inferior border of the rib. Aim slightly posterior and towards the apex of the lung. Entry into the pleural cavity is confirmed by aspiration of blood or air bubbles.
- Insert the guidewire through the needle. Remove the needle while keeping the guidewire in place. Make a skin incision over the needle that is slightly larger than the diameter of the chest tube. Remove needle.
- Insert the dilator over the guidewire.
- Remove dilator and insert the chest tube (8–10 cm) over the guidewire.
- Remove the guidewire, connect to the collection system, and secure the tube on the skin.
- Obtain chest X-ray.

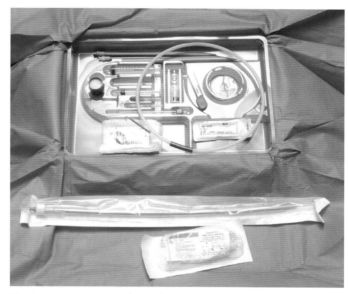

Fig. 3.7. A percutaneous chest tube tray.

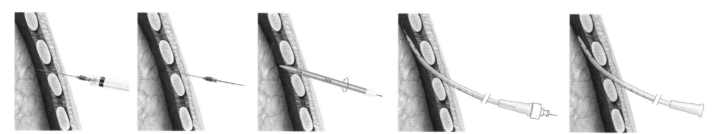

Fig. 3.8. The percutaneous dilational insertion of chest tube utilizes the Seldinger guidewire technique with progressive dilation.

(a)   (b)   (c)

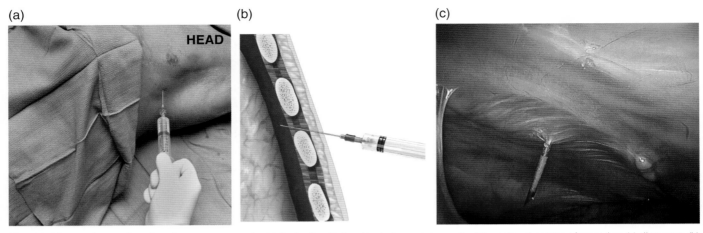

Fig. 3.9. The step-by-step insertion of a percutaneous chest tube by the dilational technique: photograph of the external portion of procedure (a), illustration (b), thoracoscopic view (c). The introducer needle with a syringe with saline is used to confirm entrance into the thorax with the return of blood or air bubbles. It is inserted in the fourth or fifth intercostal space, just above the rib to avoid injury to the neurovascular bundle.

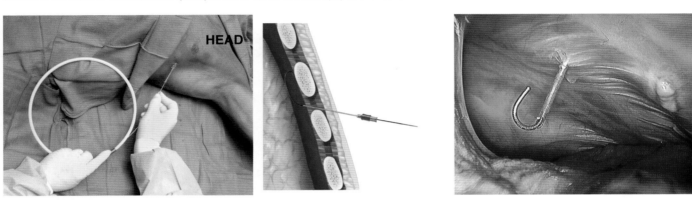

Fig. 3.10. A guidewire is inserted through the introducer needle and the needle is removed.

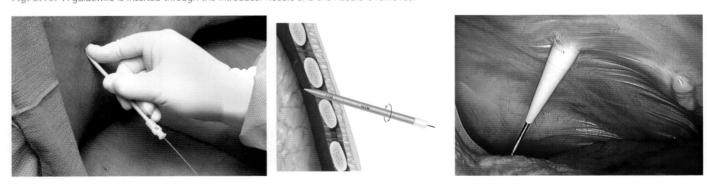

Fig. 3.11. Using the Seldinger technique, the tract is sequentially dilated after making a small skin incision for the tube.

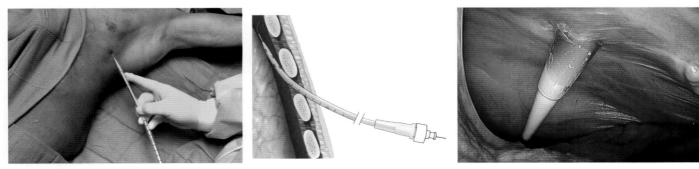

Fig. 3.12. The tube is passed into the thoracic cavity over the guidewire.

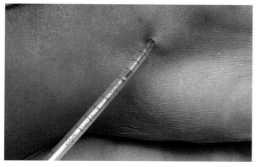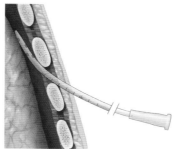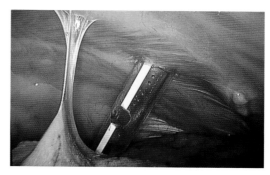

Fig. 3.13. Final position of the tube after removal of the guidewire.

Removal of the chest tube

- The chest tube can be removed once there is no air leak and the output is less than 200 mL per day. The duration of the chest tube is an independent risk factor for empyema.
- The tube can be safely removed at maximal deep inspiration or expiration.

Autotransfusion

- Blood autotransfusion is fast, inexpensive relative to banked blood product, and simple. It provides the patient with safe, matched, warm blood with coagulant factors. There are numerous autotransfusion systems available commercially.
- It is recommended for use in all patients with chest trauma, both blunt and penetrating, with large hemothoraces.
- Anticoagulant, citrate 1 mL per 10 mL of blood, can be used, but is not absolutely necessary. It should be added to the connection with the chest tube.

Tips and pitfalls

- Technical complications include bleeding secondary to injury of the intercostal vessels, the lung, heart, diaphragm, liver, or spleen. Insertion of the tube with the use of a

trocar is associated with an increased risk of injury. Digital exploration of the pleura to rule out adhesions reduces the risk of lung injury.
- Iatrogenic injuries to the diaphragm, liver, or the spleen may occur if the tube is placed too low. Avoid this serious complication by staying at or above the fourth or fifth intercostal space.
- Tube misplacement is another common complication. Insertion of the tube too far into the pleural cavity may result in kinking and poor drainage. In a normal habitus adult patient, do not insert the tube beyond 8–10 cm. Misplacement of the tube into the subcutaneous tissues is another technical complication, especially in obese patients.
- Persistent air leaks can be due to technical problems or to the injury itself. Make sure that all of the tube perforations are located within the chest cavity and that the incision around the tube is tightly sealed. All connections should be taped. If there are no technical problems, the differential diagnosis should include tracheobronchial injury or bronchopleural fistula.
- Larger size tubes do not drain more effectively. They can be more painful and more difficult to insert. In adults, do not exceed size 28–32 Fr. For pneumothoraces, use smaller size chest tubes.

4 Emergency room resuscitative thoracotomy

Demetrios Demetriades and Scott Zakaluzny

Surgical anatomy

- The major muscles, which are divided during resuscitative thoracotomy, include the pectoralis major, the pectoralis minor, and the serratus anterior muscles.
  - *Pectoralis major muscle.* It originates from the anterior surface of the medial half of the clavicle, the anterior surface of the sternum, and the cartilages of all of the true ribs. The 5-cm wide tendon inserts into the upper humerus.
  - *Pectoralis minor muscle.* It arises from the third, fourth, and fifth ribs, near their cartilages, and inserts into the coracoid process of the scapula.
  - *Serratus anterior muscle.* It originates from the first eight or nine ribs and inserts into the medial part of the scapula
- The left phrenic nerve descends on the lateral surface of the pericardium.
- The lower thoracic aorta is situated to the left of the vertebral column. The esophagus descends on the right side of the aorta to the level of the diaphragm, where it moves anterior and to the left of the aorta. The aorta is the first structure felt while sliding your fingers along the left posterior wall towards the spine.

(See Chapter 14)

General principles

- External cardiac compressions can produce approximately 20% of the baseline cardiac output and tissue perfusion. Open cardiac massage can produce approximately 55% of the baseline cardiac output. In traumatic cardiac arrest external cardiac compression has little or no role, especially in the presence of cardiac tamponade or an empty heart due to severe blood loss.
- Trauma patients arriving in the emergency room in cardiac arrest or in imminent cardiac arrest are candidates for resuscitative thoracotomy. The indications and contraindications are controversial, with many surgeons supporting strict criteria and others supporting liberal criteria for the procedure. Those supporting strict criteria cite the futility of the operation and the risks to staff. Those practicing liberal criteria cite those who do survive, the opportunity for organ donation and the educational value of the procedure.
- The emergency room resuscitative thoracotomy allows release of cardiac tamponade, control of bleeding, direct cardiac massage and defibrillation, aortic cross-clamping, and management of air embolism.
- Endotracheal intubation, intravenous line placement, and resuscitative thoracotomy can be performed simultaneously. The endotracheal tube may be advanced into the right bronchus in order to collapse the left lung and make the procedure easier. However, this may cause oxygenation problems in the presence of injuries to the right lung.

Special surgical instruments

The resuscitative thoracotomy tray should be kept simple and include only a few absolutely essential instruments, which include a scalpel, Finochietto retractor, two Duval lung forceps, two vascular clamps, one long Russian forceps, four hemostats, one bone cutter, one pair of long scissors. In addition, good lighting, working suction, and an internal defibrillator should be ready, before patient arrival. All staff should wear personal protective equipment.

Atlas of Surgical Techniques in Trauma, ed. Demetrios Demetriades, Kenji Inaba, and George Velmahos. Published by Cambridge University Press. © Cambridge University Press 2015.

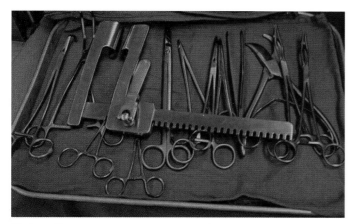

Fig. 4.1. The emergency room resuscitative thoracotomy tray should include only the absolutely essential instruments (scalpel, Finochietto retractor, two Duval lung forceps, two vascular clamps, one long Russian forceps, four hemostats, one bone cutter, long scissors).

Positioning

Supine position with the left arm abducted at 90 degrees or above the head. Antiseptic skin preparation may be performed; however, rapid entry with release of tamponade and control of hemorrhage trumps sterility and should take precedence over meticulous antiseptic precautions. Draping is not required, as it is time consuming and prevents a global view of the anatomy and patient condition.

Incision

- The left anterolateral incision is the standard incision for resuscitative thoracotomy. It provides good exposure to the heart and the left lung and allows cross-clamping of the thoracic aorta. If necessary, it can be extended as a clamshell incision into the right chest through a mirror incision and division of the sternum.
  - The incision is performed through the fourth to fifth intercostal space, at the nipple line in males or infra-mammary fold in females. It starts at the left parasternal border and ends at the sheets on the gurney. Follow the curve of the ribs by aiming towards the axilla. The pectoralis major and pectoralis minor are encountered and divided in the anterior part of the incision and the serratus anterior in the posterior part of the incision.
  - The intercostal muscles are divided close to the superior border of the rib, in order to avoid the neurovascular bundle, and the pleural cavity is entered with the use of

scissors taking care to avoid injury to the underlying inflated lung. Right mainstem intubation or holding ventilation during entry into the pleural cavity can reduce the risk of lung injury. A Finochietto retractor is then inserted and the ribs are spread. The left lower lobe of the lung is grasped with Duval forceps and retracted towards the patient's head and laterally to improve the exposure of the heart and the thoracic aorta.

(a)

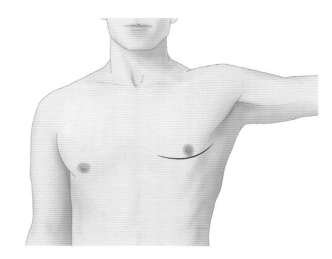

(b)

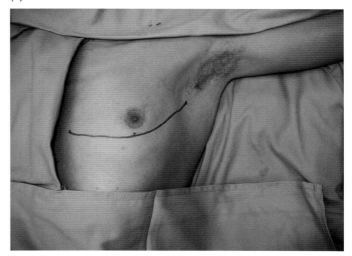

Fig. 4.2(a),(b). The resuscitative thoracotomy incision is placed just below the nipple in males or in the infra-mammary crease in females (through the fourth to fifth intercostal space). It starts at the left parasternal border and extends to the mid-axillary line, with a direction toward the axilla.

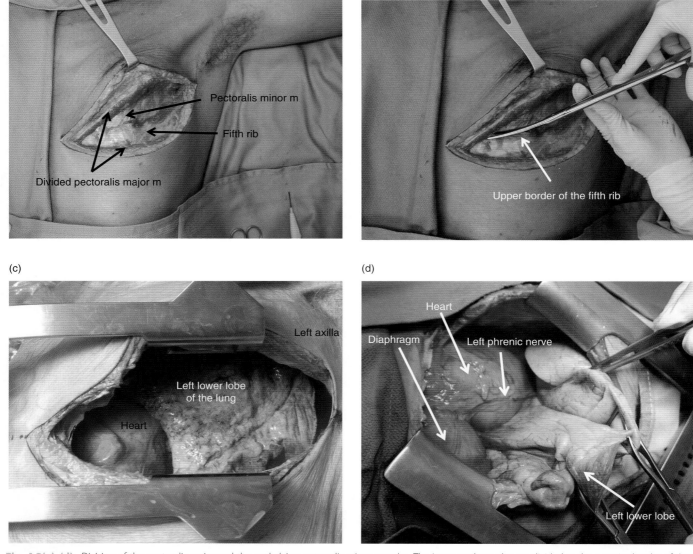

Fig. 4.3(a)–(d). Division of the pectoralis major and the underlying pectoralis minor muscles. The intercostal muscles are divided at the superior border of the rib with scissors, taking care to avoid injury to the lung. A Finochietto retractor is placed, and the left lung and the heart are exposed. The left lower lobe of the lung is grasped with Duval forceps and retracted towards the patient's head and laterally to improve the exposure of the heart and the thoracic aorta.

- In some patients with injuries to the right chest or the upper mediastinal vessels, a clamshell incision may be needed for bleeding control and improved exposure. The left thoracotomy incision is extended through a transverse division of the sternum with a bone cutter or heavy scissors into a symmetrical right thoracotomy. During the division of the sternum, both internal mammary arteries are transected, and clamping or ligation should be performed after restoration of cardiac activity and circulation.

(a)

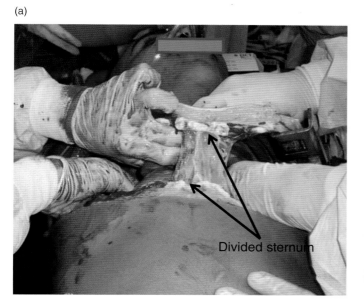

(b)

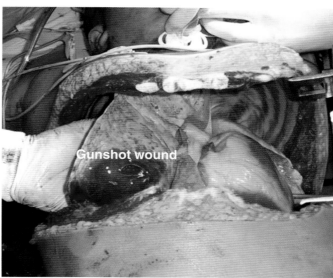

Fig. 4.4(a),(b). Clamshell incision: the left thoracotomy incision is extended through a transverse division of the sternum into a symmetrical right thoracotomy. It provides good exposure of the anterior aspect of the heart, the superior mediastinal vessels, and both lungs.

Procedure

- After entering the left pleural cavity, any free blood is evacuated and any obvious significant bleeding from the lung or thoracic vessels is controlled, initially by direct pressure, and subsequently with a vascular clamp.
- The next step is to open the pericardium to release any tamponade, repair any cardiac injury and perform direct cardiac resuscitation with cardiac massage, defibrillation, and the intracardiac injection of medication.

- The left phrenic nerve is identified along the lateral surface of the pericardium. In the absence of cardiac tamponade, the pericardium is grasped with two hemostats anterior to the nerve and a small incision is made. However, in the presence of tamponade the pericardium is tense and it may be difficult to apply a hemostat. In these cases a small pericardiotomy is performed with a scalpel and the pericardium is then opened longitudinally and parallel to the phrenic nerve.

(a)

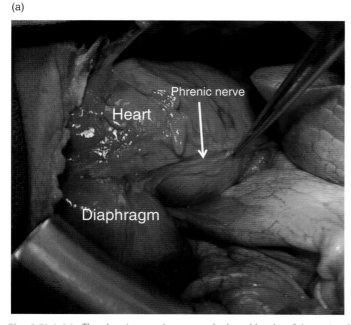

(b)

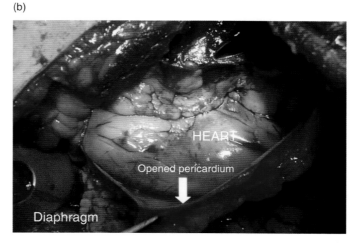

Fig. 4.5(a)–(c). The phrenic nerve is seen on the lateral border of the pericardium and should be protected. The pericardium is opened in front and parallel to the nerve.

(c)

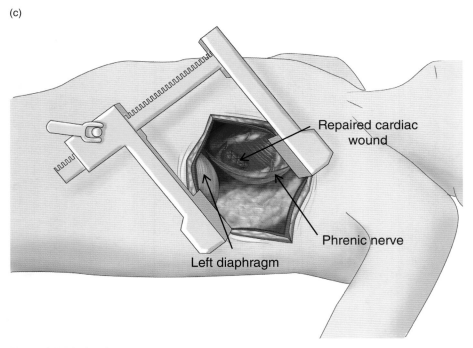

Repaired cardiac wound

Phrenic nerve

Left diaphragm

Fig. 4.5(a)–(c). *(cont.)*

- Any tamponade is then released and cardiac bleeding is controlled by finger compression between the thumb and index finger or for large atrial injuries with a vascular clamp. For small cardiac wounds, temporary bleeding control may be achieved by inserting and inflating a Foley catheter. Care should be taken to avoid accidental dislodgement of the balloon and inadvertent puncture of the balloon during suturing. Skin staples may be used temporarily for stab wounds, but will be ineffective in most cases with gunshot wounds associated with cardiac tissue loss.
- The cardiac wound is repaired with figure-of-eight, horizontal mattress or continuous sutures, using non-absorbable 2–0 or 3–0 suture on a large tapered needle. Routine use of pledgets is time consuming and unnecessary in the majority of cases and should be reserved only in cases where the myocardium tears during tying the sutures. The technical details of cardiac repair are demonstrated in Chapter 15.

Open cardiac massage

Cardiac massage should always be performed using both hands. Squeezing the heart with only one hand is less effective and may result in rupture of the heart with the thumb. The heart should be held between the two palms and compression should proceed from the apex towards the base.

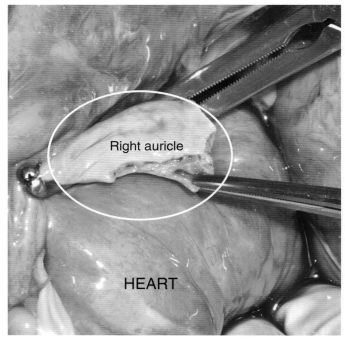

Right auricle

HEART

Fig. 4.6. Atrial injuries can temporarily be controlled with a vascular clamp.

(a)

(b)

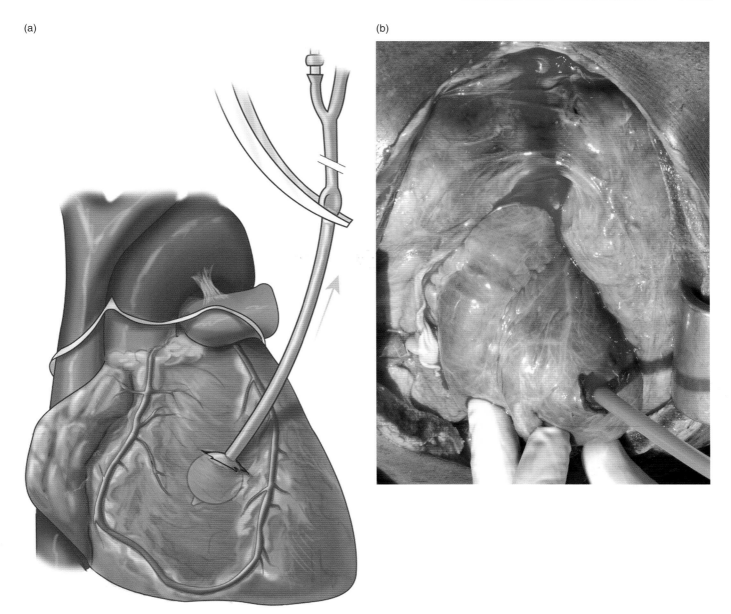

Fig. 4.7(a),(b). In some cases with small cardiac wounds, temporary bleeding control may be achieved by inserting and inflating a Foley catheter.

Internal cardiac defibrillation

Internal cardiac defibrillation should be used in cases with ventricular fibrillation or pulseless ventricular tachycardia. The two internal cardiac paddles are placed on the anterior and posterior wall of the heart and the heart is shocked with 10–50 joules.

Pharmacological treatment of cardiac arrest

Medications such as epinephrine, calcium, magnesium, and sodium bicarbonate can be injected into the left ventricle as needed.

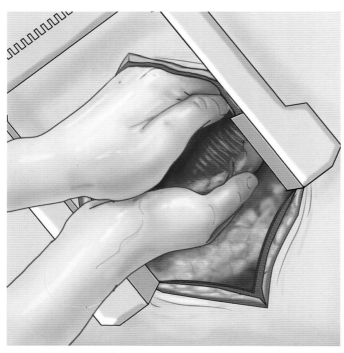

Fig. 4.8. Technique of internal cardiac massage: the heart is held between the two palms, squeezing from the apex towards the base of the heart.

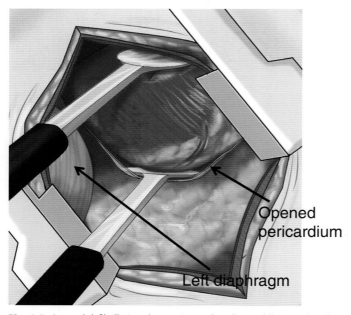

Opened pericardium

Left diaphragm

Fig. 4.9. Internal defibrillation: the two internal cardiac paddles are placed on the anterior and posterior walls of the heart.

Epicardial pacing

- Intraoperative and early postoperative temporary epicardial pacing should be considered in patients with arrhythmias, in order to improve haemodynamic function and suppress tachyarrhythmias.

- Epicardial pacing wires are usually placed on the upper part of the anterior wall of the right ventricle, one at the top of the ventricle and the second approximately 1 cm below. Alternatively, the wires can be placed on the left ventricle.
- Epicardial wires have a small needle on one end. This needle is used to embed the wires superficially in the myocardium, after which the needle is cut off. Some wires are slightly coiled to prevent easy dislodgement. A larger needle on the other end of the wire is used to pierce the chest wall and bring the wire to the skin surface. The exteriorized wires are then connected to the pacer. The usual settings for the pacer are a heart rate of 70–90 per minute and a maximal current output of 10 mA.

(a)

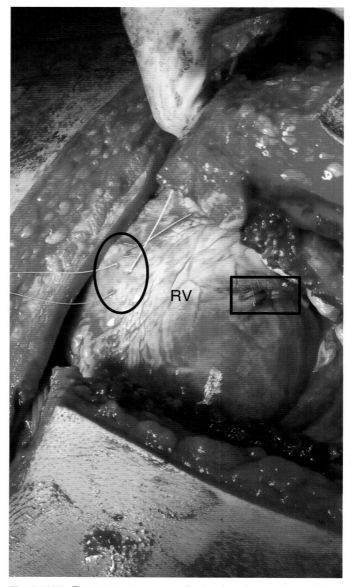

RV

Fig. 4.10(a). The pacing wires are usually placed on the upper part of the anterior wall of the right ventricle, with the second wire about 1 cm below the first (circle). Note repair of penetrating cardiac wound (box).

(b)

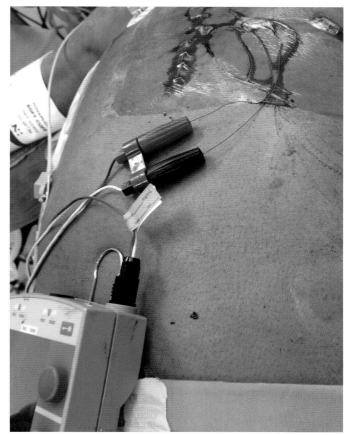

Fig. 4.10(b). The pacing wires are brought out through the skin and connected to the pacer.

Aortic cross-clamping

The most accessible site of the thoracic aorta for cross-clamping is approximately 2–4 cm above the diaphragm. The left lower lobe of the lung is grasped and retracted upwards with a Duval clamp in order to improve the exposure of the aorta. In cardiac arrest the aorta is collapsed and might be difficult to distinguish from the esophagus. The aorta is the first structure felt while sliding the fingers along the left posterior wall towards the spine. The esophagus is more anterior and medial. The inferior pulmonary ligament may be divided to improve exposure. The mediastinal pleura over the aorta is then incised with long scissors and a vascular clamp is applied. The dissection of the aorta should be kept to a minimum because of the risk of avulsion of the intercostal arteries. The aortic clamp is removed as soon as the cardiac activity returns and the carotid pulse is palpable.

Air embolism

In patients with cardiac arrest or severe arrhythmias who have injury to the low-pressure cardiac chambers, the lung or major veins, air embolism should be suspected. Sometimes, air can be

(c)

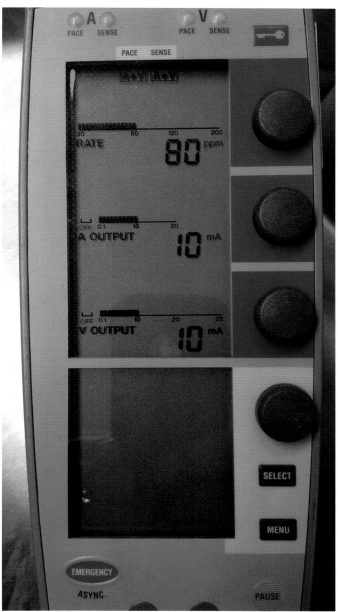

Fig. 4.10(c). Cardiac pacer: the usual settings of the pacer are: heart rate 70–90 per minute and V output 10 mA.

seen in the coronary veins. In these cases control of the source of the air should be obtained immediately, followed by needle aspiration of the air from the ventricles.

Hilar occlusion

Consider hilar occlusion in cases with lung trauma associated with severe bleeding or air embolism. Digital occlusion of the hilum can be achieved by compression of the hilar structures

(a)

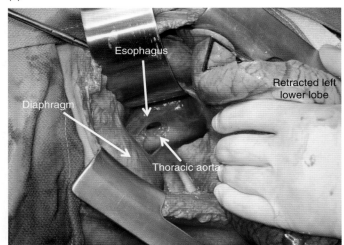

(c)

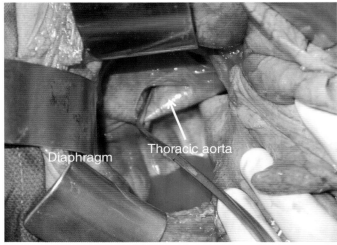

Fig. 4.11(a)–(c). (*cont.*)

(b)

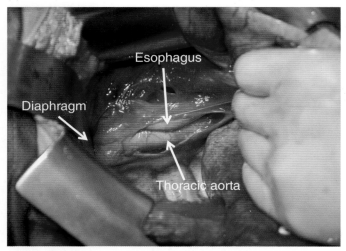

Fig. 4.11(a)–(c). Cross-clamping of the thoracic aorta. The most accessible site of the thoracic aorta for cross-clamping is about 2–4 cm above the diaphragm. The mediastinal pleura over the aorta is incised. Note the esophagus anteriorly and medially. A vascular clamp is applied to the aorta.

between the index finger and the thumb. A vascular clamp can replace the digital compression.

Hilar twist

This is an alternative approach to the digital or clamp occlusion of the hilum. The inferior pulmonary ligament, which is a double layer of pleura joining the lower lobe of the lung to the mediastinum and the medial part of the diaphragm, is divided, taking care to avoid injury to the inferior pulmonary vein.

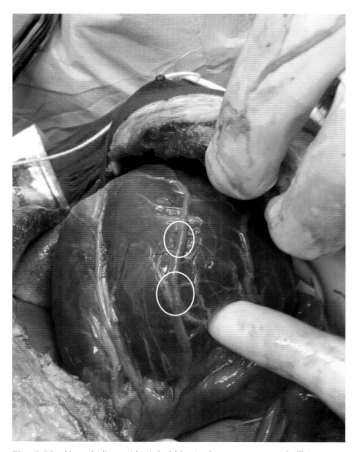

Fig. 4.12. Air embolism with air bubbles in the coronary vessels. This complication should be suspected in injuries to the low-pressure cardiac chambers, the lung, or major veins.

Incision closure

- The thoracotomy incision should be closed in the operating room, as described in Chapter 14.
- Damage control with temporary closure of the thoracotomy incision should be considered in patients with persistent arrhythmias or who are at high risk for cardiac arrest during the ICU phase of resuscitation. In these cases immediate access to the heart for cardiac massage may be life-saving. Temporary incision closure is best achieved with the VAC technique.

Tips and pitfalls

- Common errors with the incision include (a) low incision with an increased risk of injury to the elevated diaphragm and poor exposure of the upper part of the heart, (b) the incision does not follow the curve of the ribs, (c) division of the intercostal muscles with the scalpel with the potential for injury to the underlying inflated lung, (d) injury to the left internal mammary artery if the incision is too close to the sternum, which can be especially problematic if not immediately recognized.
- Common errors during aortic cross-clamping include (a) clamping the esophagus (the aorta is the first structure felt while sliding the fingers along the left posterior wall towards the spine); a nasogastric tube may help in identifying the esophagus, which is anteromedial to the aorta, (b) injury to the esophagus, (c) avulsion of intercostal arteries, and (d) attempting to clamp a collapsed aorta without any pleural dissection.

Insertion of intracranial pressure monitoring catheter

Howard Belzberg and Matthew D. Tadlock

Surgical anatomy

- The intracranial pressure can be monitored via a catheter placed in one of the lateral ventricles, or with devices placed intracranially, in the subarachnoid, subdural or epidural spaces or in the brain parenchyma.

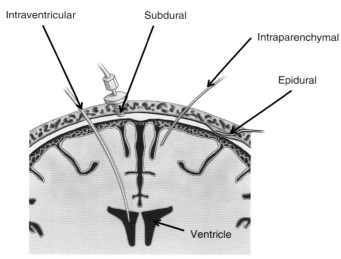

Fig. 5.1. The intracranial pressure can be monitored via a catheter placed in one of the lateral ventricles, or with devices placed in the epidural, subdural, or subarachnoid spaces, or in the brain parenchyma.

- The ICP monitor should be placed in the non-dominant hemisphere (right hemisphere in right-handed people).
- The Kocher's point is the external skin landmark for the insertion point of the catheter; at this point, the device insertion avoids the bridging veins, the superior sagittal sinus, and the motor strip, and allows the placement of the catheter in the frontal horn of the lateral ventricle. Kocher's point is at the mid pupillary line (2–3 cm lateral to midline or the sagittal line) and 2 cm anterior to the coronal suture. The coronal suture is about 11–12 cm from the base of the nose.

- Another useful point for the insertion of the catheter is the Keens point, which is about 2.5 cm posterior and superior to the top of the ear.

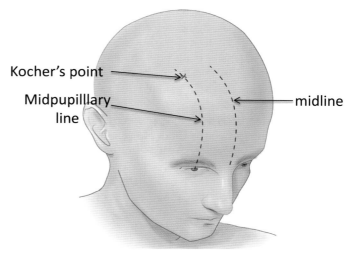

Fig. 5.2. Identification of the Kocher's point (red X) for insertion of the ICP monitor: Mid pupillary line, about 2 cm anterior to the coronal line.

General principles

- Insertion of ICP catheter may be performed in the operating room, emergency room, or intensive care unit.
- Avoid ICP placement if the INR is >1.5.
- The Brain Trauma Foundation recommends intracranial pressure (ICP) monitoring in salvageable victims of traumatic brain injury (TBI) with a Glasgow Coma Score (GCS) of 8 or less and an abnormal head computed tomography (CT) scan. With a normal CT scan, ICP monitoring is recommended after TBI in patients with two of the following criteria: (1) age over 40, (2) motor posturing (unilateral or bilateral) (3) systolic blood pressure $\leq$ 90 mm Hg.

Atlas of Surgical Techniques in Trauma, ed. Demetrios Demetriades, Kenji Inaba, and George Velmahos. Published by Cambridge University Press. © Cambridge University Press 2015.

- Cerebral perfusion pressure (CPP) is a calculated physiologic measurement defined as the difference between the mean arterial pressure (MAP) and the ICP: CPP = MAP – ICP. By affecting the MAP or the ICP, the CPP should generally be maintained above 60 mm Hg.

Types of ICP monitoring

- The intraventricular catheters allow therapeutic drainage of CSF. All other types of catheters (intraparenchymal, subarachnoid, epidural, or subdural devices) do not allow drainage of CSF, but they are easier to place.

Intraventricular ICP monitor

- An external ventricular drain (EVD) or intraventricular catheter is an external flexible catheter inserted into one of the lateral ventricles. It allows for both monitoring of ICP and drainage of CSF as a therapeutic maneuver. A fluid coupled EVD catheter is the gold standard for ICP monitoring. The EVD is low cost and the most accurate. Further, it is the only ICP monitor that can be recalibrated in situ.
- Traditionally, EVDs only allowed intermittent ICP measurements (when the drain is closed), but newer catheters allow simultaneous ICP monitoring and CSF drainage.
- Different methods of the pressure transduction may be utilized during EVD ICP monitoring. The basic (and least expensive) is the fluid coupled external mechanical transducer.

Intraparenchymal ICP monitor

- Intraparenchymal monitors are usually placed as an alternative to EVD placement. A fluid coupled catheter with mechanical transducer, fiber optic transducer, or pneumatic technology catheter can be utilized.
- Intraparenchymal monitors are easier to place than the EVD and allow for continuous monitoring.

Subarachnoid bolt

- The subarachnoid screw or bolt allows for continuous fluid coupled ICP monitoring within the subarachnoid space.

Epidural or subdural ICP monitor

- These are the least accurate of the ICP monitors. Subdural monitors utilize fluid coupled, fiber optic transducers. Epidural monitors utilize either a fluid coupled or fiber optic tip catheter.
- Infection risk is lower with intraparenchymal monitors than with EVD.

Special surgical instruments

- Figure 5.3 shows the major components of a drill kit. Components required for the procedure include a marking pen, scalpel, self-retaining retractor, twist drill, spinal needle, and either a screw or catheter depending on the type of ICP monitoring desired. If a catheter is used, a tunneler (included with kit) is also needed. Kits typically have two different drill bits. The smaller drill bit is for placement of a subarachnoid screw, whereas the larger bit is for the intraventricular catheter.

(a)

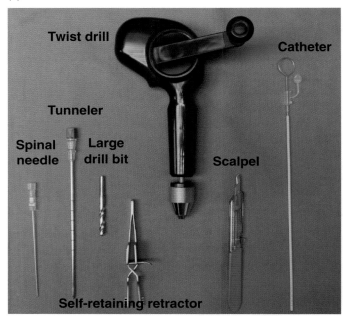

Fig. 5.3(a). Major components of a disposable twist drill kit. The ventricular drain catheter is also shown here. The large drill bit comes with the twist drill kit.

(b)

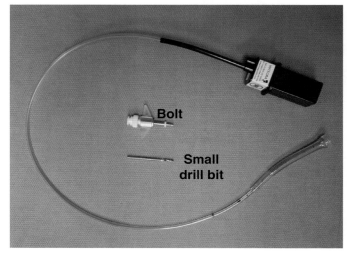

Fig. 5.3(b). Additional components required to place a subarachnoid bolt. Note that the smaller drill bit comes with the bolt kit.

Patient position

- The patient should be positioned with the head of the bed elevated at 30 degrees, with the head immobilized in a neutral position.

Procedure

Intraventricular ICP monitor

- Administer adequate analgesia and sedation.
- The hair should be clipped around the incision and exit sites. Hair should not be shaved due to increased risk of wound infection. The site should be prepared with antiseptic solution and draped in the standard sterile surgical fashion. The person performing the procedure should wear appropriate sterile gown and gloves, surgical mask, eye protection, and hair covering.
- With a marking pen, mark the mid pupillary line (with forward gaze), the sagittal line (skull midline starting at the base of the nose), and the coronal suture. The coronal suture is located at about 11–12 cm from the root of the nose. Next, identify the Kocher's point, which is on the mid pupillary line, about 2 cm in front of the coronal line.

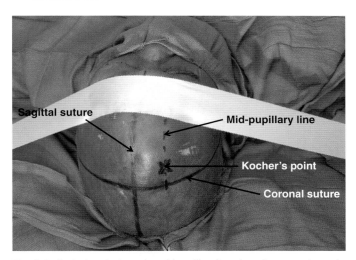

Fig. 5.4. Kocher's point is on the mid pupillary line, about 2 cm anterior to the coronal suture. The coronal suture is about 11–12 cm from the root of the nose.

- Inject 1% lidocaine with or without epinephrine in the skin and subcutaneous tissue for local anesthesia prior to incision. An approximate 1–2 cm longitudinal incision is

then made down to the bone at Kocher's point, and the skull is cleared of periosteum.

- A self-retaining retractor (comes with the drill kit) is used to expose the skull below. Holding the twist drill perpendicular to the skull, a burr hole is made, penetrating both the outer and the inner tables of the skull. The stop guard should be used to prevent accidental entry into the brain parenchyma when the inner table of the skull is breached. A probe/spinal needle is introduced through the opening to ensure that the drill completely penetrated the bone. Use saline to irrigate the bone fragments in the burr hole to expose the dura matter. Using an 11-blade, make a small cruciate incision in the dura.

(a)

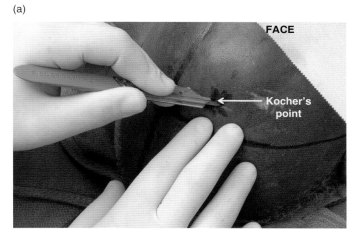

(b)

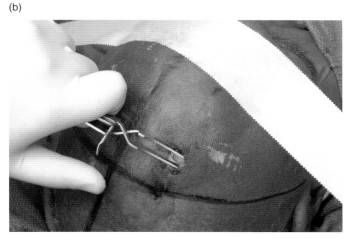

Fig. 5.5(a),(b). A 1–2 cm incision is made at Kocher's point, down to the bone, and a self-retaining retractor is placed.

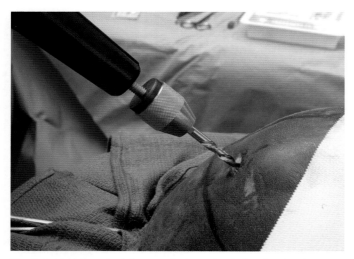

Fig. 5.6. Hold the twist drill perpendicular to the skull and make a burr hole, penetrating both the outer and the inner tables of the skull.

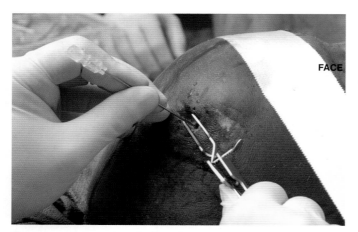

Fig. 5.7. Insert a spinal needle through the burr hole to ensure complete penetration through the bone.

- The ventricular catheter is inserted perpendicular to the brain parenchyma and aiming towards the inner canthus of the ipsilateral eye. The catheter is advanced 5–7 cm to enter the frontal horn of the lateral ventricle. Usually, a "pop" or a "give in" is felt and cerebral spinal fluid (CSF) is encountered, indicating entry into the ventricle. If CSF is not encountered, two additional attempts may be made directing the catheter slightly more medial, either toward the bridge of the nose or to the inner canthus of the contralateral eye. If no CSF

is encountered after three attempts, then an intraparenchymal monitor or subarachnoid screw should be placed.

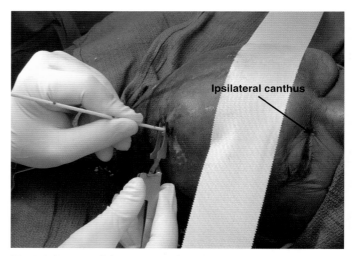

Fig. 5.8. Insertion of the intraventricular catheter. Insert perpendicular to the brain parenchyma aiming towards the inner canthus of the ipsilateral eye.

- Avoid excessive loss of CSF, as the brain may not tolerate sudden decompression of the ventricles.
- Make a separate skin incision, approximately 5 cm posterior to the insertion site, and tunnel the ventricular catheter, to reduce the risk of infection. Suture the catheter to the scalp and close the incisions with a nylon suture. Place a sterile dressing.

(a)

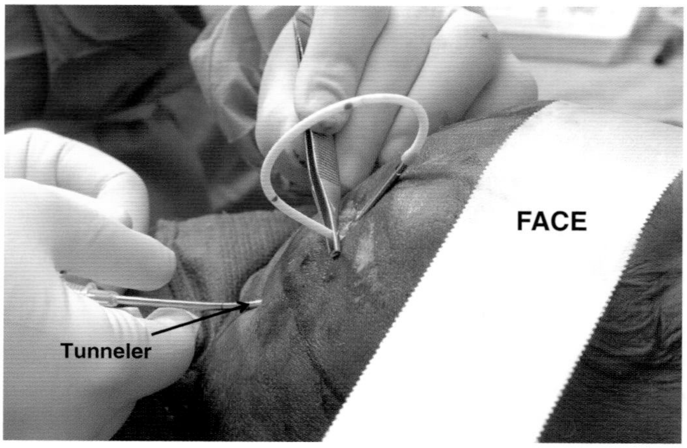

Fig. 5.9(a),(b). Using a tunneler, the catheter is tunneled through an incision 5 cm posterior to the initial incision. The primary incision is sutured with a running suture.

(b)

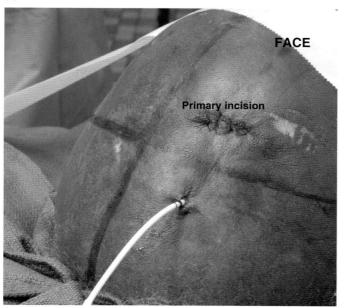

FACE

Primary incision

Fig. 5.9(a),(b). (cont.)

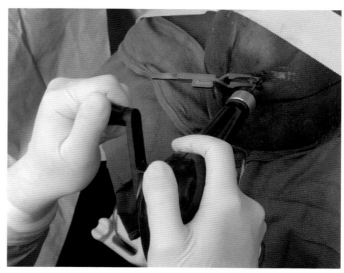

Fig. 5.10. Insertion of a subarachnoid bolt: the twist drill is used to make a burr hole. Note the smaller drill bit utilized for the subarachnoid screw.

- Zero the monitor at the level of external auditory meatus.

Intraparenchymal ICP monitor
- Kocher's point should also be utilized for the placement of intraparenchymal monitors. The depth of the insertion depends on the area to be monitored. Once the monitor is in place, it should be tunneled as described above.

Subarachnoid bolt
- The initial incision is the same as for an EVD or intraparenchymal monitor, but the bit for the twist drill is wider. Once the burr hole has been made, make a cruciate incision in the dura and open the arachnoid. The threaded bolt is placed so that it abuts the dura.

(a)

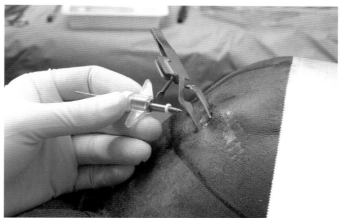

Fig. 5.11(a)–(c). The subarachnoid bolt is screwed into place through the skull so that it abuts the dura. Then the transducer is placed through the bolt.

(b)

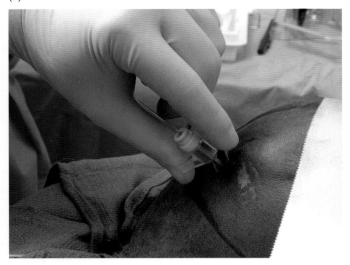

(c)

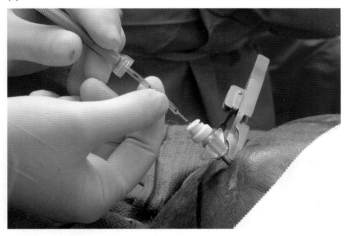

Fig. 5.11(a)–(c). (*cont.*)

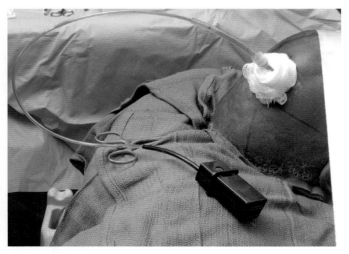

Fig. 5.12. Picture demonstrating the subarachnoid screw dressed with sterile gauze and attached to the transducer.

Epidural and subdural monitor

- The preparation and location are as listed above. The catheter is placed in either the epidural or subdural space.

Tips and pitfalls

- When ventricles are compressed or displaced because of significant brain trauma, an EVD may be difficult to place. In the event that the ventricles are too small or inaccessible, epidural or subdural monitors may be used. Be wary of blood or debris obstructing the fluid column causing inaccurate measurements. These can be flushed with 1–2 mL of normal saline using strict sterile precautions, but ultimately this increases the risk of infection.

- Contraindications to ICP monitoring include coagulopathy (INR>1.5) and thrombocytopenia. Scalp infection is a relative contraindication.

- Transfuse platelets and plasma as appropriate prior to procedure to achieve an INR of 1.6 or less and a platelet count of at least 100 000 to prevent unnecessary hemorrhage.

- Intraventricular hemorrhage is a contraindication to same side EVD placement.

- Avoid excessive loss of CSF, as the brain may not tolerate sudden decompression of the ventricles.

Head

Evacuation of acute epidural and subdural hematomas

Gabriel Zada and Kazuhide Matsushima

Surgical anatomy

- There are three meninges covering the brain: the dura mater, the arachnoid mater, and the pia mater.

  ○ The dura mater is the thickest and strongest membrane and is firmly attached to the inner surface of the cranial bone, especially along the sutures. It contains the meningeal arteries.

  ○ The arachnoid mater is a thin membrane under the dura mater. Its inner surface has numerous thin trabeculae extending downward, into the subarachnoid space.

  ○ The pia mater is a thin membrane that covers the surface of the brain, entering the grooves and fissures.

- Due to the tight adhesion of the dura mater to the inner skull, significant force is required to separate them. In contrast, separation of the dura from the subarachnoid mater can occur with relatively little force.

- The middle meningeal artery arises from the external carotid artery. It enters the foramen spinosum and branches into the anterior, middle, and posterior branches with various patterns. It is a common source of bleeding in acute epidural hematomas (EDH).

- The bridging veins connect the cortical superficial veins to the sagittal sinus in the dura. They are a common source of bleeding in acute subdural hematomas (SDH).

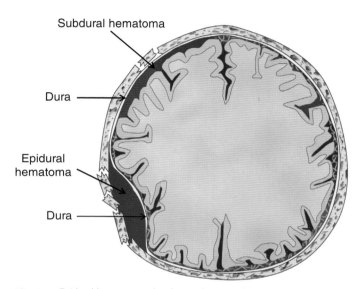

Fig. 6.1. Epidural hematomas develop in the space between the inner table of the skull and the dura. Subdural hematomas develop in the space between the dura and arachnoid.

General principles

- Acute epidural hematomas (EDH) and subdural hematomas (SDH) are commonly caused by blunt mechanisms (e.g. motor vehicle accident, fall, assault).

Atlas of Surgical Techniques in Trauma, ed. Demetrios Demetriades, Kenji Inaba, and George Velmahos. Published by Cambridge University Press. © Cambridge University Press 2015.

- EDHs develop when blood collects in the space between the inner table of the skull and the dura; SDHs occur when blood collects between the dura and arachnoid.
- The majority of EDHs are due to injury to the meningeal arteries, usually the middle meningeal artery, associated with skull fractures in the temporal region. A torn dura venous sinus or bleeding from a skull fracture may also result in an EDH. The hematoma is located between the inner plate of the skull and the dura mater.
- Although the temporal region is the most common site for EDHs, they may occur almost anywhere in the cranial cavity.

(a)

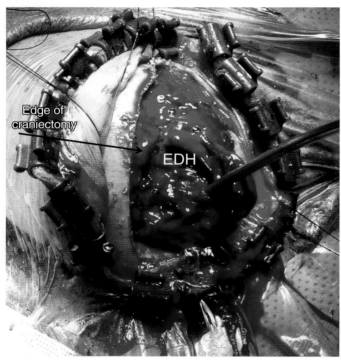

Fig. 6.2(a). Appearance of a large epidural hematoma (EDH) after craniectomy.

(b)

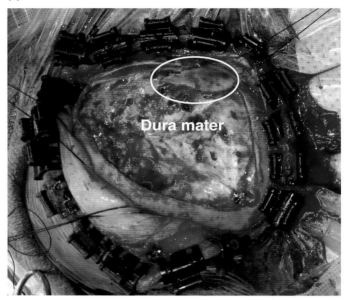

Fig. 6.2(b). Appearance of the intact dura mater after evacuation of the EDH. Note the fracture of the skull, which was the primary cause of the bleeding.

- Acute SDHs are commonly caused by bleeding from brain parenchyma injury or from torn bridging veins, which connect the cortical superficial veins to the sagittal sinus in the dura. The hematoma is located between the dura mater and the arachnoid mater.

(a)

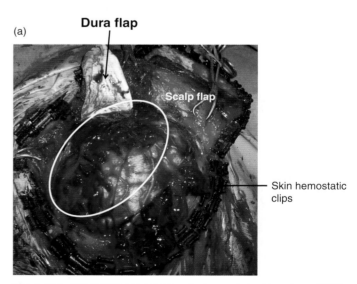

Fig. 6.3(a). Intraoperative appearance of a large subdural hematoma (SDH) (white circle) after craniectomy and opening of the dura mater.

(b)

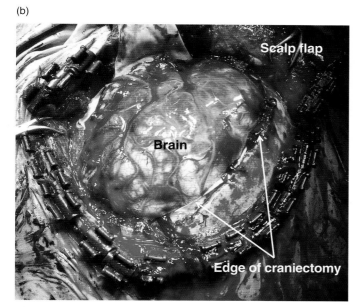

Fig. 6.3(b). Intraoperative appearance after evacuation of the SDH. Note the exposed and edematous brain.

- The acute EDH appears as a hyperdense lenticular (biconvex)-shaped lesion, often associated with an overlying skull fracture. It usually does not cross suture lines. The acute SDH appears as a crescent-shaped lesion that may cross suture lines.

(a)

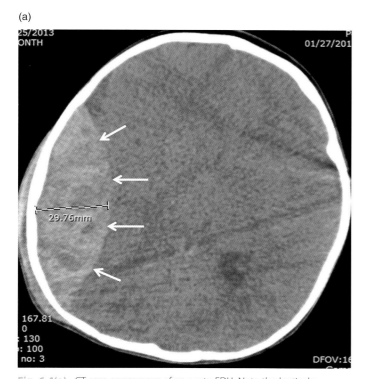

Fig. 6.4(a). CT scan appearance of an acute EDH. Note the lenticular (biconvex) shape of the hematoma (arrows).

(b)

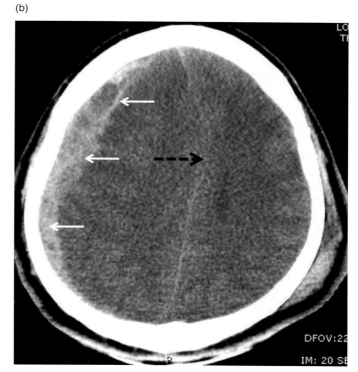

Fig. 6.4(b). CT scan appearance of an acute SDH. Note the crescent shape of the hematoma (white arrows). There is a significant midline shift (black arrow).

- Patients with EDH/SDH may present with a wide array of clinical manifestations from mild headache to coma. A classic "lucid interval" (brief loss of consciousness with recovery followed by neurological deterioration) is seen in only half of patients with acute EDH.
- EDHs are typically caused by arterial sources of bleeding, and therefore often have a more rapid time course to neurological deterioration. Many SDHs, on the other hand, are caused by venous sources, and may accumulate and exert neurological effects via a slower progression pattern.
- Emergency surgical evacuation of EDHs or SDHs by craniotomy is often required to prevent death and long-term functional disability.
- Acute SDHs, are commonly caused by bleeding from brain parenchyma trauma or by the bridging veins that cross the subdural space. The bridging veins connect the cortical superficial veins to the sagittal sinus in the dura.
- Elderly people are more likely to develop SDHs due to cerebral atrophy associated with increased fragility and tension of the bridging veins. On the other hand, elderly people are less likely to develop EDH because of the fibrosis and firmer attachment of the dura mater to the skull.

Indications for surgical intervention

- The decision for surgical evacuation of an EDH or SDH is typically based on an assessment of a variety of clinical, systemic, and imaging findings. The neurological examination, including the Glasgow coma scale (GCS), pupillary findings, and motor function is a major consideration. Systemic considerations may include restrictions due to polytrauma, hemodynamic instability, hypocoaguable states, and comorbidities. Other objective information that weighs on this decision-making process includes CT imaging findings (i.e., large EDH in a patient with only headache) and intracranial pressure (ICP) concerns in patients with ICP monitors.
- Medical management in patients with EDH or SDH, and a concern for elevated ICPs include elevating the head of the bed, sedation/intubation as needed, mild hyperventilation, hyperosmolar therapy, reversal of hypocoagulable state, seizure control, and potentially local or systemic hypothermia.
- Surgical evacuation is generally recommended for adult patients with an EDH volume >30 cm³ on CT scan, regardless of GCS. In many patients with GCS<9, anisocoria on pupillary exam, thickness of hematoma >15 mm, or midline shift >5 mm on CT scan, surgical evacuation may also be warranted. In pediatric patients with acute EDH, the threshold for surgery is often lower than in adult patients. Location of the EDH also plays an important role, with temporal and posterior fossa EDHs often warranting a lower threshold for evacuation because of their propensity to cause uncal herniation and hydrocephalus or brainstem compression, respectively.
- The indication for surgical evacuation of acute SDHs often includes hematoma thickness >10 mm or midline shift >5 mm on the CT scan (regardless of GCS), anisocoria, sustained ICP>20 mmHg, or decreased GCS by ≥ 2 points from injury to admission.

Special surgical instruments

- A setup for emergency craniotomy should include: Raney scalp clips, Hudson brace hand-drill or air-powered (pneumatic) drill, burrs, and Gigli wire saw, or electric bone saw (craniotome).
- Head lights and surgical loupes are recommended.
- Hemostatic products (e.g., oxidized cellulose, gelatin sponge, etc.).

(a)

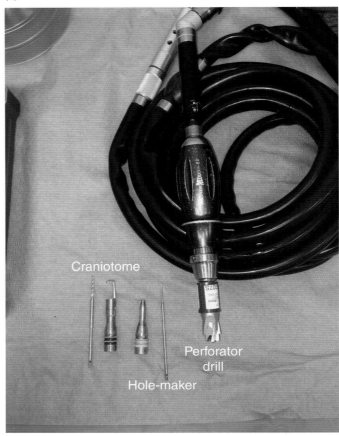

Fig. 6.5(a), (b). Essential instruments for craniectomy.

(b)

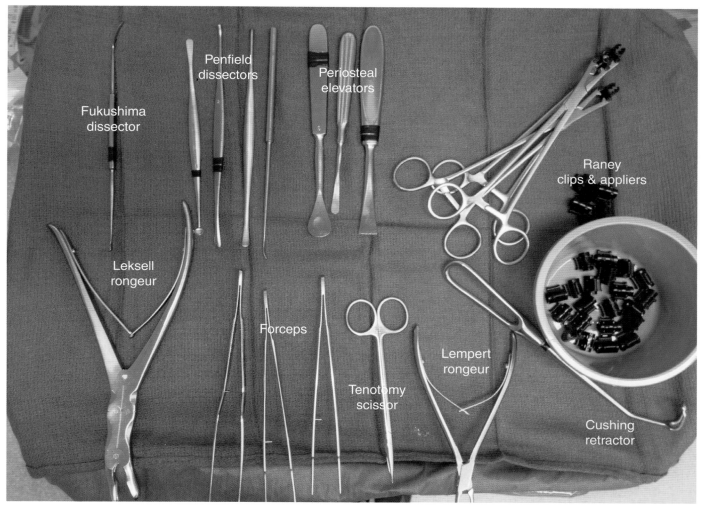

Fig. 6.5(a), (b). (cont.)

Patient positioning

- The patient is placed in the supine position under general anesthesia with both arms tucked. The head is usually elevated above the level of the heart (typically with reverse Trendelenburg position) to promote venous outflow and reduce ICPs. For a posterior fossa or occipital hematoma, prone position may be required.
- The patient's head is rotated to the contralateral side of craniotomy, 0–15 degrees from the horizontal plane. A shoulder roll is placed to facilitate head turning. This is especially required for patients with potential cervical spine injury who must remain in rigid collar fixation.
- The patient's head is supported with a donut pillow or horseshoe headholder. Mayfield pin fixation systems are not required for most cases in supine position.

Incision for craniectomy

- The entire scalp or the ipsilateral region of interest is shaved, prepped, and draped. A dose of antibiotics should be administered prior to skin incision.
- The exact position of the incision varies and depends on the location of the hematoma, but it should never reach the midline, at the top of the skull.
- The usual incision starts at the zygomatic arch, anterior to the tragus. This is extended to (1) the summit of the pinna, (2) the external occipital protuberance, (3) the vertex ending at the hairline. Careful consideration (and avoidance) of midline structures must be maintained at all times.

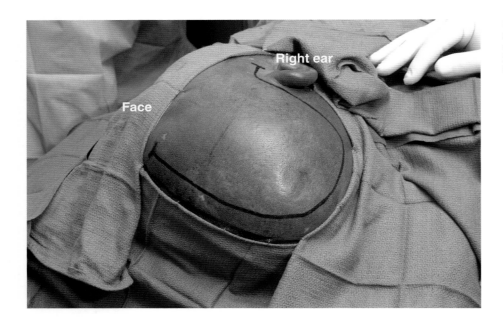

Fig. 6.6. Skin incision is made starting at the zygomatic arch anterior to the tragus to the vertex, ending at the hairline (question mark incision). The incision should avoid the midline, at the top of the skull.

- Major scalp bleeding is controlled with the electrocautery, and Raney clips are applied to achieve hemostasis along the edge of the scalp incision. The temporalis fascial and muscle are split, and the scalp/temporalis musculocutaneous flap are elevated together to avoid injury to the frontalis branch of the facial nerve.

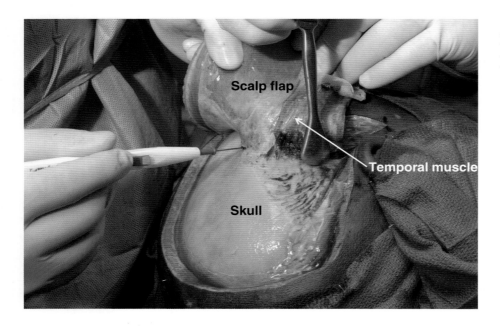

Fig. 6.7. A musculocutaneous flap is made to expose the skull for craniotomy. The scalp/temporalis musculocutaneous flap are opened together to avoid injury to the frontalis branch of the facial nerve.

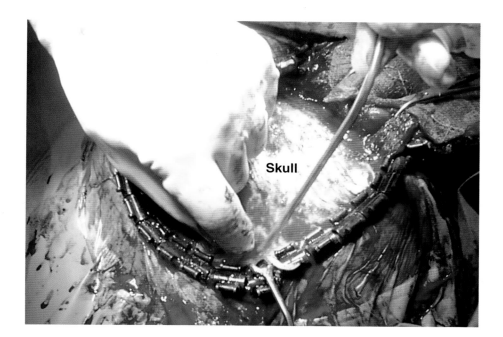

Fig. 6.8. Application of Raney clips on the edges of the incised scalp achieves hemostasis.

Tips and pitfalls

- Maintain awareness of the location of the midline at all times. Avoid midline at the top of the skull to prevent injury to the sagittal sinus.
- Be careful to avoid injury to the frontal branch of the facial nerve, located 1 cm anterior to the tragus.

Burr holes and bone flap removal

- For patients with large, hemispheric lesions (usually SDH), four burr holes are created using either a hand drill or a pneumatic/electric drill. Burr holes are placed in the (1) temporal squama, (2) parietal area, (3) frontal area, (4) pterion (area behind the zygomatic arch of the frontal bone).

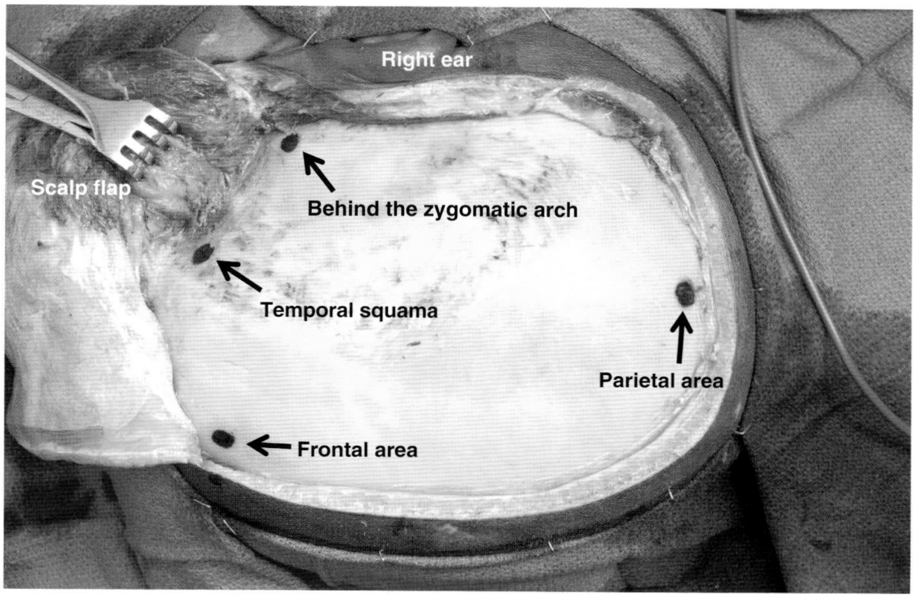

Fig. 6.9. Sites of the burr holes for large, hemispheric lesions.

- In patients with localized/confined EDH (i.e., temporal EDH), three burr holes can be placed surrounding the confines of the hematoma. (In cases of EDH, the hematoma is often encountered immediately following placement of the burr hole.)
- The Burr holes can be created using a hand-held or a pneumatic drill. The drill is always placed perpendicular to the skull.
  - The hand-held drill should be advanced carefully with a pointed bit (first bit) until the inner table is penetrated and the dura is barely exposed. Then the drill bit with more of a curvature (second/third bit) is used to widen the hole.

  - The pneumatic drill bit stops spinning on penetrating the inner table of the skull. A curette or rongeur is used to remove the remaining bone fragments.
- The dura is dissected off the inner table of the skull using a Penfield dissector or angled Fukushima instrument to prevent the violation of the dura and brain tissue underneath. Bony bleeding is controlled with bone wax.
- The burr holes are then connected using an air-powered bone saw (craniotome). A thin metal strip can be placed between the skull and the dura. The craniotome also has a protective footplate. The bone flap is subsequently removed carefully from the underlying dura. Again, great care should be taken to avoid midline structures (sagittal sinus) with this step. The bone flap is preserved in a sterile location.

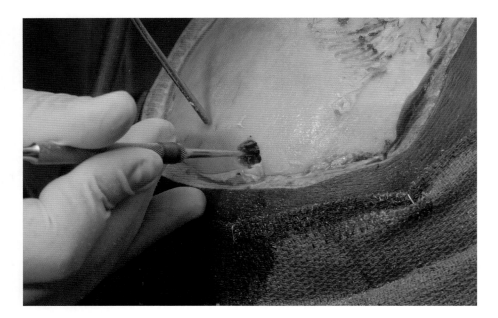

Fig. 6.10. The dura is dissected off the inner skull using a dissector.

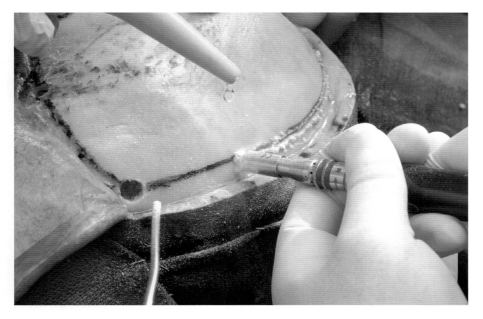

Fig. 6.11. Burr holes are connected with a bone saw to create a bone flap.

(a)

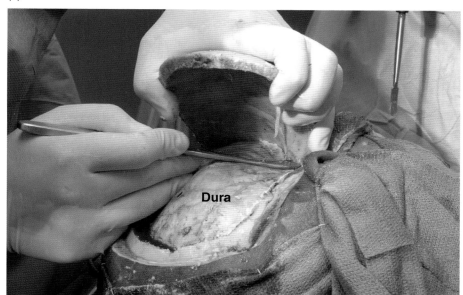

Fig. 6.12(a). A bone flap is removed with attention to avoid injury to sagittal midline

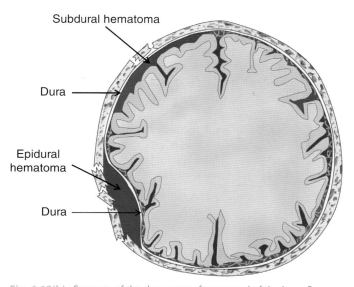

Fig. 6.12(b). Exposure of the dura mater after removal of the bone flap.

- In patients with EDH, the hematoma can be evacuated at this time. The offending (bleeding) vessel can be identified and coagulated at this time. The dura is tacked up to the surrounding bone to prevent reaccumulation of hematoma.
- In cases of SDH, the durotomy is created in a cruciate, stellate, or semicircular fashion. The dura is tacked up, and the hematoma is evacuated using gentle suction and irrigation.

Tips and pitfalls

- To avoid injury of the superior sagittal sinus or arachnoid granulation by making the burr holes in the frontal and parietal area, these holes should be created at least 1–2 cm off the midline.
- Additional bone removal at the temporal base may be performed using a single-action or double-action rongeur to achieve complete decompression of the medial temporal structures (uncus), ambient cisterns, and brainstem.

(a)

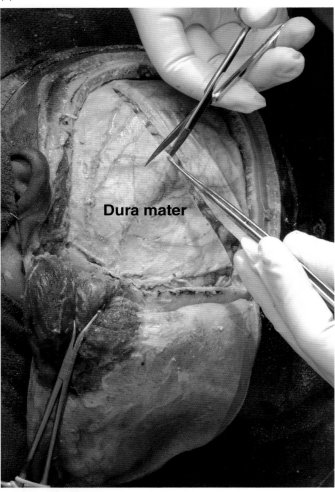

Dura mater

Evacuation of hematoma and bleeding control

- The main purposes of surgery for this particular indication are evacuation of hematoma, establishment of hemostasis, and prevention of reaccumulation of hematoma.
- Aggressive reversal of coagulopathy using blood products (e.g., fresh frozen plasma, recombinant factor VIIa, prothrombin complex concentrate, platelets) should be considered.
- Once the hematoma is encountered, the clot is removed with forceps, irrigation, and/or suction. The source of bleeding can be from (1) arterial injury, (2) venous injury, (3) brain parenchymal injury, (4) bony bleeding, (5) venous sinus bleeding. The bleeding site may not always be identified at the time of surgery (particularly venous bleeding that has thrombosed/clotted by the time of surgery).
- Arterial bleeding can be cauterized using a bipolar coagulator. Avoid cauterizing intact veins, as extensive venous infarction may occur. Several types of topical hemostatic agents (e.g., oxidized cellulose, gelatin sponge) can be used to achieve hemostasis.

Tips and pitfalls

- Great care must be taken to avoid the iatrogenic injury to the brain parenchyma when hematoma is evacuated using a suction tip or any other instruments. Any variety of cottonoids can be used to protect the brain.
- To control bleeding outside the area of exposure, additional removal of bone may be required. Attempting to achieve hemostasis without direct observation (i.e. under surrounding bone), which may cause further injury to vessels or brain parenchyma, should be avoided.

Closure

- Once the hematoma is evacuated and bleeding is stopped, a Valsalva maneuver can be performed to verify that hemostasis has been achieved.
- In EDH cases, a small durotomy may be made to rule out the presence of SDH.
- When possible, the dura is closed in a watertight manner. In cases with significant brain edema, the bone flap is often not replaced (craniectomy), and a dural substitute overlay is often used to protect the brain prior to scalp closure.
- A decision should be made whether to replace the bone flap, and whether any epidural drains would be of benefit to the patient. Our preference is to use round drains (Blake or round Jackson–Pratt drains) when necessary, which are more easily removed at the bedside. Drains can be tunneled out of a burr hole and through the scalp lateral to the incision.

(b)

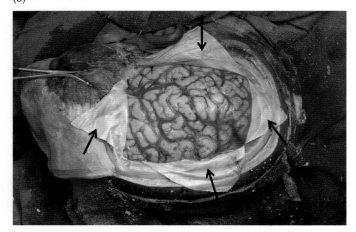

Fig. 6.13(a), (b). For evacuation of a subdural hematoma, the dura is opened in a cruciate, stellate, or semi-circular fashion.

- To prevent the development or recurrence of EDH postoperatively, the dura can be tacked up to the surrounding bone in a circumferential manner by drilling small holes in the surrounding bony edges, and suturing the dura to these holes using 4–0 Neurilon sutures.
- Intracranial cerebral pressure (ICP) monitoring may be a useful adjunct, and a monitor can be placed (often contralateral to the operative site) prior to, during, or following the operation.
- When indicated, the bone flap is replaced and secured using standard bone fixation plates. This is not possible in the presence of severe brain swelling.

- A separate drain can be placed underneath the galea as needed. The temporalis fascia is reapproximated. Following irrigation, closure of scalp proceeds in two layers (galea aponeurotica, skin).

Tips and pitfalls
- In cases of significant brain edema, the bone flap should not be replaced (decompressive craniectomy).

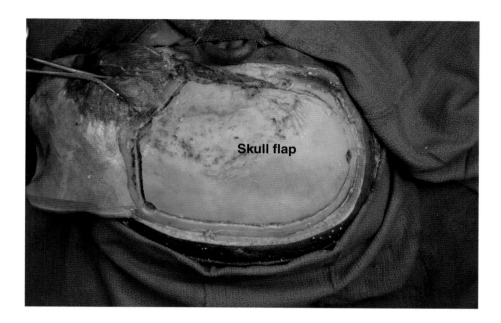

Fig. 6.14. The bone flap is placed after the evacuation. For severe swelling of the brain, the bone flap is left out.

Neck operations for trauma: general principles

Emilie Joos and Kenji Inaba

Surface anatomy

- For trauma purposes, the neck is divided into three distinct anatomical zones. Although these zones do not directly impact clinical decision making, they are important for documentation and communication purposes.

  - *Zone I*: from the sternal notch to the cricoid cartilage.
  - *Zone II*: from the cricoid to the angle of the mandible.
  - *Zone III*: from the mandible to the base of the skull.

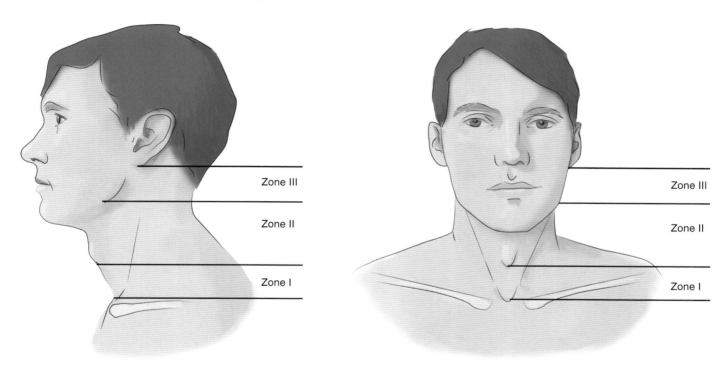

Fig. 7.1. For trauma purposes, the neck is divided into three distinct anatomical zones: Zone I, from the sternal notch to the cricoid cartilage; Zone II, from the cricoid to the angle of the mandible; Zone III, from the mandible to the base of the skull.

Atlas of Surgical Techniques in Trauma, ed. Demetrios Demetriades, Kenji Inaba, and George Velmahos. Published by Cambridge University Press. © Cambridge University Press 2015.

- At the level of the superior border of the thyroid cartilage the common carotid artery bifurcates into the internal and external carotid arteries.
- At the level of the angle of the mandible, the internal and external carotid arteries are crossed superficially by the hypoglossal nerve and the posterior belly of the digastric muscle.
- The external landmark of the pharyngoesophageal and laryngotracheal junctions is the cricoid cartilage. On esophagoscopy, this is located 15 cm from the upper incisor teeth.
- The inferior border of the middle of the clavicle is the external landmark for the transition of the subclavian artery to the axillary artery.

General principles

- Overall, approximately 35% of all gunshot wounds and 20% of stab wounds to the neck result in significant injuries to vital structures. Transcervical gunshot wounds are associated with the highest incidence of significant injuries.
- In penetrating trauma, the most commonly injured structures are the vessels, followed by the spinal cord, aerodigestive tract, and nerves.

- Overall, approximately 20% of gunshot wounds and 10% of stab wounds require operation. The remaining patients can be managed non-operatively.
- Patients with hard signs of vascular injury (pulsatile bleeding, large or expanding hematoma, bruit or thrill, and shock) or aerodigestive tract injury (hemoptysis, hematemesis, air bubbling), should proceed directly to the OR.
- Asymptomatic patients can be observed with local wound care. All remaining patients with soft signs of vascular or aerodigestive tract injury should undergo CT angiography with the selective use of catheter-based angiography, endoscopy, and contrast swallow for equivocal CT results.
- About 10% of patients with penetrating neck trauma present with airway compromise due to direct trauma to the larynx or trachea or due to external compression by a large hematoma. Airway establishment can be a difficult and potentially dangerous procedure. The surgeon should be ready to perform a surgical airway.
- Bleeding from a deep penetrating injury to the neck may be controlled by direct digital pressure in the wound or placement of a Foley catheter into the wound and inflation of the balloon with sterile water.

(a)

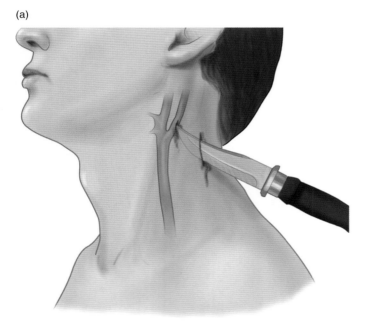

(b)

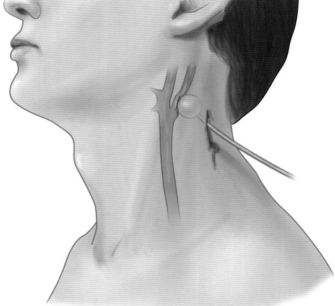

Fig. 7.2(a), (b).

(c)

(d)

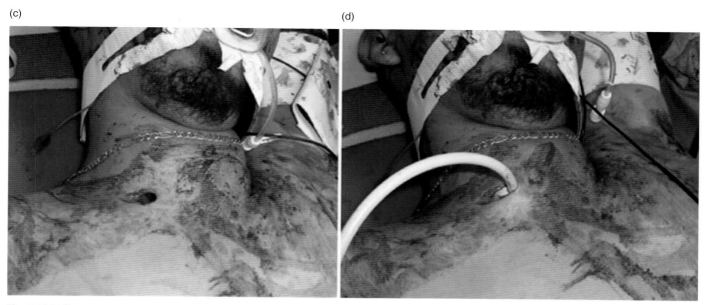

Fig. 7.2(c),(d).
Fig. 7.2(a–d). Bleeding from a deep penetrating injury to the neck may be controlled by placement of a Foley catheter into the wound and inflation of the balloon with sterile water.

- Always place intravenous lines in the arm opposite the injury, especially in periclavicular injuries with suspected subclavian vein injury.
- In suspected major venous injury, place patient in the Trendelenburg position and occlude the wound with gauze, in order to reduce risk of air embolism.

Positioning

- The patient should be in the supine position.
- If the cervical spine has been cleared, a roll should be placed under the shoulders to provide extension of the neck.
- If a sternocleidomastoid incision is planned, the head is slightly extended with the placement of a shoulder roll and turned to the opposite side of the injury. For a collar incision the head is kept in the midline position.

(a)

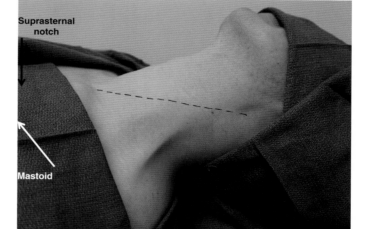

Suprasternal notch

Mastoid

Fig. 7.3(a). Position of patient for a sternocleidomastoid incision: the head is slightly extended with the placement of a shoulder roll and turned to the opposite side of the injury.

(b)

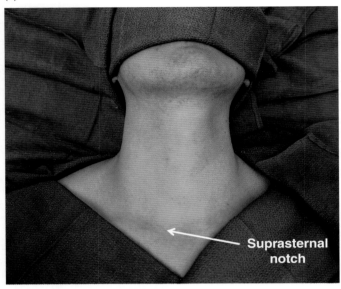

Fig. 7.3(b). Position of patient for a collar incision: the head is kept in the midline position and slightly extended with the placement of a shoulder roll.

Special instruments

- A rigid or flexible endoscope should be available for intraoperative esophagoscopy if necessary.

Skin preparation

- Prepare the patient's neck from ear to ear including chin, chest for possible sternotomy or thoracotomy, and both groins for possible vein harvesting.
- Peri-operative antibiotics should be given.
- Towels should be placed in the recesses above the shoulders.
- A clear drape should be placed from the chin upwards, so that the airway is visible and accessible to the surgeon and to facilitate joint airway manipulation with anesthesia.

Incisions

Three major incisions allow access to the neck: the anterior sternocleidomastoid, the clavicular, and the collar incision. The former is versatile and used in most cases. The collar incision is used in limited circumstances for central injuries. The clavicular incision is used for exposure of the subclavian vessels. A median sternotomy may be added to the sternocleidomastoid or the clavicular incisions for more proximal control of the common carotid or subclavian arteries.

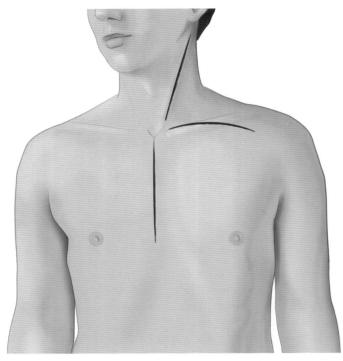

Fig. 7.4. Anterior sternocleidomastoid, clavicular, and median sternotomy incisions.

Anterior sternocleidomastoid incision

- This incision is made over the anterior border of the sternocleidomastoid muscle and extends from just below the mastoid to the suprasternal notch.
- This versatile incision can be extended down to the sternum for access to the thoracic inlet and up to the mastoid process to expose the vertebral artery and the distal internal carotid artery. Bilateral incisions can be joined with a collar incision, providing complete access to all neck structures.
- This incision provides good access to the carotid arteries, the jugular vein, the vertebral artery, and the cervical aerodigestive tract.

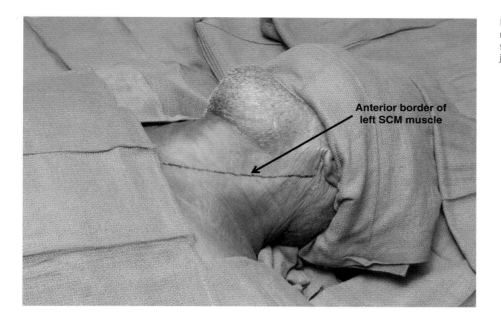

Anterior border of left SCM muscle

Fig. 7.5. The sternocleidomastoid incision is made over the anterior border of the sternocleidomastoid muscle, and extends from just below the mastoid to the suprasternal notch.

Collar incision

- The collar incision is made approximately two finger breadths above the sternal notch, extending to the medial borders of the sternocleidomastoid muscles.
- This is the preferred incision if the injury is central.
- It is commonly used for repair of a central airway injury.
- When a skin wound exists, it can be incorporated into the incision.
- This incision can also be extended to either side.

Clavicular incision

- This is the standard incision for the exposure of the subclavian vessels on both the right and the left. It may be combined with a median sternotomy, for exposure of the proximal subclavian vessels or upper mediastinal vascular structures.
- It begins at the sternoclavicular junction, extends over the medial half of the clavicle, and at the middle portion of the clavicle it curves downwards into the deltopectoral grove.
- The clavicle may be divided near the sternum and retracted to expose the proximal subclavian artery. Further details can be found in the chapter addressing subclavian injuries.

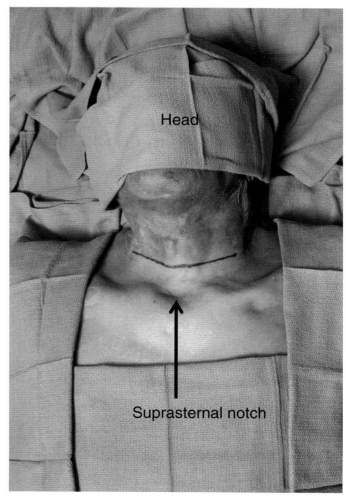

Head

Suprasternal notch

Fig. 7.6. The collar incision is made approximately two finger breadths above the sternal notch, extending to the medial borders of the sternocleidomastoid muscles.

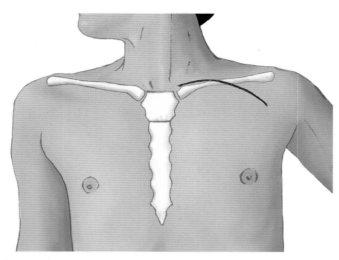

Fig. 7.7. The clavicular incision begins at the sternoclavicular junction, extends over the medial half of the clavicle, and at the middle portion of the clavicle it curves downwards into the deltopectoral groove.

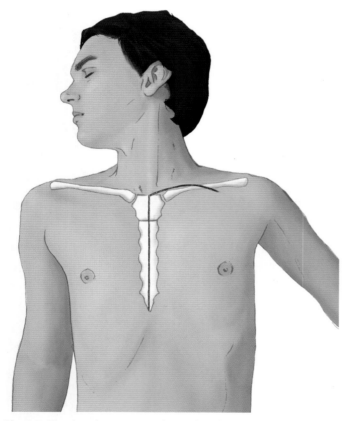

Fig. 7.8. The clavicular incision can be combined with a median sternotomy for improved exposure of the proximal left subclavian artery and upper mediastinal vessels.

Tips and pitfalls

- Airway compromise due to direct trauma to the larynx or trachea or due to external compression by a large hematoma is an emergency. The surgeon should be ready to perform a surgical airway.
- Never place an intravenous line in the arm on the same side as a periclavicular injury, because of the possibility of the presence of a subclavian venous injury.
- Air embolism may occur in patients with major venous injury. To prevent this potentially lethal complication, place the patient in the Trendelenburg position and occlude the wound with gauze.
- Always prepare the chest, as injuries in the neck may track down towards the mediastinal structures, requiring a sternotomy for control and repair. Specifically, a sternotomy can be extremely helpful for proximal control of the great vessels.
- All of the access incisions are extensible and can be combined, maximizing exposure and facilitating a high quality repair and decreasing the rate of missed or iatrogenic injuries.
- For the esophagus and trachea, take care to avoid missing a second backwall injury, as it can be difficult to detect with a lateral incision.

Carotid artery and internal jugular vein injuries

Edward Kwon, Daniel J. Grabo, and George Velmahos

Surgical anatomy

- The right common carotid artery originates from the innominate (brachiocephalic) artery. The external landmark is the right sternoclavicular joint. The left common carotid artery originates directly from the aortic arch in the superior mediastinum.
- The carotid sheath contains the common and internal carotid arteries, the internal jugular vein, and the vagus nerve. The internal jugular vein lies lateral and superficial to the common carotid artery and vagus nerve. The vagus nerve lies posteriorly, between the artery and the vein. On occasion, the vagus nerve may be located anterior to the vessels.

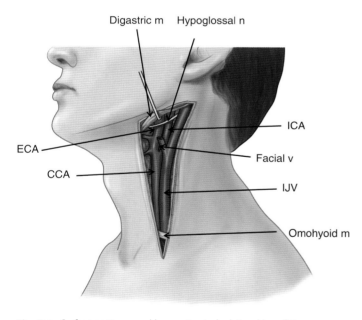

Fig. 8.1. Surface anatomy and key anatomical relationships of the carotid artery.

- The carotid sheath and its contents are covered superficially by the platysma, the anterior margin of the sternocleidomastoid muscle, and the omohyoid muscle. Deep to the vessels are the longus colli and longus capitis muscles. Medial to the carotid sheath are the esophagus and the trachea.
- At the level of the superior border of the thyroid cartilage, the common carotid artery bifurcates into the internal and external carotid arteries.
- The facial vein crosses the carotid sheath superficially to enter the internal jugular vein at the level of the carotid bifurcation.
- The external carotid artery lies medial to the internal carotid artery for the majority of their course. The first branch of the external carotid artery is the superior thyroid artery located near the carotid bifurcation.
- The internal carotid artery does not have any extracranial branches.
- At the level of the angle of the mandible, the internal and external carotid arteries are crossed superficially by the hypoglossal nerve (cranial nerve XII) and the posterior belly of the digastric muscle. The glossopharyngeal nerve (cranial nerve IX) passes in front of the internal carotid artery, above the hypoglossal nerve.
- The external carotid arteries terminate in the parotid gland, where they divide into the superficial temporal and maxillary arteries.
- At the level of the skull base, the internal carotid arteries cross deep and medial to the external carotid arteries to enter the carotid canal behind the styloid process.

Atlas of Surgical Techniques in Trauma, ed. Demetrios Demetriades, Kenji Inaba, and George Velmahos. Published by Cambridge University Press. © Cambridge University Press 2015.

Common carotid artery   **Vagus nerve**

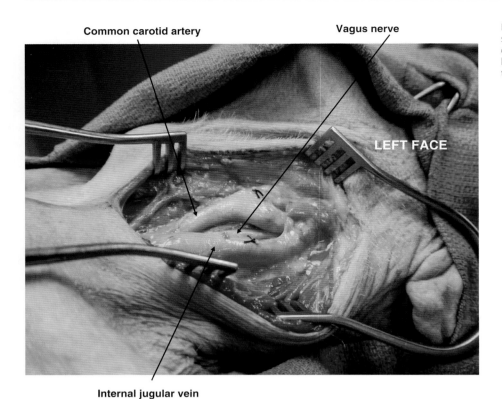

LEFT FACE

Internal jugular vein

Fig. 8.2. Carotid sheath contents. The carotid sheath contains the common carotid and internal carotid arteries medially, the internal jugular vein laterally, and the vagus nerve posteriorly between the vessels.

Internal jugular vein   **Facial vein**

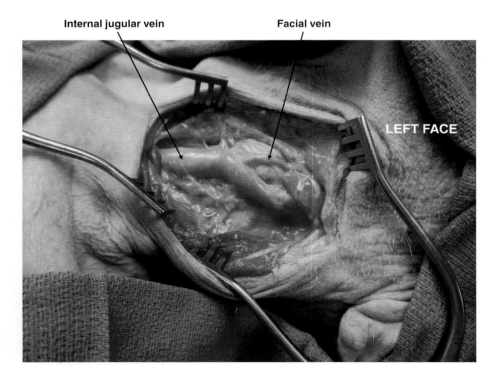

LEFT FACE

Fig. 8.3. The facial vein is the anatomical landmark approximating the location of the carotid bifurcation deep to it. The facial vein is ligated and divided in order to mobilize the internal jugular vein laterally and provide exposure to the underlying carotid bifurcation.

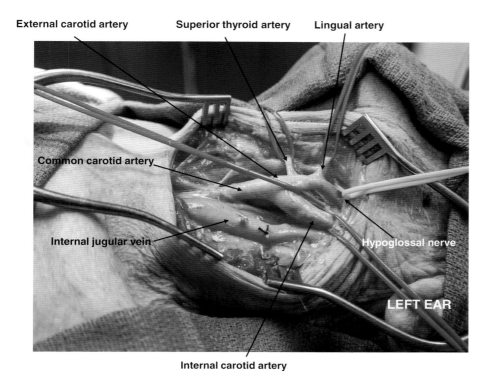

External carotid artery   Superior thyroid artery   Lingual artery

Common carotid artery

Internal jugular vein

Hypoglossal nerve

LEFT EAR

Internal carotid artery

Fig. 8.4. The external carotid lies medial to the internal carotid artery and gives several branches (the first branches are the superior thyroid and lingual arteries). The internal carotid artery has no extracranial branches. Note the hypoglossal nerve (yellow loop) crossing over the two arteries.

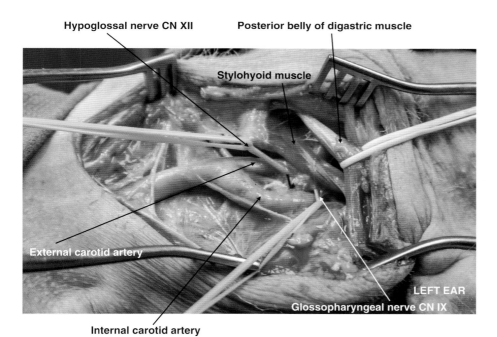

Hypoglossal nerve CN XII   Posterior belly of digastric muscle

Stylohyoid muscle

External carotid artery

LEFT EAR

Glossopharyngeal nerve CN IX

Internal carotid artery

Fig. 8.5. Distal carotid artery anatomy. At the angle of the mandible, the carotid arteries are crossed superficially by the hypoglossal nerve, the posterior belly of the digastric muscle, and the glossopharyngeal nerve.

General principles

- A preoperative neurologic examination should always be performed and documented.
- Patients with neurologic deficits secondary to carotid artery injury have a poor prognosis. If the diagnosis is made early (within 4–6 hours), revascularization should be performed. Delayed revascularization can convert an

ischemic infarct into a hemorrhagic infarct leading to increased morbidity and should therefore be avoided.
- If technically possible, all common and internal carotid artery injuries should be repaired, as ligation is associated with a significant risk of stroke. Ligation may be considered in the comatose patient with delayed operation (>6 hours from injury) or if there is uncontrollable

hemorrhage. Temporary shunt placement is a preferred method of damage control for these injuries.

- Prophylactic shunting of the common or internal carotid arteries should be considered intraoperatively in patients requiring reconstruction with grafts.
- Minor carotid injuries, such as small intimal tears, may be managed non-operatively with antithrombotic therapy and imaging to document resolution.
- Select patients with extremely proximal or distal carotid injuries may be best managed with angiographically placed stents.
- The external carotid artery can be ligated without significant sequelae.
- Systemic heparinization (100 u/kg) should be considered in patients with no other injuries. Alternatively, heparin saline solution (5000 units in 100 mL normal saline) can be injected locally, both proximal and distal into the injured vessel.
- Unilateral internal jugular vein injuries can be repaired if the patient condition allows and if there is no significant stenosis (<50%). However, unilateral ligation is well tolerated. If there are bilateral internal jugular vein injuries, at least one vein should be repaired.
- Vascular repairs should be protected in the presence of tracheal or esophageal injuries with interposed tissue, usually the strap muscles.

Special surgical instruments

- Complete vascular tray, Fogarty catheters, a carotid shunt, and rummel tourniquets. As exposure of the mediastinal

segment of the carotid arteries or internal jugular veins may be required, a chest tray, sternal saw, and sternal retractor should always be available. 1% lidocaine should also be readily available for possible injection of the carotid body if necessary, as well as prosthetic graft materials (PTFE or Dacron) in the event that reconstruction requires a conduit.

- Headlights and surgical loupes are strongly recommended.

Positioning

- The patient is positioned supine on the operating room table with adduction of the ipsilateral arm or bilateral arms if the neck injuries are bilateral.
- The neck should be slightly extended and the head turned to the contralateral side. If possible, elevation of the shoulders with a shoulder roll will facilitate extension of the neck.
- The patient should be prepped to include the entirety of the neck from the earlobes to the base of the skull and extending to the inferior aspect of the mandible down to the chest. The chest should be included to facilitate proximal control. The groins should also be included in the field, in case a saphenous vein graft is required.

Incisions

- The standard incision for exposure to the cervical carotid arteries and internal jugular veins is a longitudinal incision along the anterior border of the sternocleidomastoid muscle, extending from the suprasternal notch to just below the mastoid process.

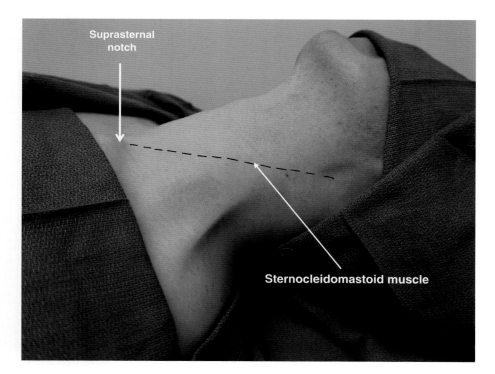

Fig. 8.6. The patient is positioned with the neck extended and the head rotated contralateral. A roll under the shoulders may be helpful to achieve maximal extension of the neck. The standard incision is placed along the anterior border of the sternocleidomastoid muscle from the suprasternal notch to the mastoid process.

- For proximal common carotid artery or internal jugular vein injuries, the combination of a sternocleidomastoid incision and median sternotomy provides the optimal exposure (see Chapter 16).

Operative technique

Exposure

- A longitudinal incision is made along the anterior border of the sternocleidomastoid muscle from the mastoid process to the suprasternal notch. The incision is carried through the platysma to expose the anterior border of the sternocleidomastoid muscle.
- The anterior border of the sternocleidomastoid muscle is then dissected free along its length and retracted laterally. At the upper part of the incision, the accessory nerve (cranial nerve XI) enters the sternocleidomastoid muscle and care should be taken to avoid injury.
- The carotid sheath is now visible and is incised along its length. If more proximal exposure is required, the omohyoid muscle may be divided.
- The contents of the carotid sheath are now exposed. The internal jugular vein is then mobilized and retracted laterally and the common carotid artery is retracted anteromedially. The vagus nerve, located posteriorly between the vessels, is identified and protected. Vessel loops are placed around the artery, vein, and nerve. For exposure of the carotid bifurcation, the facial vein is identified and ligated.

(a)

Platysma

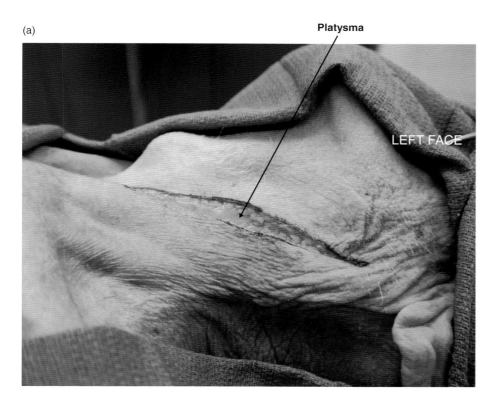

LEFT FACE

Fig. 8.7(a). The skin is incised along the anterior border of the sternocleidomastoid muscle to expose the underlying platysma.

(b)

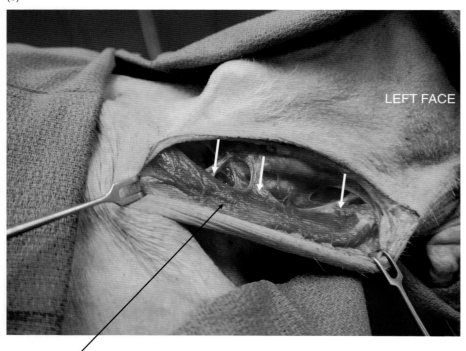

Fig. 8.7(b). The sternocleidomastoid is dissected along its anterior border and retracted laterally. Small branches of the external carotid artery (white arrows) are ligated and divided to adequately mobilize the sternocleidomastoid muscle and expose the carotid sheath.

Sternocleidomastoid muscle reflected posterior

(a)

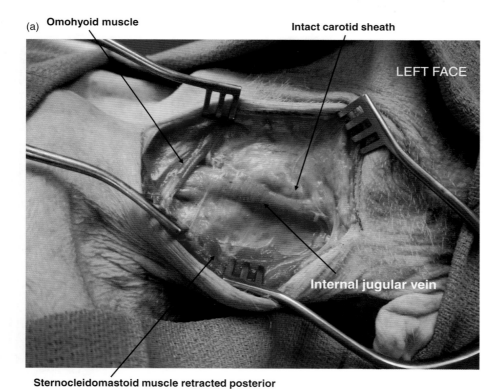

Fig. 8.8(a). Carotid sheath and omohyoid. The sternocleidomastoid muscle is retracted posterior to reveal the underlying carotid sheath and its contents. The omohyoid muscle at the inferior border of the incision may be divided if more proximal exposure is required.

Sternocleidomastoid muscle retracted posterior

(b)

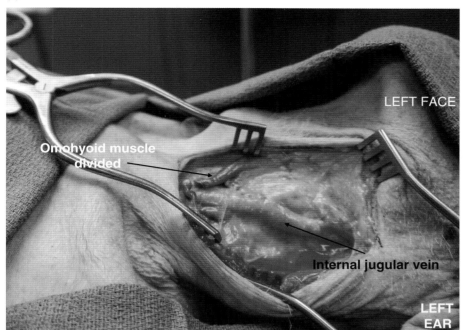

Fig. 8.8(b). Exposure to the proximal common carotid artery and internal jugular vein may be improved with division of the omohyoid muscle.

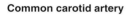

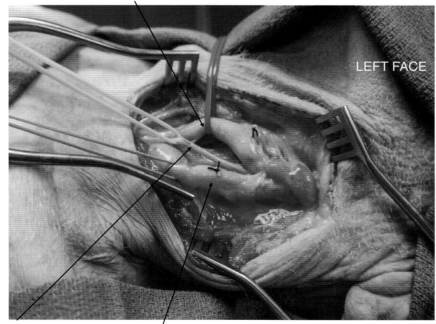

Fig. 8.9. Carotid sheath contents. The common carotid artery and internal jugular vein are identified and looped. The vagus nerve is identified posterior and between the vessels (yellow loop).

- During dissection of the carotid bifurcation, the carotid body may be stimulated causing hemodynamic instability (hypotension and bradycardia). If this is encountered, the carotid body may be injected with 1% lidocaine. The external and internal carotid arteries are then dissected and isolated using vessel loops.

- The ansa cervicalis should be visible anterior to the carotid bifurcation and can be followed to the hypoglossal nerve. Once the hypoglossal nerve (cranial nerve XII) is identified and protected, the ansa cervicalis may be divided if necessary for exposure.

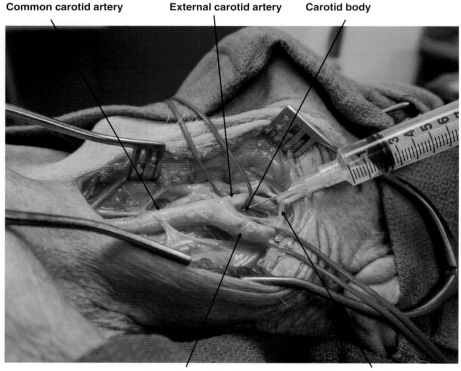

Common carotid artery **External carotid artery** **Carotid body**

Internal carotid artery **Hypoglossal nerve**

(a)

Fig. 8.10. Carotid body injection. During the dissection of the carotid bifurcation, the carotid body may become stimulated causing hypotension and bradycardia. If this situation is encountered, 1% lidocaine may be injected into the carotid body located in the crotch of the bifurcation.

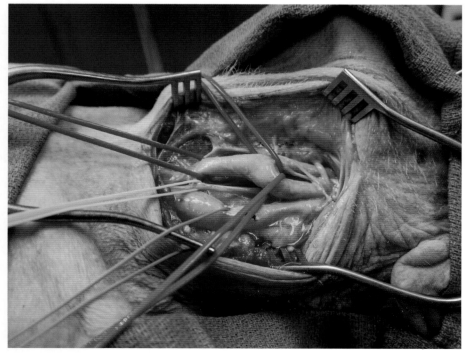

Fig. 8.11(a). The carotid bifurcation is carefully dissected and the common, internal, and external carotid arteries are isolated and looped. Note that the external carotid artery is medial to the internal carotid artery at the bifurcation.

(b)

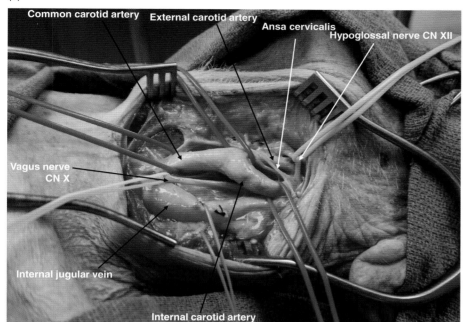

Common carotid artery   External carotid artery
Ansa cervicalis
Hypoglossal nerve CN XII
Vagus nerve CN X
Internal jugular vein
Internal carotid artery

Fig. 8.11(b). Hypoglossal nerve and ansa cervicalis. The ansa cervicalis overlies the carotid bifurcation and may be followed to identify the hypoglossal nerve. The hypoglossal nerve crosses the internal and external carotid arteries distal to the bifurcation.

- Exposure of the distal internal carotid artery is challenging and may require techniques such as subluxation of the mandible and possibly mandibular osteotomy.
  - Subluxation of the mandible may be achieved by grasping the lower teeth with two hands and pulling the mandible downward and anteriorly. An assistant may hold the jaw in position as the surgeon exposes the vessel.

  - Exposure to internal carotid at the base of the skull is achieved by extending the surgical incision posteriorly around the ear and dividing the posterior belly of the digastric, stylohyoid, stylopharyngeus, and styloglossus muscles. The styloid process is then removed. Care should be taken to avoid injury to the glossopharyngeal nerve (cranial nerve IX) deep to the posterior digastric and along the stylohyoid muscle.

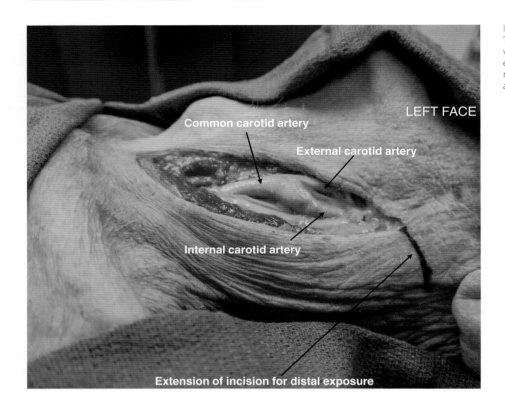

Fig. 8.12. Left distal carotid artery exposure. To expose the carotid artery and internal jugular vein close to the base of the skull the incision is extended in a postauricular fashion and the mandible is then subluxed and wired or held by an assistant to maintain subluxation.

Common carotid artery

External carotid artery

Internal carotid artery

LEFT FACE

Extension of incision for distal exposure

(a)

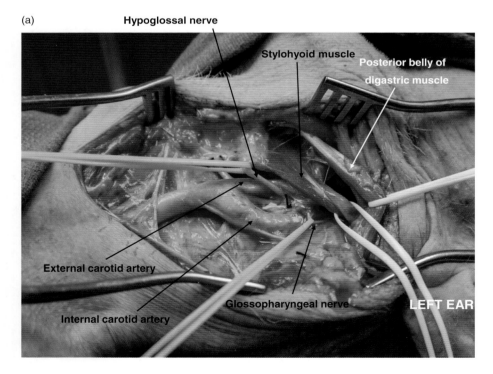

Hypoglossal nerve

Stylohyoid muscle

Posterior belly of digastric muscle

External carotid artery

Internal carotid artery

Glossopharyngeal nerve

LEFT EAR

Fig. 8.13(a). Distal carotid exposure. Subluxation of the mandible is achieved, allowing more distal exposure of the internal carotid artery. The posterior belly of the digastric muscle and stylohyoid muscles overlie the distal internal carotid artery. Deep to the muscle lies the glossopharyngeal nerve.

(b)

Division of the posterior belly of digastric muscle

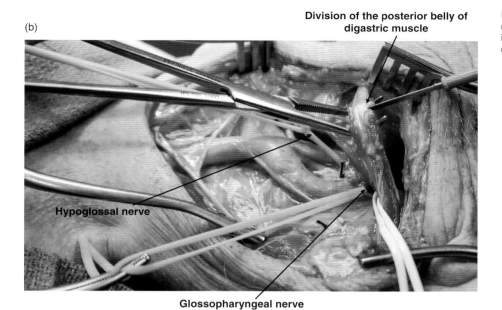

Fig. 8.13(b). Division of the posterior belly of the digastric muscle. Care should be taken to avoid injury to the underlying glossopharyngeal nerve during division.

Hypoglossal nerve

Glossopharyngeal nerve

(a)

Division of stylopharyngeus muscle

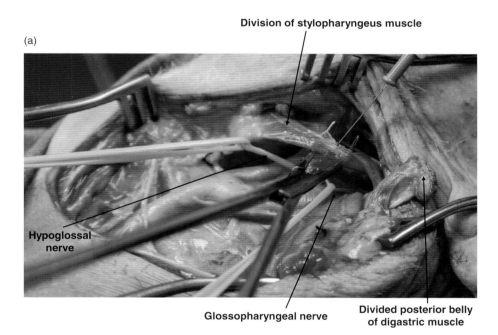

Fig. 8.14(a). Division of the stylopharyngeus. The stylopharyngeus muscle is divided to continue exposure to the distal carotid artery. Care should be taken to avoid injury to the underlying glossopharyngeal nerve.

Hypoglossal nerve

Glossopharyngeal nerve

Divided posterior belly of digastric muscle

(b)

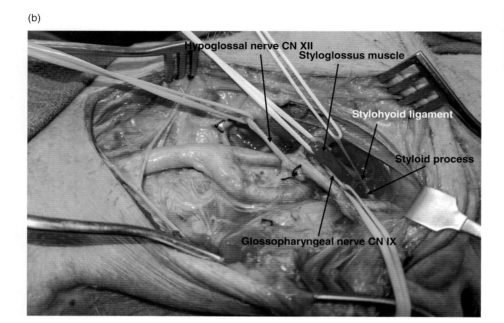

Fig. 8.14(b). Once the stylopharyngeus is divided, the underlying styloglossus and stylohyoid ligaments are identified and divided. Care should be taken to avoid injury to the underlying glossopharyngeal nerve.

(a)

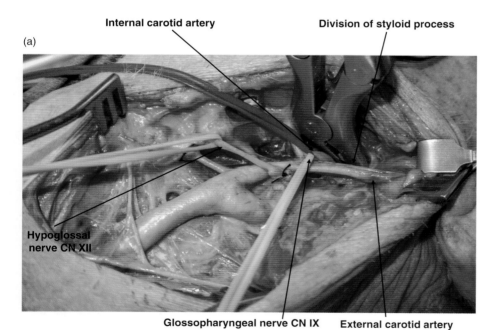

Fig. 8.15(a). Styloid process. Once the muscles are divided, the styloid process is divided with a rongeur to gain exposure to the internal carotid artery at the carotid canal.

(b)

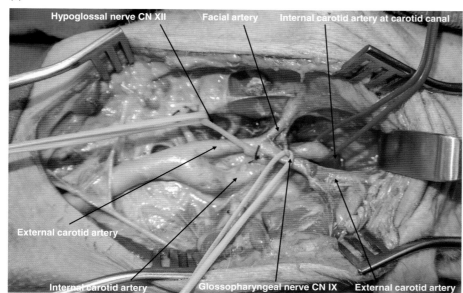

Fig. 8.15(b). Internal carotid artery at carotid canal. With the jaw subluxed and the styloid muscles and process divided, the internal carotid artery is exposed as it enters the carotid canal. Note the course of the internal carotid as it crosses deep and medial to the external carotid artery. The termination of the external carotid artery into the parotid gland is also well exposed.

- Exposure to proximal cervical carotid or jugular injuries may require the addition of a sternotomy to the standard sternocleidomastoid incision. This technique is described in the chapter on mediastinal vascular injuries.

Repair

- Small carotid artery injuries without significant tissue loss (usually secondary to knife wounds) may be repaired by

mobilization and primary suturing with 5–0 monofilament non-absorbable suture. The intima should be inspected through the injury to ensure back wall integrity prior to closure.

- Carotid shunts should be utilized during more complex repairs to protect against ischemic stroke.

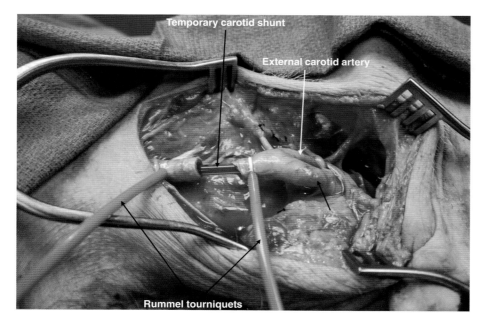

Fig. 8.16. Temporary carotid shunt. A temporary carotid shunt should be used for repairs of the carotid artery more complex than lateral arteriorrhaphy. The shunt may be secured with rummel tourniquets, allowing continued cerebral perfusion during reconstruction to prevent ischemia.

- If the repair is not possible without causing stenosis, a patch angioplasty can be performed using either a vein patch (saphenous vein or external jugular vein) or prosthetic material (Dacron, PTFE, bovine pericardium) sutured in a running continuous fashion circumferentially around the defect using a 5–0 monofilament non-absorbable suture.

- For destructive injuries with significant tissue loss (usually secondary to firearm injuries or blunt trauma), an interposition graft with either reverse saphenous vein or prosthetic material (Dacron, PTFE) should be used. Alternatively, transposition of the external carotid artery may be possible in select circumstances to reconstruct the internal carotid artery injury.

(a)

Graft in progress with shunt in place

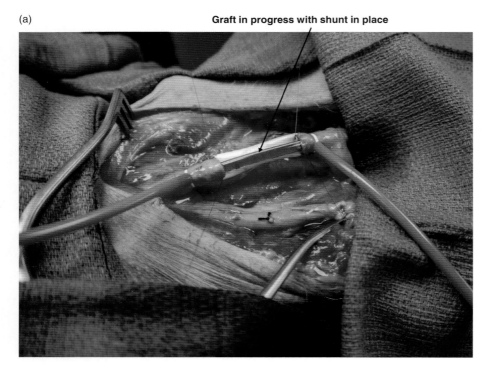

Fig. 8.17(a). Graft reconstruction with temporary shunt. A temporary shunt is placed in the lumen of the injured vessel to maintain cerebral perfusion, while a graft is sutured in place. Note that the same technique may be used during a patch angioplasty reconstruction.

(b)

Completed graft

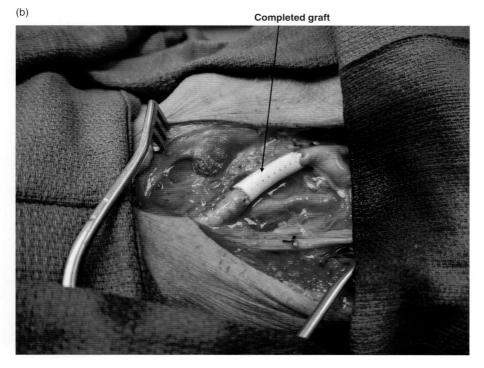

Fig. 8.17(b). Interposition graft. Once the graft is anastomosed, the temporary shunt is removed. Possible conduits include reverse saphenous vein, PTFE, and dacron.

Proximal external carotid artery   **Anastomosis**

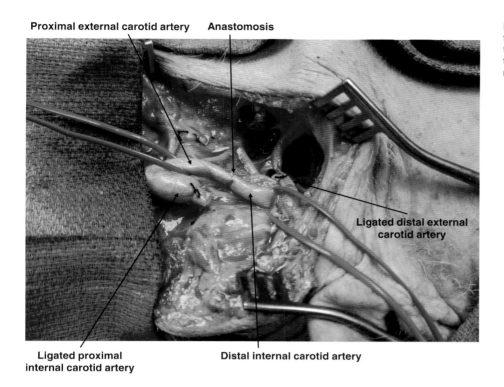

Ligated distal external carotid artery

Ligated proximal internal carotid artery   **Distal internal carotid artery**

Fig. 8.18. External to internal carotid transposition. In rare circumstances transposition of the external carotid artery proximal to the injury to the distal internal carotid artery may be used to reconstruct the injured vessel.

- If the patient is not stable enough to undergo definitive repair of the carotid vessels, a carotid shunt may be placed to maintain cerebral blood flow during the resuscitative period with delayed reconstruction.

Damage control shunt

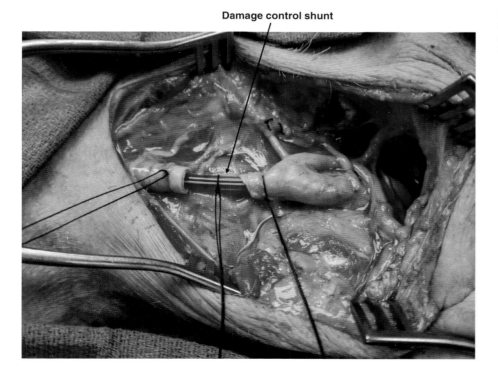

Fig. 8.19. Damage control carotid shunt. The shunt is secured with silk ties around the proximal and distal arterial segments as well as the shunt itself, to prevent migration of the shunt.

- Internal jugular vein injuries may be repaired if technically feasible and if repair does not result in stenosis greater than 50%. If there is unilateral injury and the patient is unstable, then ligation is appropriate. If there are bilateral injuries to the internal jugular veins, then attempts should be made to repair one side if at all possible.

Wound closure

- The wound should be closed in layers with reapproximation of the sternocleidomastoid muscle, platysma, and skin over a closed suction drain.

Tips and pitfalls

- In patients with neurologic deficits secondary to carotid artery injury, revascularization should be performed within 4–6 hours of the injury. Delayed revascularization after this time period can convert an ischemic brain infarct into a hemorrhagic infarct.
- Subluxation of the mandible is not difficult and may improve the exposure of the distal internal carotid artery by an additional 2–3 cm.
- Distal control of internal carotid injuries at the level of the base of the skull may require balloon catheter tamponade and thrombosis or ligation as the definitive management if it is not possible to revascularize distally secondary to anatomical barriers.

9

Subclavian vessels

Demetrios Demetriades and Jennifer Smith

Surgical anatomy

- On the right side, the subclavian artery originates from the innominate (brachiocephalic) artery, which branches into the right subclavian and right common carotid arteries. On the left side, it originates directly from the aortic arch. In some individuals the left subclavian artery may have a common origin with the left common carotid artery.

- The subclavian artery courses laterally, passing between the anterior and middle scalene muscles. This is in contrast to the subclavian vein, which is located superficial to the anterior scalene muscle.

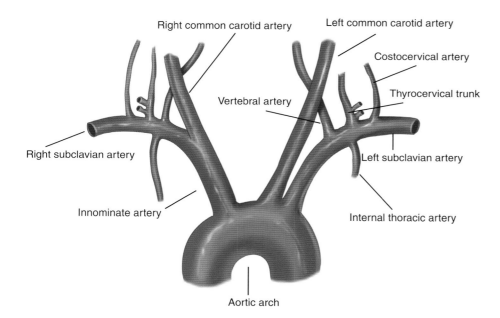

Right common carotid artery

Left common carotid artery

Costocervical artery

Vertebral artery

Thyrocervical trunk

Right subclavian artery

Left subclavian artery

Innominate artery

Internal thoracic artery

Aortic arch

Fig. 9.1. The right subclavian originates from the innominate artery and the left subclavian directly from the aortic arch. Note the major branches of the subclavian artery.

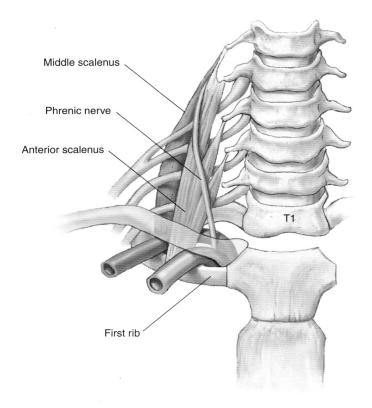

Fig. 9.2. The subclavian vein is anterior to the anterior scalene muscle and the artery is posterior. Notice the phrenic nerve on the anterior surface of the muscle. The brachial plexus is between the anterior and middle scalene muscles.

sternocleidomastoid and the strap muscles. It gives rise to the vertebral, internal mammary (internal thoracic), and thyrocervical arteries. The second part lies deep to the anterior scalene muscle and superficial to the upper and middle trunks of the brachial plexus. Here, it gives rise to the costocervical artery (on the left side the costocervical artery comes off the first part of the subclavian artery). The third part is located lateral to the anterior scalene muscle, and courses over the lower trunk of the brachial plexus, usually giving rise to the dorsal scapular artery, although its branches are not constant.

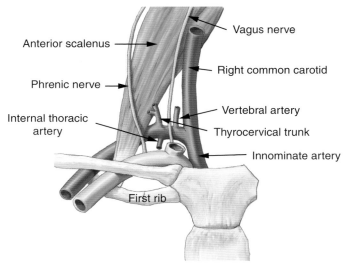

Fig. 9.3. Anatomy and branches of the right subclavian artery. Note the three branches of the first part of the artery (vertebral and thyrocervical arteries coursing superiorly, and the internal thoracic artery coursing inferiorly). The phrenic nerve crosses over the anterior scalenus muscle and lies lateral to the internal thoracic artery. The vagus nerve is medial to the internal thoracic artery.

- The subclavian artery is divided into three parts on the basis of its relationship to the anterior scalene muscle. The first part extends from its origin to the medial border of the anterior scalene muscle, coursing deep to the

Fig. 9.4. Branches of the first part of the left subclavian artery, shown after division of the anterior scalene muscle: vertebral a., internal thoracic a., and thyrocervical trunk.

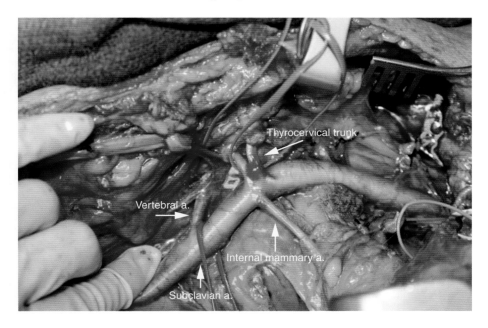

- The subclavian artery continues as the axillary artery, as it passes over the first rib. The external landmark for this transition is the lower border of the middle of the clavicle. The external landmark for the axillary artery is a curved line from the middle of the clavicle to the deltopectoral grove.
- The subclavian vein is the continuation of the axillary vein and originates at the level of the outer border of the first rib. It crosses in front of the anterior scalene muscle, and at the medial border of the muscle it joins the internal jugular vein to form the innominate (brachiocephalic) vein. The left thoracic duct drains into the left subclavian vein at its junction with the left internal jugular vein. The right thoracic duct drains into the junction of the right subclavian vein and right internal jugular vein.

- The vagus nerve is in close proximity to the first part of the subclavian artery and it lies medial to the internal thoracic artery. On the right side, it crosses in front of the artery and immediately gives off the recurrent laryngeal nerve (RLN), which loops behind the subclavian artery and ascends behind the common carotid artery into the tracheoesophageal groove. On the left side, the vagus nerve travels between the common carotid and subclavian arteries and immediately gives rise to the RLN, which loops around the aortic arch and ascends into the tracheoesophageal groove.

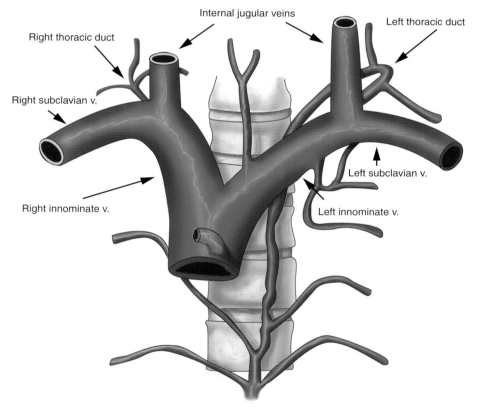

Internal jugular veins
Left thoracic duct
Right thoracic duct
Right subclavian v.
Right innominate v.
Left subclavian v.
Left innominate v.

Fig. 9.5. Anatomical relationship between the subclavian vein and the thoracic duct. The duct drains at the posterior junction of the subclavian vein with the internal jugular vein.

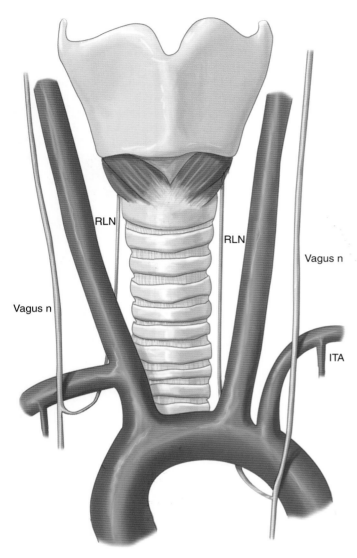

Fig. 9.6. Anatomical relationship between the vagus and recurrent laryngeal nerves and the subclavian artery. The vagus nerve crosses over the first part of the subclavian artery, medial to the internal thoracic artery. On the left, the recurrent nerve loops around the aortic arch and on the right, around the subclavian artery.

General principles

- Ligation of the subclavian artery is associated with a high incidence of limb loss and should not be performed. In critically unstable patients, temporary shunting with delayed reconstruction should be considered.
- Vascular reconstruction usually requires a 6 mm or 8 mm polytetrafluoroethylene graft. A saphenous

vein graft may be possible in some cases if the size match is adequate.

Special surgical instruments

The surgeon should have readily available a standard vascular tray, sternal saw, Gigli saw, Finochietto retractor, periosteal elevator, Doyen Raspatory, and a selection of Fogarty catheters.

Positioning

The patient is placed supine on the operating room table with the ipsilateral arm abducted to 30 degrees. Avoid excessive abduction. The patient's head should be turned to the contralateral side. Ensure that the patient is prepped from the chin to the knees and include the entire ipsilateral arm within the surgical field.

Incisions

- Depending on the site of the subclavian vascular trauma (left or right, proximal or distal) and on surgeon preference, a variety of incisions and exposures can be used, the most common being the clavicular incision with or without a median sternotomy, and the trap door incision.
- Generally, for injuries to the middle or lateral part of the subclavian vessels, a clavicular incision provides good exposure. For more proximal injuries, the clavicular incision can be combined with a median sternotomy, facilitating excellent exposure of both the left and right subclavian arteries.
- For proximal injuries on the left side, classically a "trap door" incision has been described; however, it does not improve surgical exposure and is associated with greater postoperative morbidity.
- In rare cases, if the injury is located at the mid or distal subclavian artery, exposure can be obtained through a supraclavicular incision made directly over the site of injury. The proximal and distal exposures are severely limited, however, and not generally recommended.

Exposure through a clavicular incision

- This is the preferred starting incision and provides good exposure of the second and third parts of the subclavian artery. It begins at the sternoclavicular junction, extends over the medial half of the clavicle, and at the middle portion of the clavicle it curves downward into the deltopectoral groove.

(a)

(b)

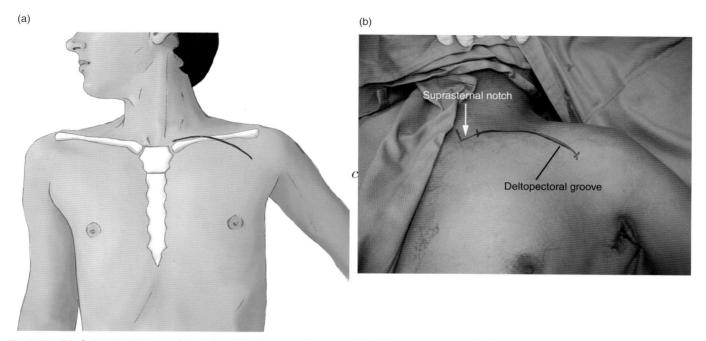

Fig. 9.7(a),(b). Patient positioning and clavicular incision for surgical exposure of the left subclavian artery. The head is turned to the opposite site and the arm is abducted to 30 degrees. The clavicular incision begins at the sternoclavicular junction, extends over the medial half of the clavicle, and at the middle of the clavicle it curves downward into the deltopectoral groove. The axillary vessels are deep to this groove.

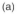 Each of the muscles attached to the medial half of the clavicle (platysma and clavicular head of the sternocleidomastoid muscle superiorly, pectoralis major and subclavius muscles inferiorly) are detached with a combination of cautery, periosteal elevator, and Doyen Rasp. The proximal half of the clavicle is now exposed and stripped of all muscular attachments.

(a)

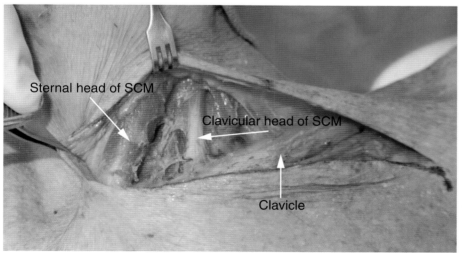

Fig. 9.8(a)–(e). Subclavian vascular exposure through a clavicular incision. All the muscles attached to the medial half of the clavicle (platysma and clavicular head of the SCM superiorly, and pectoralis major and subclavius inferiorly, are divided, using cautery and the periosteal elevator. Note the deltopectoral groove, deep to which are the axillary vessels.

(b)

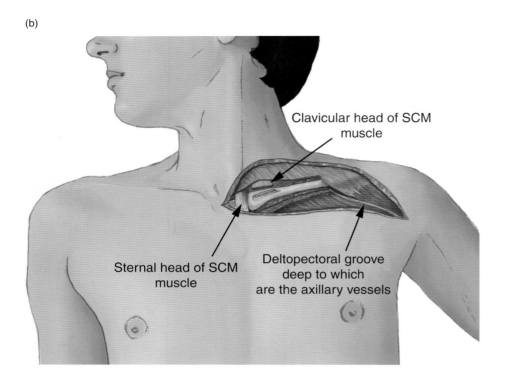

Clavicular head of SCM muscle

Sternal head of SCM muscle

Deltopectoral groove deep to which are the axillary vessels

(c)

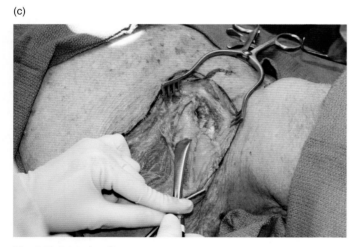

(d)

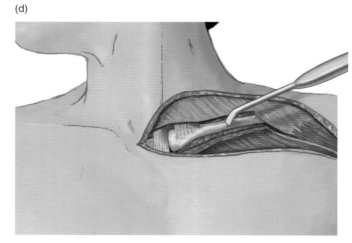

Fig. 9.8(a)–(e). *(cont.)*

(e)

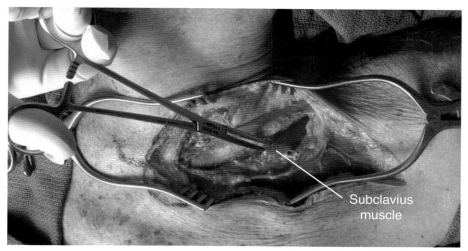

Subclavius
muscle

Fig. 9.8(a)–(e). (*cont.*)

- The subclavian vessels lie deep to the clavicle, and their exposure requires the dislocation or division or excision of the clavicle.

  o The fastest approach is division of the clavicle with the Gigli saw close to the sternoclavicular junction. At the end of the procedure, the anatomic integrity of the clavicle can be restored by wiring together the divided ends.

  o Disarticulation of the sternoclavicular joint is another option, but it takes significantly longer than division of the clavicle.

  o Excision of the medial half of the clavicle is also an acceptable option. It does not result in any functional disability but the cosmetic results are inferior to clavicular reconstruction.

  o In clavicle-sparing procedures, the clavicle is grasped with a towel clamp and retracted upward or downward to expose the underlying tissues.

(a)

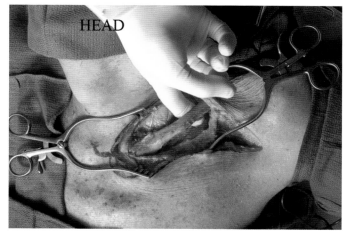

HEAD

(b)

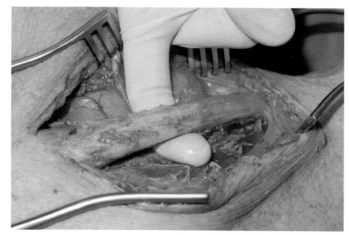

Fig. 9.9(a)–(d). The medial part of the clavicle has been freed from all muscle attachments. The clavicle is divided with a Gigli saw, close to the sternoclavicular junction. The clavicle is retracted and the underlying tissues are exposed (circle). These fatty tissues need to be dissected in order to identify the vessels.

(c)

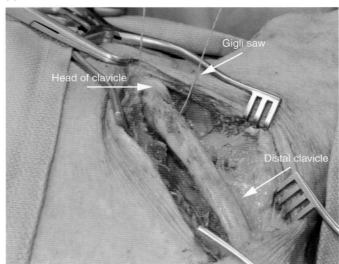

(d)

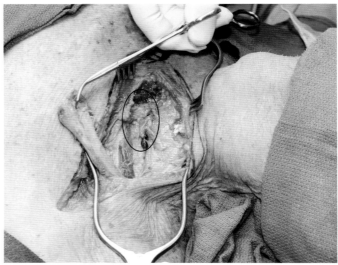

Fig. 9.9(a)–(d). *(cont.)*

- The subclavian vessels, especially the artery, lie deep under the clavicular bed and their identification requires extensive dissection of the surrounding tissues. The vein is located superficial and inferior to the artery and is the first vessel to come into view. The artery is significantly deeper than most surgeons think.

- Exposure of the first and second part of the artery requires division of the strap muscles and the anterior scalene muscle. The phrenic nerve, which lies anterior to the anterior scalene muscle, should be identified and preserved.

(a)

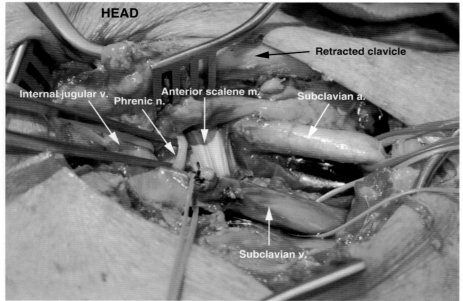

Fig. 9.10 (a)–(d). Exposure of the left subclavian vessels after division and superior retraction of the clavicle. The subclavian vein is in front of the anterior scalene muscle and the artery behind it. Note the phrenic nerve crossing over the muscle (a). The anterior scalene muscle is divided to expose the proximal subclavian artery. The phrenic nerve is retracted and protected (yellow loop) (b),(c). Exposure of the subclavian vessels after division of the anterior scalene muscle (circles). TCT = thyrocervical trunk, ITA = internal thoracic artery, IJV = internal jugular vein (d).

(b)

Fig. 9.10 (a)–(d). *(cont.)*

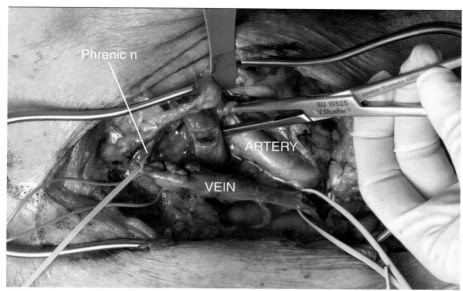

(c)

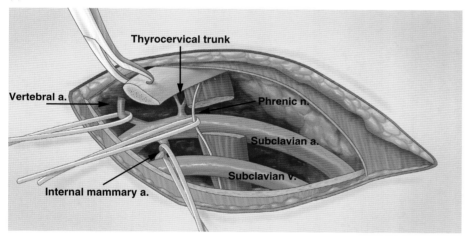

- Identification of the artery may be difficult if there is no pulsation because of proximal injury, thrombosis, or retraction of the transected ends. In these cases, it is easier to expose the axillary artery first (see Chapter 10) and proceed proximally.

Exposure through a combined clavicular incision and median sternotomy

- After successfully performing the clavicular exposure, a standard median sternotomy should be performed to obtain proximal control of either a left or right subclavian artery injury.
- For very proximal control, the artery can be dissected at its origin from the brachiocephalic artery on the right or from the aortic arch on the left. This can be done by dissecting and lifting the thymic remnant and surrounding fat in the upper mediastinum. This exposes the left innominate vein and the aortic arch with its branches. The origin of the subclavian artery (innominate artery on the right and aortic arch on the left side) is then identified and isolated. This approach is described in detail in Chapter 16.

(d)

Fig. 9.10 (a)–(d). (*cont.*)

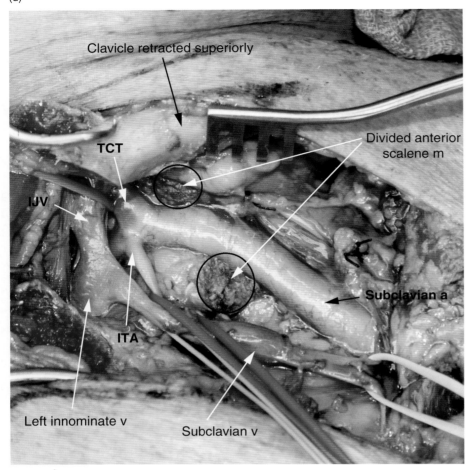

Clavicle retracted superiorly

Divided anterior scalene m

TCT

IJV

Subclavian a

ITA

Left innominate v

Subclavian v

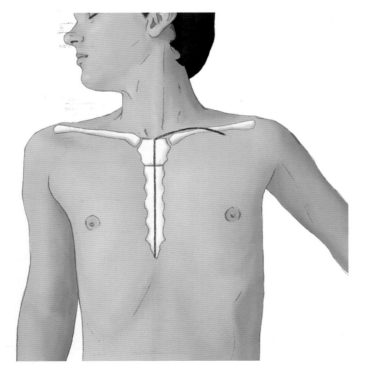

Fig. 9.11. Combined clavicular and sternotomy incisions for exposure of the very proximal subclavian artery.

(a)

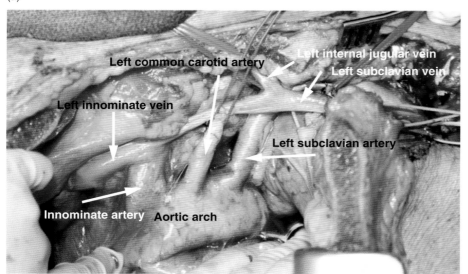

Left common carotid artery

Left internal jugular vein

Left subclavian vein

Left innominate vein

Left subclavian artery

Innominate artery Aortic arch

Fig. 9.12(a)–(c). Combined clavicular and sternotomy incisions. The aortic arch with the innominate artery, left common carotid artery, and the left subclavian artery exposed. The left innominate vein is seen retracted superiorly (a). Complete exposure of the left subclavian artery. (IJV = internal jugular vein, VA = vertebral artery). (b). Exposure of the left proximal subclavian artery and its major branches. Note the phrenic nerve, which is lateral to the internal thoracic artery and the vagus nerve, which is medial (c).

(b)

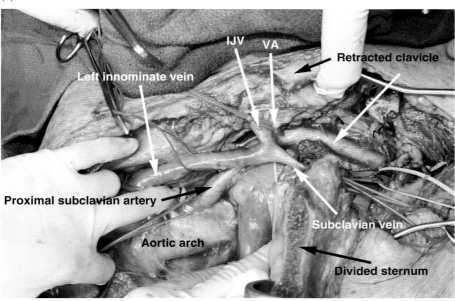

IJV VA

Retracted clavicle

Left innominate vein

Proximal subclavian artery

Subclavian vein

Aortic arch

Divided sternum

(c)

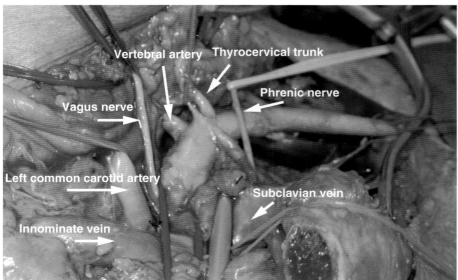

Vertebral artery Thyrocervical trunk

Phrenic nerve

Vagus nerve

Left common carotid artery

Subclavian vein

Innominate vein

Exposure through a supraclavicular incision

- This incision is rarely used in trauma, because of the limited exposure and poor proximal and distal control it provides. It may be considered in stable patients with distal subclavian arterial injuries.
- A 6-cm transverse skin incision is made 1 cm above the medial half of the clavicle. The platysma is then divided. The clavicular head of the sternocleidomastoid muscle is divided approximately 1 cm from its clavicular insertion.

- The subcutaneous tissue above the clavicle is dissected to expose and identify the subclavian vein, which courses more superficial and inferior relative to the artery.
- The anterior scalene muscle is then divided 1 cm above its insertion onto the first rib. The vein is located in front of the artery. Identify and preserve the phrenic nerve located on the anterior surface of the muscle. The subclavian artery is then identified and isolated.

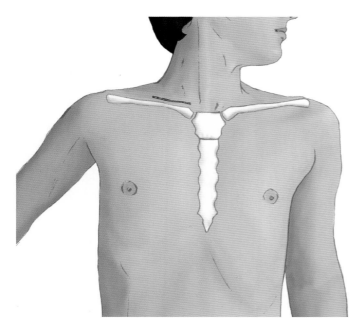

Fig. 9.13. Supraclavicular incision for exposure of the subclavian artery. A 6-cm transverse skin incision about 1 cm above the medial half of the clavicle.

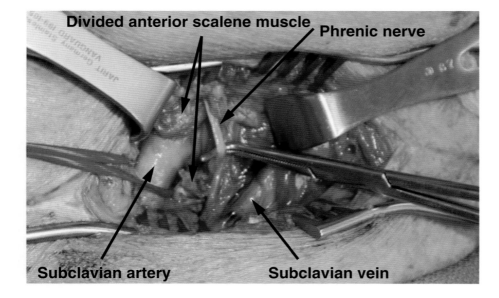

Fig. 9.14. Exposure of the right subclavian artery through a supraclavicular incision. Division of the anterior scalene muscle, with protection of the phrenic nerve.

Exposure through a "trap door" incision

This incision has been used by some surgeons to expose the proximal left subclavian artery. The "trap door" approach combines a clavicular incision, an upper median sternotomy, and an anterior left thoracotomy through the third or fourth intercostal space. This exposure is, however, associated with greater morbidity including bleeding, iatrogenic rib fractures, severe postoperative pain and more common respiratory complications when compared to the above described clavicular/median sternotomy approach.

Vascular reconstruction

- Primary arterial repair is rarely possible. In the majority of cases reconstruction using a synthetic or an autologous saphenous vein graft is necessary. The choice of graft (autologous or synthetic) is a matter of personal preference, the general condition of the patient, and the availability of an appropriately sized saphenous vein. Standard vascular techniques are used.
- The subclavian artery should not be ligated, even in clinically unstable patients, because of the significant risk of limb ischemia. For patients requiring damage control, a temporary shunt with subsequent semi-elective definitive reconstruction is recommended.
- The subclavian vein can be ligated without any significant complications. Repair should be considered only if it can be done with simple techniques and without producing significant stenosis. Stenosis greater than 50% increases the risk of thrombosis and pulmonary embolism.
- At the completion of the operation, assess for a palpable peripheral pulse and for any evidence of compartment syndrome. On-table angiography should be considered in cases with only a Doppler signal present. Routine prophylactic fasciotomies are not necessary; however, therapeutic fasciotomies should be performed without delay.

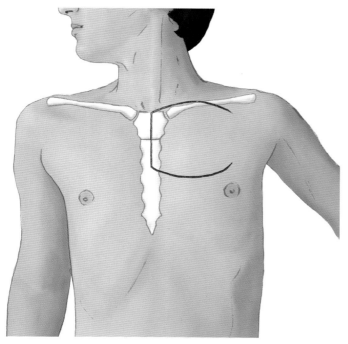

Fig. 9.15. Trap door incision combines a clavicular incision, upper median sternotomy, and a third or fourth intercostal space left thoracotomy.

Fig. 9.16. The divided clavicle is wired at the end of the vascular procedure.

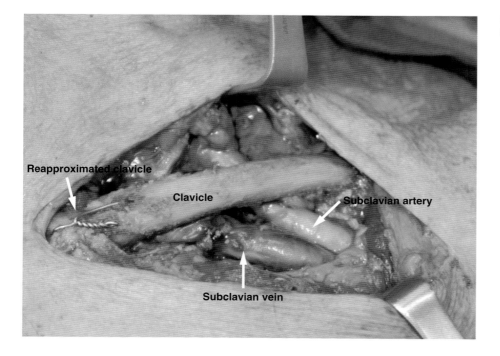

Reapproximated clavicle

Clavicle

Subclavian artery

Subclavian vein

Wound closure

- The continuity of the divided clavicle can be re-established with wiring or plating. In cases of disarticulation, the periosteum and ligaments around the sternoclavicular joint are repaired.
- The platysma should be reapproximated separately for good cosmetic results. Failure to do so can result in retraction of the muscle and poor aesthetics.

Tips and pitfalls

The subclavian artery lies deep behind the clavicle and its exposure can be challenging. Its proximal segment is approximately 5–6 cm from the skin and extensive dissection of the surrounding pre-scalene muscle fat is required.

- Intraoperative use of ultrasound may be helpful to identify the artery.
- In the absence of pulsation (thrombosis or complete transection), start with the much easier exposure of the axillary artery and proceed proximally towards the injury.
- For very proximal injuries, start with the isolation of the origin of the subclavian artery, through the combined clavicular incision/median sternotomy, and proceed distally.

Postoperatively, monitor for peripheral pulses and for the development of compartment syndrome.

- There is no role for routine prophylactic fasciotomy.
- Administration of mannitol intraoperatively and postoperatively in hemodynamically stable patients may reduce the risk of developing compartment syndrome.

The phrenic nerve is at risk of transection during the division of the anterior scalene muscle for proximal injuries. This will result in paralysis of the ipsilateral diaphragm. Identify and protect it prior to the division of the muscle.

During dissection of the right subclavian artery, isolate and preserve the recurrent laryngeal nerve, which loops around the proximal subclavian artery anteriorly prior to ascending (posteriorly) into the neck.

During dissection of the subclavian vein near its junction with the internal jugular vein, protect the thoracic duct, which drains into this part of the vein. If injured, ligate both ends. Failure to recognize and ligate the injured duct results in a troublesome postoperative chyle leak.

Axillary vessels

10

Demetrios Demetriades and Emilie Joos

Surgical anatomy

- External landmarks: the axillary vessels start at the middle of the clavicle, course deep, under the deltopectoral groove and end at the lateral border of the axilla.
- The axillary artery is divided by the pectoralis minor into three parts: the first part is proximal to the muscle and gives one branch. The second part is under the muscle, is surrounded by the cords of the brachial plexus, and gives two branches. The third part lies lateral to the muscle, is surrounded by the nerves of the brachial plexus, and gives three branches.
- The axillary vein is the continuation of the basilic vein. Prior to its transition to the subclavian vein, the cephalic vein joins it. Its middle segment lies under the pectoralis minor muscle, inferior to the axillary artery.

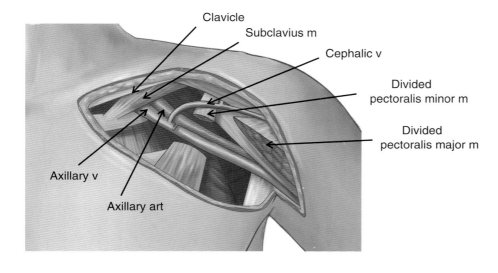

Clavicle
Subclavius m
Cephalic v
Divided
pectoralis minor m
Divided
pectoralis major m
Axillary v
Axillary art

Fig. 10.1. The axillary vessels start under the middle of the clavicle and curve downwards, deep under the deltopectoral groove. Part of the vessels are under the pectoralis minor muscle. The vein is below and more superficial to the artery. Note the cephalic vein crossing over the pectoralis minor muscle and draining into the proximal axillary vein.

Atlas of Surgical Techniques in Trauma, ed. Demetrios Demetriades, Kenji Inaba, and George Velmahos. Published by Cambridge University Press. © Cambridge University Press 2015.

General principles

- Ligation of the axillary artery is associated with a high incidence of limb loss and should not be performed. In critically unstable patients, temporary shunting with delayed reconstruction should be considered.
- Vascular reconstruction can be done with either a saphenous vein graft or a synthetic graft.

Special surgical instruments

- A standard vascular tray.
- Periosteal elevators and Doyen Raspatory may be needed for clavicular resection and exposure of the distal subclavian vessels (see Chapter 9).

Positioning

- The patient should be in the supine position, with the injured arm abducted from the body at about 30 degrees. The head is slightly turned to the opposite side.
- The neck, arm, and entire chest should be fully prepped. The groin should be included in the surgical field in case a vein harvest is needed.

Incision

- The incision starts just below the middle of the clavicle, and courses over the deltopectoral groove.
- In very proximal injuries the incision should start at the sternoclavicular junction, course directly over the medial half of the clavicle and, at the middle of the clavicle, curve downward into the deltopectoral groove. The clavicle may have to be divided to allow proximal vascular control (see Chapter 9).

(a)

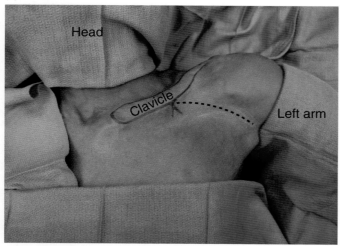

Fig. 10.2(a),(b). The standard incision for the exposure of the axillary vessels starts just below the middle of the clavicle, and courses over the deltopectoral groove. The cephalic vein courses superficially in the groove and should be avoided.

(b)

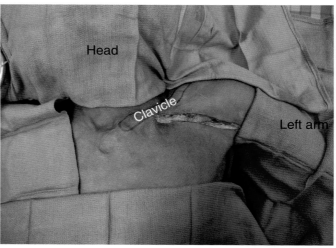

Fig. 10.2(a),(b). (cont.)

Vascular exposure

- The subcutaneous tissue under the incision is dissected into the deltopectoral groove. The cephalic vein will come into view and can be retracted or ligated.
- The lower skin flap is mobilized to allow good exposure of the pectoralis major and its insertion into the humerus.
- The pectoralis major muscle fibers are split and retracted, exposing the underlying pectoralis minor muscle. However, in severe active bleeding or if the exposure is not satisfactory, the pectoralis major is divided about 2–3 cm from its insertion into the humerus and retracted medially. The underlying pectoralis minor muscle comes into full view.

(a)

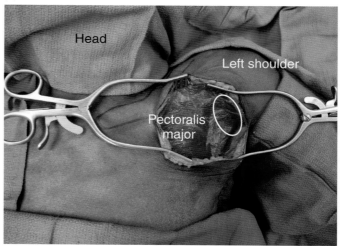

Fig. 10.3(a),(b). The lower skin flap is mobilized to allow good exposure of the pectoralis major and its insertion into the humerus (circle). The muscle might be split to expose the underlying pectoralis minor. However, for faster and better exposure its insertion into the humerus may be divided 2–3 cm from the bone.

(b)

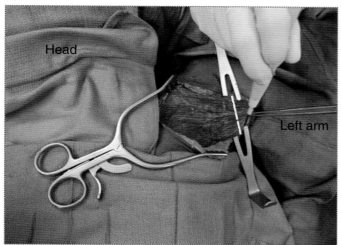

Fig. 10.3(a),(b). *(cont.)*

- The pectoralis minor is then retracted laterally or divided near its insertion into the coracoid process and retracted medially.
- The vein will first come into view, inferior and anterior to the artery.
- The axillary vessels are now fully exposed, with the brachial plexus roots and nerves surrounding them.

(a)

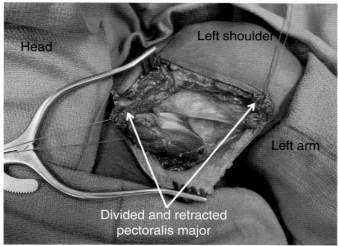

Fig. 10.4(a). Heavy absorbable sutures are placed on the divided edges of the pectoralis major. The edges are retracted to expose the underlying pectoralis minor muscle. At the completion of the operation, the sutures are tied together to reconstruct the muscle.

(b)

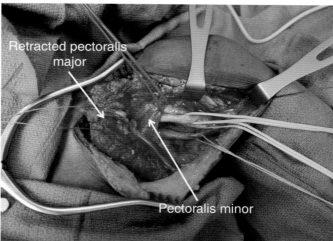

Fig. 10.4(b). Retraction of the divided pectoralis major exposes the underlying pectoralis minor and the distal subclavian vessels and brachial plexus. Note the roots of the brachial plexus (artery in red vessel loop, vein in blue, and nerves in yellow). The middle part of the axillary vessels are underneath the pectoralis minor muscle.

(a)

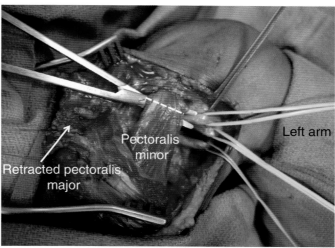

Fig. 10.5(a). Division of the pectoralis minor exposes the middle part of the subclavian vessels.

(b)

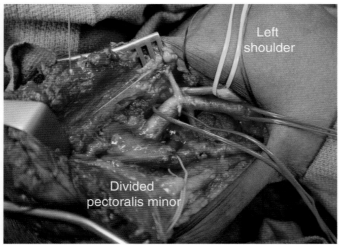

Fig. 10.5(b). After division of the pectoralis minor muscle, the axillary vessels are completely exposed (artery in red vessel loop, vein in blue, and nerves in yellow).

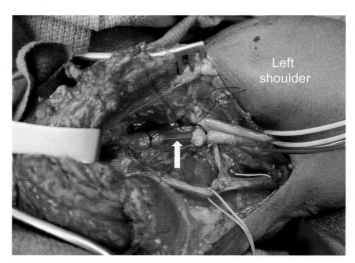

Fig. 10.7. Damage control with temporary shunt (arrow). The sutures securing the tube proximally and distally are tied together to prevent accidental dislodgement (vein in blue loop and nerves in yellow).

Vascular injury management

- The axillary artery should always be repaired or reconstructed. Damage control with temporary shunting and delayed reconstruction should be considered in patients in extremis.
- The arterial reconstruction can be done with either a synthetic or an autologus saphenous vein graft.
- The axillary vein should be repaired only if it can be done with simple suturing. Complex graft reconstruction is not advisable. Ligation of the vein is well tolerated.
- The divided pectoralis major muscle should be reapproximated using absorbable sutures.

Closure

- Reconstruction of the pectoralis minor is likewise performed.

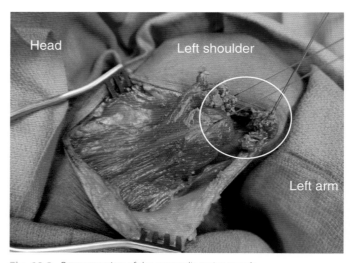

Fig. 10.8. Reconstruction of the pectoralis major muscle.

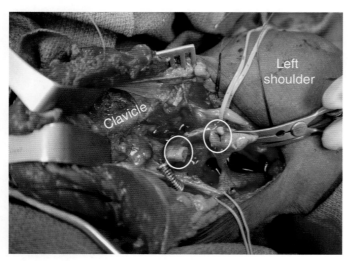

Fig. 10.6. The injured part of the axillary artery is debrided to healthy tissues (circles). Reconstruction usually requires a synthetic size 6 or 8 graft (vein in blue, vessel loop and nerves in yellow).

Tips and pitfalls

- Positioning: Excessive abduction of the arm distorts the anatomy and makes the exposure more difficult.
- To obtain proximal control of the subclavian artery, resection of the proximal clavicle may be required.

- If there is ongoing bleeding and rapid exposure is needed, the pectoralis major and minor muscles should be divided, as described above.
- Care must be taken not to injure the brachial plexus, which is intimately associated with the axillary vessels.

In cases where there was prolonged ischemia due to an arterial injury, monitor closely for compartment syndrome. There is no need for routine prophylactic arm fasciotomy. Intraoperative administration of mannitol in stable patients may reduce the risk of compartment syndrome.

Vertebral artery injuries

Demetrios Demetriades and Nicholas Nash

Surgical anatomy

- The vertebral artery (VA) is the first cephalad branch of the subclavian artery. From the trauma surgery perspective, it is divided into three parts: Part I, from its origin at the subclavian artery to C6, where it enters the vertebral foramen; Part II, which courses in the vertebral bony canal, formed by the transverse foramen, from C6 to C1; Part III, which runs outside the vertebral canal, from C1 to the base of the skull. The VA enters the skull through the foramen magnum, piercing the dura mater. It joins the opposite VA to form the basilar artery, which is part of the circle of Willis.
- The first part of the VA courses superiorly and posteriorly between the anterior scalenus and the longus colli muscles, before entering the vertebral canal at the C6 level.
- The carotid sheath is anterior and medial to the first part of the VA.
- The first part of the VA is located in the triangle formed by the sternal and clavicular insertions of the sternocleidomastoid muscle and the clavicle.
- The external landmark of C6, where the VA enters into the vertebral canal, is the cricoid cartilage.
- The VA is surrounded by a venous plexus.

General principles

- Many vertebral artery (VA) injuries can be effectively managed with angioembolization. Due to the difficult anatomy and complex operative exposure, angiographic intervention remains the preferred therapeutic modality. Operative management and direct surgical control of the bleeding are reserved only for cases with severe active bleeding or if interventional radiology is not available.
- Ligation or endovascular occlusion of the VA is tolerated well and rarely causes neurological deficits.
- Gunshot wounds to the VA are often associated with spinal fractures and spinal cord injuries.

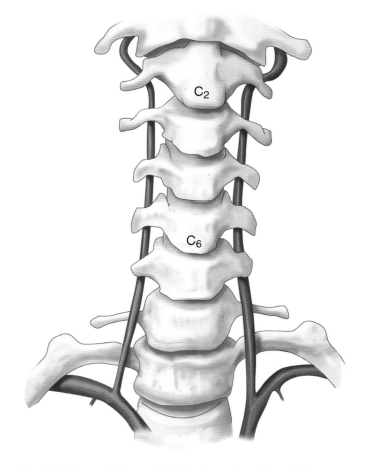

Fig. 11.1. The vertebral artery (VA) is the first cephalad branch of the subclavian artery. It enters the vertebral canal at the C_6 level and exits the canal at the C_2 level.

Special surgical instruments

- Equipment for the operation should include a major vascular tray for trauma, periosteal elevator, and bone rongeurs.

Positioning

- Supine with head turned away from the injured side and if the cervical spine has been cleared, the neck should be slightly extended, with a folded towel placed between the patient's shoulders.

Exposure of the first part of the VA

Incision

- A supraclavicular transverse incision may be used in rare occasions for exposure of the proximal VA, outside the vertebral canal. This is a limited exposure and does not allow satisfactory exploration of the carotid sheath or the aerodigestive tracts.
- Mark the sternal and clavicular heads of the sternocleidomastoid (SCM) muscle. Perform a transverse skin incision, extending between the medial border of the sternal head and the lateral border of the clavicular head of the SCM muscle, approximately two finger breadths above the clavicle.

Exposure

- Continue the dissection deep into the base of the triangle. Place a self-retaining retractor in the wound, retracting the sternal head of the SCM muscle medially and the clavicular head laterally. If necessary, divide the clavicular head of the SCM muscle near the clavicle or split the muscle heads superiorly.
- The scalene fat pad is then visualized and dissected to expose the anterior scalene muscle. The phrenic nerve will be running on the surface of the anterior scalene and the inferior thyroid artery. The muscle is retracted laterally or divided.
- The carotid sheath is the first vascular structure to be identified in the medial part of the triangle. The jugular vein is lateral, the common carotid artery medial, and the vagus nerve posterior. The structures of the carotid sheath are dissected and retracted medially. The first part of the VA is located deeper and more laterally, between the anterior scalenus laterally and longus colli muscle medially. Identification of the vessel is greatly facilitated by palpating, with the tip of the index finger, the groove between the vertebral body of C7 and the transverse process. The VA lies immediately anterior to this groove. A right-angled clamp is used to dissect the VA. Care should be taken not to injure the vertebral venous plexus, which is located in front of the artery.
- The phrenic nerve is seen laterally, on the surface of the anterior scalenus muscle, and should be protected.

(a)

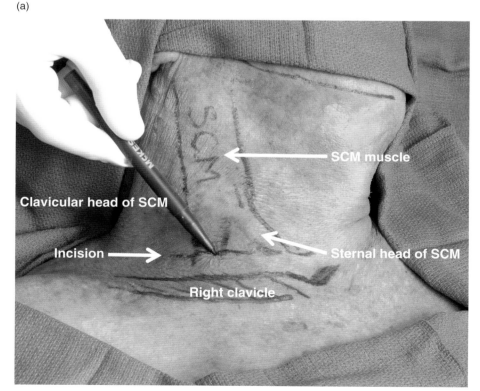

Fig. 11.2(a)–(c). Exposure of the first part of the right VA through a supraclavicular transverse incision. The incision extends between the medial border of the sternal head and the lateral border of the clavicular head of the SCM muscle, about two finger breadths above the clavicle. Following the division of the platysma, the sternal and clavicular heads of the SCM muscle are exposed. The clavicular head of the SCM can be divided and retracted superiorly for better exposure.

(b)

Fig. 11.2(a)–(c). *(cont.)*

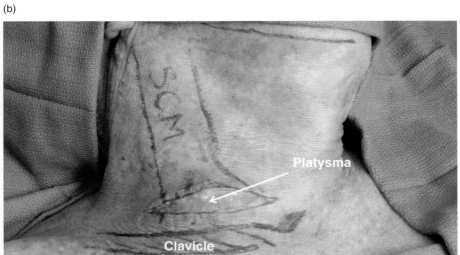

(c)

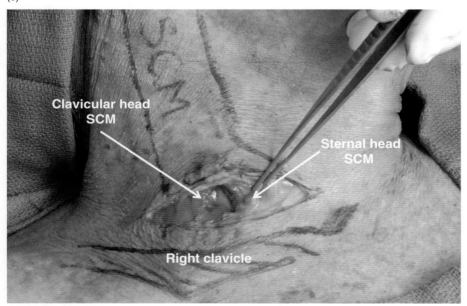

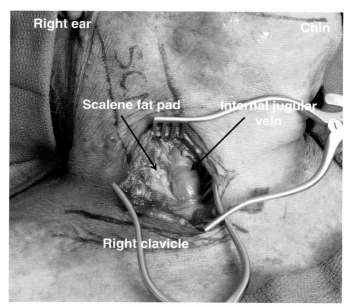

Fig. 11.3. The internal jugular vein with the carotid sheath is retracted medially and the scalene fat pad is exposed. Dissection in this area exposes the anterior scalene muscle, which is retracted laterally or divided (protect the phrenic nerve crossing over the anterior scalene).

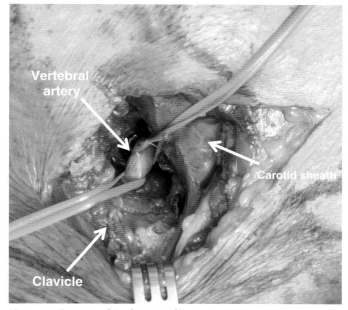

Fig. 11.4. Exposure of the first part of the VA, prior to its entry into the vertebral canal. The anterior scalene muscle along with the phrenic nerve have been retracted laterally and the VA is exposed just deep to it.

Sternocleidomastoid incision approach

Incision

- This is the preferred incision in trauma. It allows exploration of the carotid artery, the internal jugular vein, the aerodigestive tract, and the first and second parts of the VA.

- The incision is placed over the anterior border of the SCM muscle, extending from just below the mastoid process to the suprasternal notch.

Exposure

- The dissection is continued through the subcutaneous tissues and platysma, until the anterior border of the SCM is encountered. The SCM is retracted laterally to expose the carotid sheath. The jugular vein is more superficial and lateral, the common carotid artery medial, and the vagus nerve will lie posterior.

- The contents of the carotid sheath are all identified and retracted medially. The midline structures of the neck, which include the esophagus, trachea, and larynx, may also be encountered during this portion of the dissection and should be gently retracted medially as necessary.

- The anterior scalene muscle is retracted laterally or divided while protecting the phrenic nerve which lies on the surface of the muscle. The longus colli muscle, which is on the anterolateral surface of the vertebra, and the prevertebral fascia, are swept off the bone with a periosteal elevator, exposing the anterior rim of the vertebral foramen. The rim is located between the vertebral body and the anterior tubercle of the transverse process and is best identified by palpation with the tip of the index finger. This rim is excised

(a)

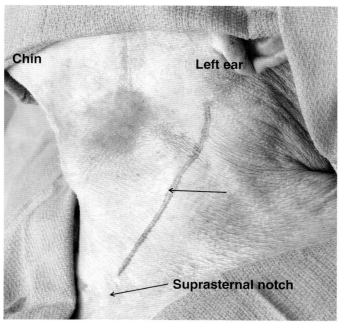

Fig. 11.5(a)–(c). Exposure of the left VA in the vertebral canal through an SCM incision. An incision is made along the anterior border of the SCM, and extends from below the mastoid process to the suprasternal notch (arrow) (a), (b). (b) The anterior border of the SCM is mobilized and SCM is retracted laterally to expose the carotid sheath (c).

(b)

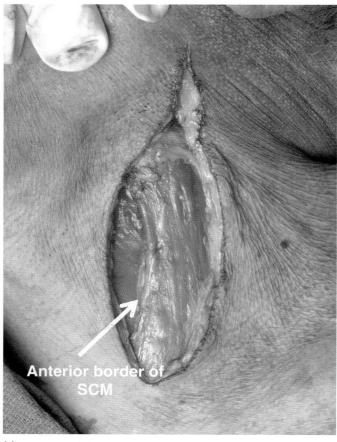

Anterior border of SCM

(c)

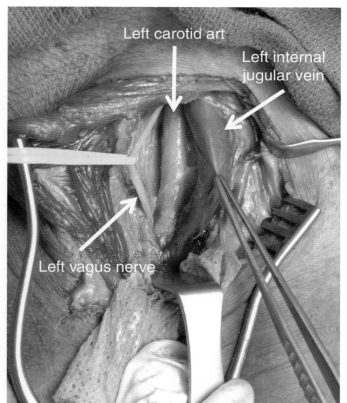

Left carotid art

Left internal jugular vein

Left vagus nerve

with bone rongeurs, and the VA is exposed and ligated or clipped. If necessary, the same process is repeated at the adjacent vertebrae. The anterior nerve root is posterior to the VA and not at risk of injury if the unroofing is done properly. Troublesome bleeding from the surrounding venous plexus can be controlled with local hemostatic agents and compression.

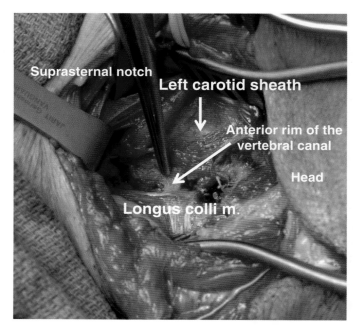

Suprasternal notch

Left carotid sheath

Anterior rim of the vertebral canal

Head

Longus colli m.

Fig. 11.6. The carotid sheath structures have been retracted medially. The forceps and arrow are pointing to the anterior rim of the vertebral foramen, that has already been cleared of its longus colli muscle attachments with a periosteal elevator. The vertebral artery lies in the canal, directly below this bony rim.

(a)

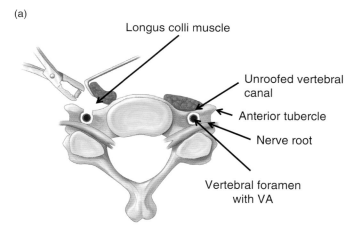

Longus colli muscle

Unroofed vertebral canal

Anterior tubercle

Nerve root

Vertebral foramen with VA

Fig. 11.7(a),(b). The longus colli muscle is detached and retracted. With the help of bone rongeurs, the vertebral canal is unroofed by excising the anterior rim to expose the VA. The rim can easily be palpated with the tip of the finger, and is located between the body of the vertebra and the anterior tubercle of the transverse process (a). The vertebral canal is unroofed (arrows) and the VA is exposed (b).

(b)

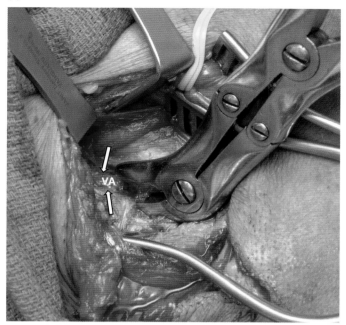

Tips and pitfalls

- In stable patients angioembolization is the procedure of choice.
- The anatomy of the VA is difficult and the surgeon should consult an atlas before the operation.
- Proximal ligation of the VA does not effectively control bleeding from a distal injury because of retrograde blood flow.
- For distal VA injuries, above C2, the exposure is difficult and a suboccipital craniectomy by a neurosurgical team may be necessary.
- For penetrating injuries that require emergent exploration due to bleeding, if direct visualization and ligation of the VA is not possible, damage control packing of the area with local hemostatic agents with postoperative angioembolization is a viable option.

Fig. 11.7(a),(b). *(cont.)*

(a)

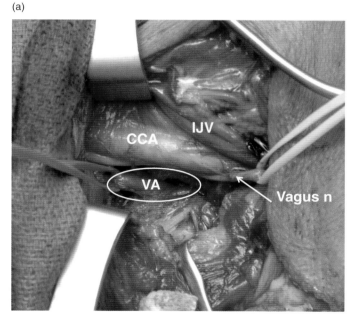

(b)

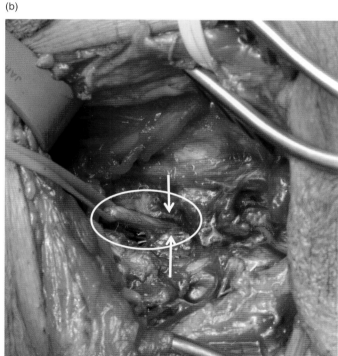

Fig. 11.8(a),(b). Following unroofing of the vertebral canal (circle), the VA (red vessel loop) is exposed. (CCA = common carotid artery, IJV = internal jugular vein, VA = vertebral artery.) Arrows in Fig. 11.8(b) show the edges of the unroofed canal. Note the carotid sheath contents retracted medially (yellow vessel loop is around the vagus nerve).

Trachea and larynx

Elizabeth R. Benjamin and Kenji Inaba

Anatomy

- The trachea is 10–12 cm long and 2–2.5 cm wide, extending from C6 to T5.
- The trachea is composed of 16–20 incomplete rings with a flattened posterior wall of muscle and fibrous tissue.
- The anatomic borders of the trachea include the isthmus of the thyroid and paired strap muscles anteriorly, the common carotid arteries, thyroid lobes, and recurrent laryngeal nerves laterally and the esophagus posteriorly.

- The paired strap muscles lie in front of the trachea and larynx. These include superficially the sternohyoid muscles and the underlying sternothyroid and thyrohyoid muscles.
- The thyroid cartilage is suspended from the hyoid bone by the thyrohyoid membrane. The cricothyroid ligament connects the inferior portion of the thyroid cartilage to the cricoid cartilage. Inferior to this is the first tracheal ring.
- The larynx is composed of three paired (arytenoid, corniculate, and cuneiform), and three unpaired (cricoid, thyroid, and epiglottic) cartilages.

(a)

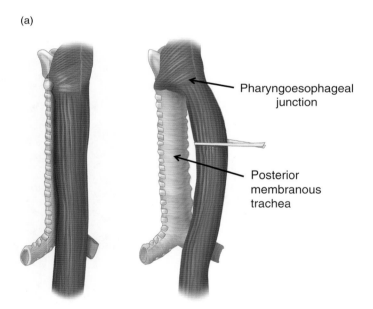

Fig. 12.1(a). The trachea is composed of 16–20 incomplete rings. The posterior membranous portion of the trachea lies just anterior to the esophagus.

(b)

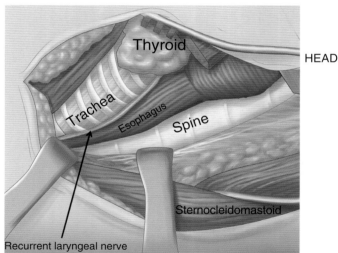

Fig. 12.1(b). Lateral view of the midline neck structures from a left sternocleidomastoid incision. The trachea is the most anterior structure. The posterior membranous portion of the trachea abuts the anterior surface of the esophagus and the recurrent laryngeal nerve runs in the trachea–esophageal groove. Posterior to the esophagus is the spine. The carotid sheath and sternocleidomastoid muscle are retracted laterally to provide this exposure.

Atlas of Surgical Techniques in Trauma, ed. Demetrios Demetriades, Kenji Inaba, and George Velmahos. Published by Cambridge University Press. © Cambridge University Press 2015.

(c)

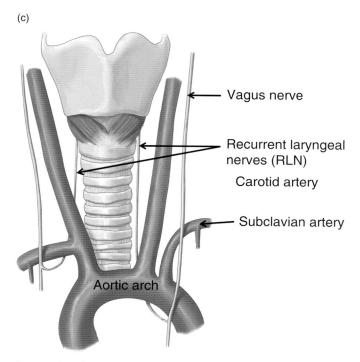

Vagus nerve

Recurrent laryngeal nerves (RLN)

Carotid artery

Subclavian artery

Aortic arch

Fig. 12.1(c). The recurrent laryngeal nerves (RLN) run laterally along the trachea–esophageal groove.

General principles

- Stridor, respiratory distress, blowing neck wound, hemoptysis, and subcutaneous emphysema are all signs and symptoms of a tracheolaryngeal injury. Patients with hard signs of injury which include hemoptysis, air bubbling, and respiratory distress can proceed directly to the operating room. CT is an excellent screening test.
- Direct laryngoscopy can be used to confirm laryngeal injury, and bronchoscopy can be used to identify tracheal injury.
- In the presence of tracheal trauma, there is a high incidence of associated injury including vascular injury.
- In suspected airway injury, a definitive secure airway obtained by an expert anesthesiology team should be the highest priority. This is best achieved in the operating room with the surgical team ready to intervene. If the patient is maintaining an airway, do not attempt prophylactic intubation in the emergency department.

Instruments

- A standard instrument tray can be used for tracheal and laryngeal dissection. Weitlaner or cerebellar retractors and a tracheal hook are helpful for exposure, especially in the deep neck.
- A size 6 and 8 tracheostomy tube should be available in the event of a large tracheal injury or lost airway.

Patient positioning

- In a patient with isolated injury and a cleared cervical spine, it is ideal to place a bump or shoulder roll underneath the upper back and allow the patient's head to extend, thus opening up the neck for improved exposure.
- If there is concern for cervical spine injury, the patient must be kept in spinal precautions and no shoulder roll should be used. Cervical spine stabilization can be accomplished using bilateral sandbags.

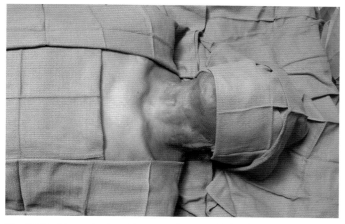

Fig. 12.2. A bump is placed between the patient's shoulder blades to allow hyperextension of the neck and improved exposure of the underlying structures.

Incisions

- The choice of incision depends on the mechanism of injury (blunt or penetrating), the location of the injury, and the suspected presence of associated injuries (i.e., esophagus or major vessel).

Collar incision

- For tracheal injuries, a collar incision is made approximately two finger breadths above the sternal notch, extending to the medial borders of the sternocleidomastoid muscles.
- After the collar skin incision is made, the platysma is divided, and subplatysmal flaps are created superiorly and inferiorly to expose the strap muscles.
- The strap muscles are split in the avascular plane along the midline to expose the trachea, larynx, and thyroid gland.
- The thyroid isthmus will often need to be divided in order to fully expose the underlying trachea and larynx. This can be accomplished using electrocautery or suture ligation.
- The larynx may also be accessed from the collar incision, provided a generous superior extension of the subplatysmal flap is performed.

(a)

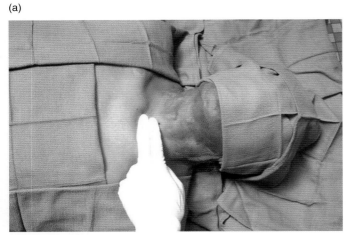

(b)

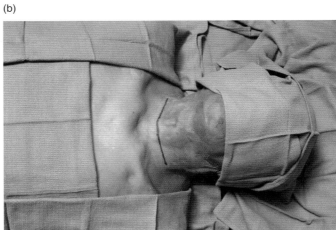

(c)

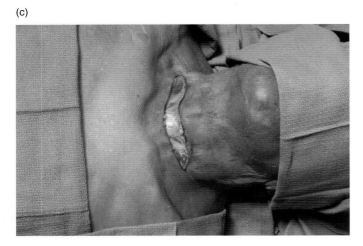

Fig. 12.3. A curvilinear incision is made two finger breadths above the sternal notch and extending laterally to the sternocleidomastoid muscles (a), (b). This incision is carried through the platysma (c).

Fig. 12.4. Subplatysmal flaps are dissected superiorly and inferiorly to expose the underlying strap muscles.

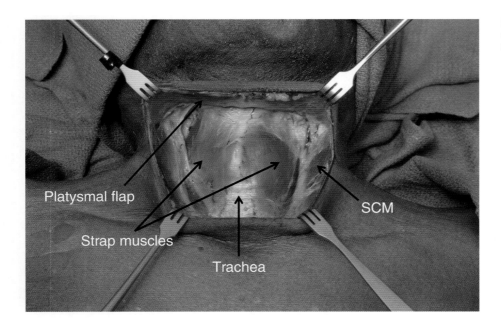

Platysmal flap

Strap muscles

Trachea

SCM

(a)

(b)

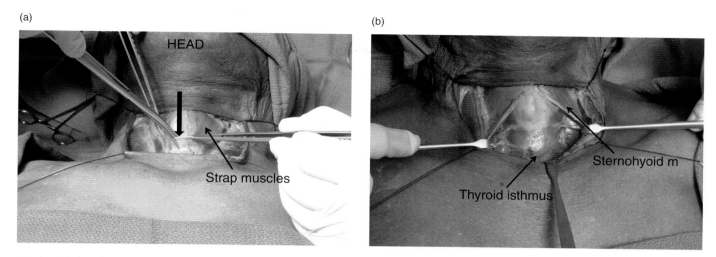

Fig. 12.5(a),(b). The paired strap muscles are split at the midline to expose the trachea, larynx, and thyroid. The most superficial strap muscle encountered is the sternohyoid muscle.

(a)

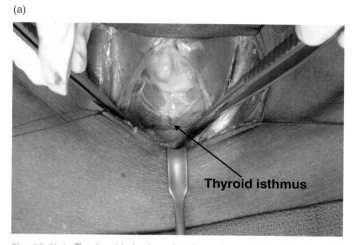

Fig. 12.6(a). The thyroid gland overlies the trachea and might interfere with adequate exposure of the underlying trachea.

(b)

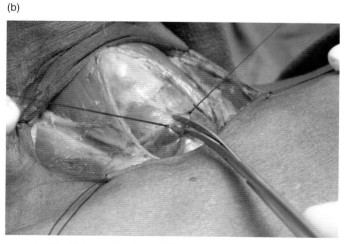

Fig. 12.6(b). Division of the thyroid isthmus for better exposure of the trachea.

(c)

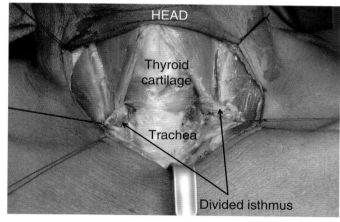

Fig. 12.6(c). Exposure of the trachea after division of the isthmus of the thyroid.

Sternocleidomastoid incision

- In patients with suspected associated injuries to the esophagus or major vessels, an incision over the anterior border of the sternocleidomastoid is preferable (see Chapter 7).
- A neck incision is made through the skin and the platysma is divided.
- The sternocleidomastoid muscle is retracted laterally to expose the carotid sheath.
- Division of the omohyoid muscle allows for exposure of the deep structures of the neck.
- The carotid sheath is then retracted laterally with the sternocleidomastoid muscle to expose the trachea and esophagus.

(a)

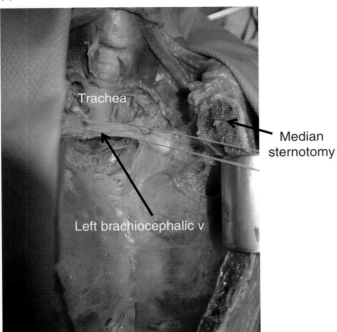

Fig. 12.7(a). Exposure of the lower trachea requires addition of a median sternotomy. The left brachiocephalic vein may need to be divided to provide additional exposure.

(b)

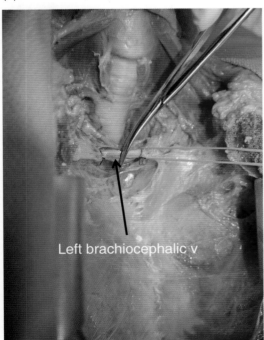

Fig. 12.7(b). Ligation and division of the left brachiocephalic vein.

(a)

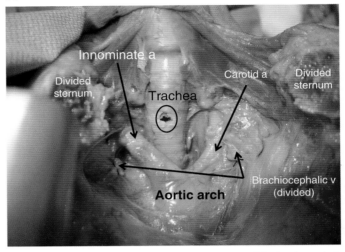

Fig. 12.8(a). The addition of a sternotomy and division of the brachiocephalic vein provide excellent exposure to lower tracheal injuries. The aortic arch and brachiocephalic artery can be gently retracted to access the lower trachea.

(b)

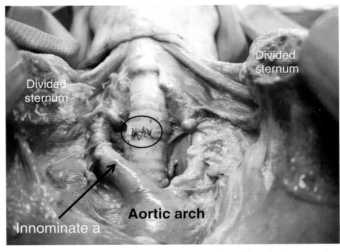

Fig. 12.8(b). Repair of simple penetrating wound (circle) to the lower trachea, through a combined collar incision and median sternotomy.

- Bilateral sternocleidomastoid incisions may be necessary for penetrating transcervical wounds.
- For lower tracheal injuries, a median sternotomy may be necessary. This will usually be an inferior extension of the sternocleidomastoid or collar incision.
- A midline incision is made from the sternal notch to the xiphoid process.
- The midpoint of the sternum is identified and scored using electrocautery.
- Superiorly, the interclavicular ligament is divided and the undersurface of the sternum is bluntly dissected away from the pericardial sac.

- The sternum is divided using an electric saw or Lebsche knife, providing exposure to the substernal trachea.
- For inferior tracheal injuries, rarely the brachiocephalic vein may need to be divided for additional exposure.

Repair

- Most penetrating laryngotracheal injuries without significant tissue loss can safely be managed by primary repair and without a tracheostomy.
- All devitalized tissue must be debrided prior to repair or reconstruction.
- Most injuries to the cervical trachea can be primarily repaired using simple interrupted absorbable suture.
- In complex injuries, the repair should be buttressed with an adjacent muscle flap. A protective tracheostomy should be considered.

- Prior to placing sutures through the trachea, it is important to deflate the endotracheal balloon in order to avoid damage or inclusion of the balloon in the repair.
- In rare cases, when the injury is not amenable to primary repair, a tracheal resection and anastamosis is performed.

  o If resection is to be performed, the trachea is mobilized superiorly and inferiorly using sharp dissection to minimize potential recurrent laryngeal nerve injury.
  o The injured section of trachea is sharply debrided.
  o The trachea is reapproximated using interrupted 3–0 absorbable sutures.
  o The endotracheal tube cuff is advanced and inflated distal to the repair or, in the event of a complex repair, a tracheostomy may be performed.
  o All efforts should be made for early postoperative extubation.

(b)

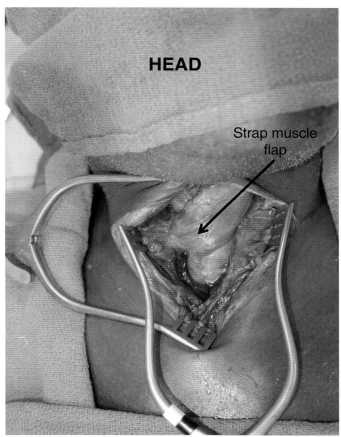

(a)

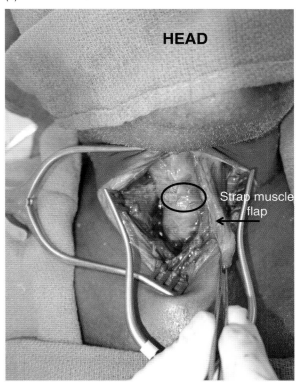

Fig. 12.9(a). Buttressing of the tracheal repair (circle) with muscle flap: preparation of strap muscle flap.

Fig. 12.9(b). Strap muscle flap sutured over the tracheal repair.

(c)

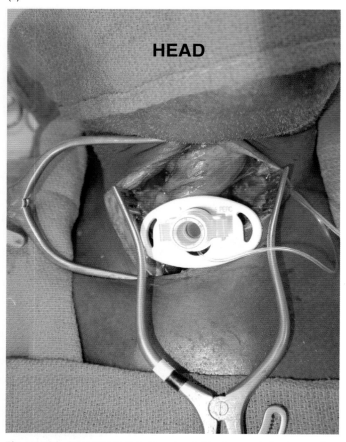

Fig. 12.9(c). Protective tracheostomy in addition to muscle flap buttressing.

- In extensive injuries with large mucosal lacerations, displaced fractures, unstable laryngeal cartilaginous skeleton, or complete laryngotracheal separation, a head and neck surgical team should be involved. Many of these patients may require endolaryngeal stents or other complex repairs.

Tips and pitfalls

- Once the platysma is divided, care must be taken to avoid or ligate the paired anterior jugular veins to avoid excess blood loss or staining of the operative field.
- A septum exists along the midline between the anterior strap muscles that identifies the avascular plane. Failure to identify this anatomic marker can lead to additional blood loss and damage to the muscle that may be needed later to buttress a repair.
- The recurrent laryngeal nerve runs vertically on either side of the trachea along the tracheoesophageal groove. Injury to this nerve is more common with the local use of electrocautery or if the dissection planes are unclear.
- During mobilization of the trachea, it is important to minimize the superior and inferior extent of dissection in order to preserve tracheal blood supply.
- In most major laryngotracheal injuries, the patient aspirates significant amounts of blood. It is strongly recommended that fiberoptic bronchoscopy be performed to clear the bronchial tree at the end of the operation.

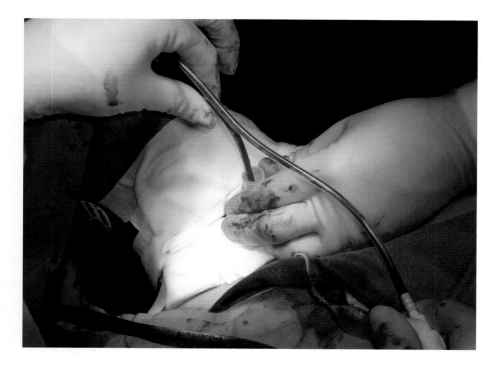

Fig. 12.10. In most major laryngotracheal injuries, the patient aspirates significant amounts of blood. It is strongly recommended that suctioning and fiberoptic bronchoscopy are performed to clear the bronchial tree at the end of the operation.

Cervical esophagus

13

Elizabeth R. Benjamin and Kenji Inaba

Surgical anatomy

- The cervical esophagus extends from the cricopharyngeus muscle into the chest to become the thoracic esophagus.
- The external landmark of the pharyngoesophageal junction is the cricoid cartilage. On esophagoscopy, this is at 15 cm from the upper incisors.
- The esophagus lacks a serosal layer and consists of an outer longitudinal and inner circular muscle layer.
- The cervical esophagus is approximately 5–7 cm long and lies posterior to the cricoid cartilage and trachea and anterior to the longus colli muscles and vertebral bodies. It is flanked by the thyroid gland and carotid sheath on either side.
- Blood supply is primarily from the inferior thyroid artery, although significant collateral circulation exists.
- The recurrent laryngeal nerves lie on either side of the esophagus in the tracheoesophageal groove.

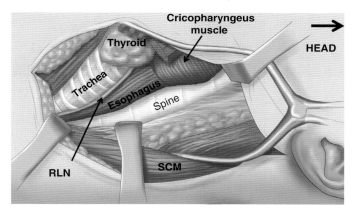

Fig. 13.1. Surgical anatomy of the cervical esophagus. RLN, recurrent laryngeal nerve.

General principles

- Esophageal trauma often presents with other associated injuries including carotid, jugular, tracheal, and thyroid injury. As such, neck exploration for suspected injury of

any of these structures must always include evaluation of the cervical esophagus.
- Early clinical signs and symptoms of cervical esophageal injury include odynophagia, hoarseness, hematemesis, and subcutaneous air. Late signs include fever, erythema, leukocytosis, swelling and/or abscess formation, and ultimately spreading of the infection along the precervical plane leading to mediastinitis.
- Workup of a stable patient with potential esophageal injury includes a neck CT, gastrograffin followed by barium swallow study, and/or esophagoscopy. CT is an excellent screening examination, however, it often requires direct confirmation with a swallow or esophagoscopy.
- Management of esophageal injuries hinges on early debridement and repair or, if delayed, drainage, broad spectrum antibiotics, and nutritional support.

Special instruments

- In addition to a standard instrument tray, for the neck exploration, a self-retaining Weitlaner or cerebellar retractor will be necessary.
- If there is concern for thoracic extension of the esophageal injury, the surgeon should be prepared to perform a high right thoracotomy to expose the proximal thoracic esophagus.
- A rigid and flexible endoscope should be available for intraoperative esophagoscopy if necessary.

Patient positioning

- Provided cervical spine injury has been ruled out, the patient is positioned in a supine position with the head turned to the right. A bump is placed under the patient's shoulder to allow gentle neck extension for improved exposure. When possible, the arms are tucked.

Atlas of Surgical Techniques in Trauma, ed. Demetrios Demetriades, Kenji Inaba, and George Velmahos. Published by Cambridge University Press. © Cambridge University Press 2015.

Incision

- Standard exposure of the cervical esophagus is through a left-sided oblique neck incision running along the anterior border of the sternocleidomastoid muscle and extending from the mastoid to the suprasternal notch.

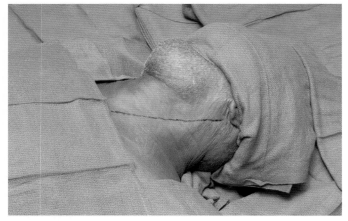

Fig. 13.2. To access the cervical esophagus, the patient's head is turned to the right and the neck is extended. The incision is made along the anterior border of the sternocleidomastoid muscle.

Esophageal exposure

- An incision is made through the skin and dermis and the platysma is divided.
- The sternocleidomastoid muscle is retracted laterally to expose the carotid sheath.
- Division of the omohyoid muscle allows for exposure of the deep structures of the neck.

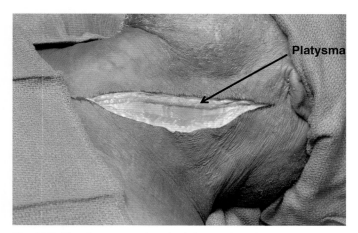

Fig. 13.3. The platysma muscle is divided using sharp dissection or electrocautery. This layer is reapproximated with absorbable suture upon closure.

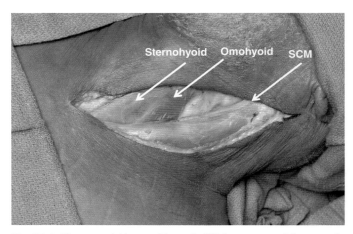

Fig. 13.4. The sternocleidomastoid muscle (SCM) runs tangentially across the neck and must be retracted laterally to expose the vascular and aerodigestive structures of the neck. The omohyoid and sternohyoid muscles are medial and just deep to the SCM.

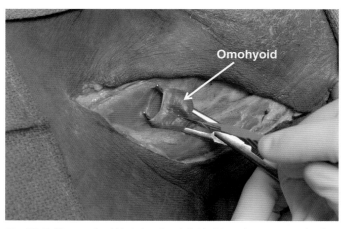

Fig. 13.5. The omohyoid is isolated and divided in order to expose the deep structures of the neck.

- The carotid sheath is then retracted laterally, while the trachea and thyroid are retracted medially to expose the cervical esophagus.
- A nasogastric tube, if in place, can be of assistance in palpating the esophagus.
- The middle thyroid vein and often the inferior thyroid artery may be ligated and divided to gain better access to the esophagus.
- Retraction alone may provide adequate exposure for injury identification and repair. If further mobilization is required, with the aid of a nasogastric tube or bougie, the esophagus can be bluntly dissected circumferentially and manipulated by passing a ½ inch Penrose drain or vessel loop around the structure for additional retraction.

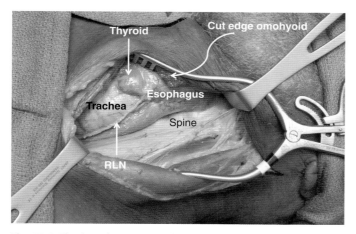

Fig. 13.6. The thyroid is anterior on the trachea and can be retracted medially. With the omohyoid divided, the tracheal–esophageal groove is exposed. The recurrent laryngeal nerve (RLN) runs in this groove, anterior to the cervical esophagus. From this exposure, the esophagus is directly posterior and left lateral to the trachea and anterior to the spine.

Repair

- Traumatic cervical esophageal injury can often be identified on gross inspection. Intraoperative endoscopy or esophageal insufflation with air or methylene blue can also be useful adjuncts to identify an injury.
- The majority of injuries can be repaired primarily without tension. The wound edges are first debrided of any devitalized tissue and the mucosal defect is identified. The injury can be closed in one or two layers however, when possible, a two-layer closure using absorbable suture is recommended. The inner layer should reapproximate mucosal edges.
- Neighboring strap muscle can be used to buttress the esophageal repair and isolate the suture line from associated tracheal or vascular injuries.
- A closed suction drain is typically placed outside the esophageal repair. This drain is removed on POD #5–7 after anastamotic leak is ruled out by contrast study.

(a)

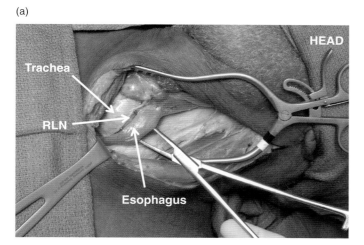

(b)

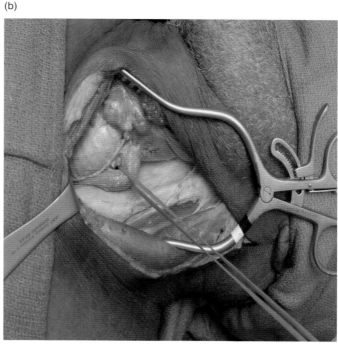

Fig. 13.7(a),(b). Additional exposure can be obtained by mobilization and gentle retraction of the esophagus.

(a)

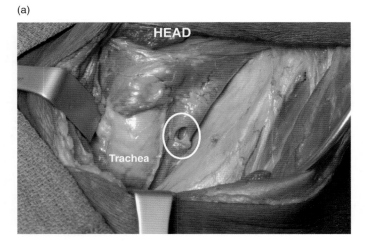

(b)

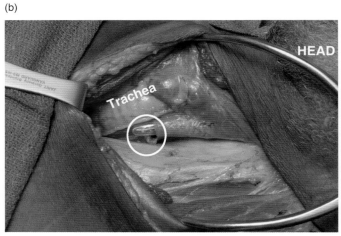

Fig. 13.8(a),(b). A full thickness defect of the left lateral wall of the cervical esophagus (circle).

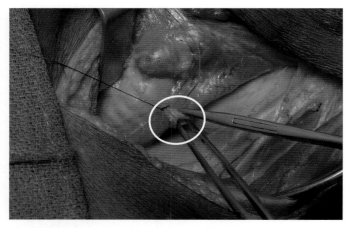

Fig. 13.9. Esophageal injuries are repaired with absorbable suture in one or two layers. Repair must include reapproximation of the mucosa.

- For destructive injuries that are unable to be primarily repaired, wide drainage, possible cervical esophagostomy, and delayed interposition graft are treatment options.
- In some cases, local resection with one- or two-layer anastomosis may be necessary.
- In rare occasions with destructive injuries and damage control, a proximal esophagostomy with distal stapling may be necessary. Semi-elective reconstruction with gastric pull-up or colon bypass may be done at a later stage.

(a)

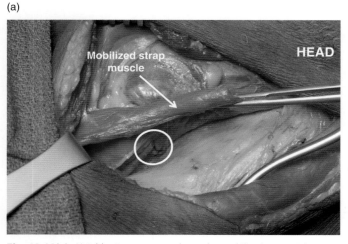

Fig. 13.10(a). Neighboring strap muscle can be mobilized to provide a buttress or be used to isolate the esophageal repair.

(b)

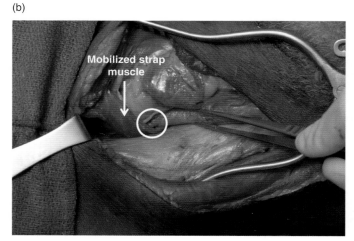

Fig. 13.10(b). Mobilized strap muscle placed over esophageal repair (circle).

Tips and pitfalls

- The recurrent laryngeal nerve runs in the tracheoesophageal groove and can easily be injured during exposure of the esophagus.
- The posterior membranous portion of the trachea is very delicate, and injury can easily occur with dissection of the trachea off the anterior esophagus.
- The inner layer of the esophageal repair must reapproximate the mucosal edges to minimize the rate of postoperative leak.

- Care must be taken with the outer layer not to cause narrowing of the esophagus. It is often helpful to close these injuries over a nasogastric tube or bougie.
- Care should be taken to avoid missing a second esophageal injury on the opposite site. Check carefully with appropriate circumferential mobilization of the esophagus or on table endoscopy.

Chest

Section 5

Chapter

14

General principles of chest trauma operations

Demetrios Demetriades and Rondi Gelbard

Surgical anatomy

The following are the major muscles that will be encountered and may be divided during thoracic operations for trauma:

Anterior chest wall

Pectoralis major muscle. It originates from the anterior surface of the medial half of the clavicle, the anterior surface of the sternum, and the cartilages of all the true ribs. The 5 cm wide tendon inserts into the upper humerus.

Pectoralis minor muscle. It arises from the third, fourth, and fifth ribs, near their cartilages, and from the aponeuroses over the intercostal muscles. It inserts into the coracoid process of the scapula.

Lateral chest wall

Serratus anterior muscle. It originates from the lateral part of the first eight to nine ribs and inserts into the medial aspect of the scapula.

Posterior chest wall

Latissimus dorsi muscle. It originates from the spinous processes of the lower thoracic spine and the posterior iliac crest and inserts into the upper portion of the humerus.

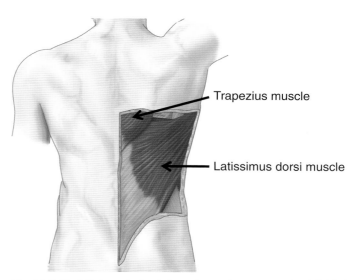

Fig. 14.2. The latissimus dorsi m is the main muscle encountered and divided during a posterolateral incision.

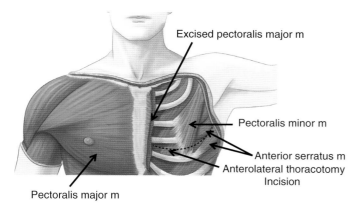

Fig. 14.1. The pectoralis major and pectoralis minor muscles in the anterior chest wall and the anterior serratus muscle on the lateral thoracic wall may be divided during anterolateral thoracotomy.

General technical principles

- In order to preserve chest wall function, muscle sparing techniques should be utilized whenever possible.
- Excessive rib retraction should be avoided to prevent rib fractures, and all ribs should be preserved when possible.
- The thoracic wall structures should be closed by re-approximating the divided muscles in multiple layers.
- Avoid over-approximating the ribs in order to reduce postoperative pain.
- Preoperative placement of a double-lumen endotracheal tube or a bronchial blocker allows isolation of the ipsilateral lung and facilitates the exposure of posterior mediastinal structures, such as the descending thoracic aorta and the esophagus.

Atlas of Surgical Techniques in Trauma, ed. Demetrios Demetriades, Kenji Inaba, and George Velmahos. Published by Cambridge University Press. © Cambridge University Press 2015.

Positioning

In hemodynamically unstable patients, often there is no time for special positioning and the patient is placed in the standard supine position.

Median sternotomy/anterolateral thoracotomy/ clamshell

- Supine position, abducted arms.

Posterolateral thoracotomy

- The patient is placed in a lateral decubitus position with the hips secured to the table by wide adhesive tape. Bean bags should be used to provide additional support.
- The lower leg is flexed at the knee, while the upper leg is straight and a pillow is placed between the knees.
- A rolled sheet is placed under the axilla to support the shoulder and upper thorax.
- The arm on the side of the thoracotomy is extended forward and upward (praying position) and placed in a padded grooved arm holder in line with the head.
  - Overextension can lead to brachial nerve injury.
- The lower arm is extended and placed on a board at 90 degrees.

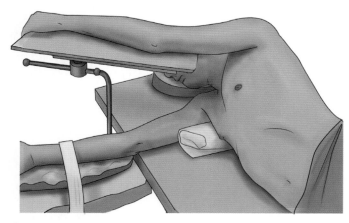

Fig. 14.3. Positioning of the patient for a posterolateral thoracotomy.

Incision(s)

The selection of incision should be based on the clinical condition of the patient, the location of the operation (emergency room versus operating room), the need for thoracic aortic cross-clamping, the location of any penetrating injuries and the suspected injured organs. Incisions such as a posterolateral thoracotomy requiring special time-consuming positioning of the patient should be avoided in the unstable patient.

Median sternotomy

- This is the preferred incision in penetrating injuries to the anterior chest.
  - It provides good exposure of the heart, the anterior mediastinal vessels, both of the lungs, the middle to distal trachea, and the left mainstem bronchus. It is quick to perform, bloodless, and causes less postoperative pain and fewer respiratory complications than a thoracotomy.
  - However, it does *not* provide good exposure of the posterior mediastinal structures and does not provide adequate access for cross-clamping of the thoracic aorta for resuscitation purposes.
- The incision is made over the center of the sternum, extending from the suprasternal notch to the xiphoid and is carried down to the sternum.
- The sternum is scored in the midline with electrocautery to direct the saw or the Lebsche knife, which is then used to divide the sternum.
- The interclavicular ligament at the suprasternal notch is cleared from its attachment to the sternum using a combination of cautery and blunt dissection, always staying close to the bone to avoid injuring the underlying vessels.
- Confirm clearance of the posterior wall of the suprasternal notch by passing the index finger behind the manubrium.
  - Note that the pneumatic saw does not work in the presence of soft tissues!
- Place the hook of the pneumatic saw or the Lebsche knife under the suprasternal notch and lift the sternum upwards.
  - Ask anesthesia to hold ventilation and divide the sternum directly in the midline, maintaining upwards traction along the entire length.
- Place the Finochietto retractor in the upper part of the sternotomy and spread the sternum.

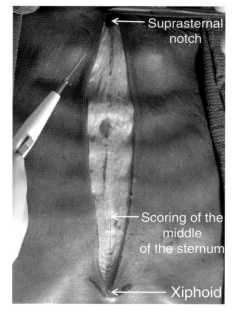

Fig. 14.4. The median sternotomy extends from the suprasternal notch to the xiphoid and is carried down to the sternum. The sternum is scored in the midline with the knife or electrocautery, to direct the saw or the Lebsche knife to stay in the middle of the sternum.

Labels in figure: Suprasternal notch; Scoring of the middle of the sternum; Xiphoid

(a)

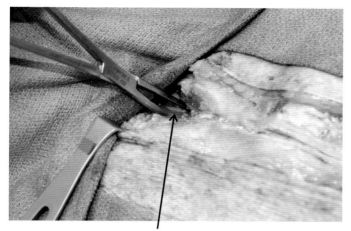

Clearance of the interclavicular ligament

(b)

Digital confirmation of the clearance of the soft tissues behind the manubrium

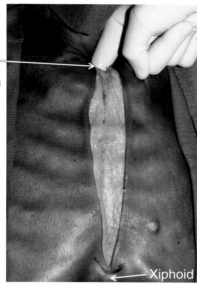

Xiphoid

Fig. 14.5(a),(b). The interclavicular ligament at the suprasternal notch is cleared from its attachment to the sternum using a combination of cautery and blunt dissection (a). The clearance is confirmed by passing the index finger behind the manubrium (b).

(a)

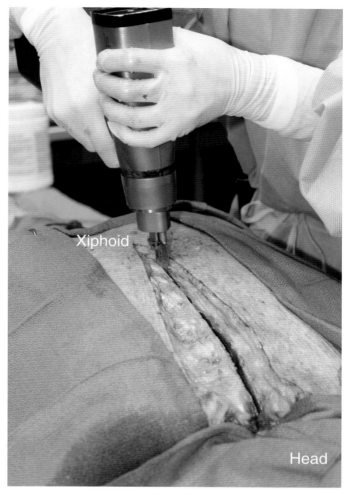

Xiphoid

Head

(b)

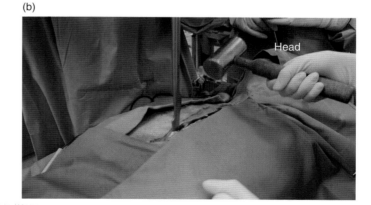

Head

Fig. 14.6(a)–(c). Division of the sternum with the pneumatic saw (a) and the Lebsche knife (b). A Finochietto retractor is placed in the upper part of the sternotomy and the sternum is spread open (c).

(c)

**Finochietto placed in the
superior sternum**

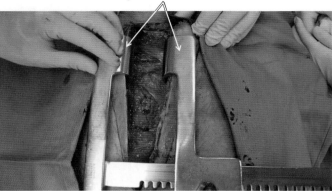

Fig. 14.6(a)–(c). *(cont.)*

Closure of median sternotomy

- Ensure good hemostasis along the divided bone edge with cautery or bone wax.
- Check for any bleeding under the sternum from the internal mammary arteries after removal of the sternal retractor.
- Place at least one waterseal chest drain under the sternum, and place additional drains in open chest cavities.
- Close the sternum with steel wires, using the heavy needle driver.
- Close the presternal fascia with heavy absorbable sutures.

(a)

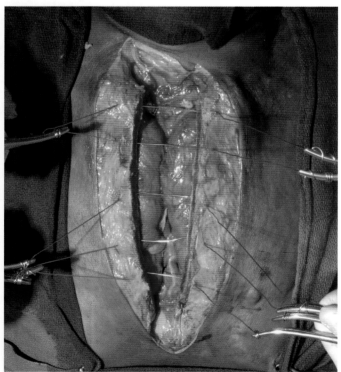

Fig. 14.7(a),(b). Closure of the median sternotomy with steel wires.

(b)

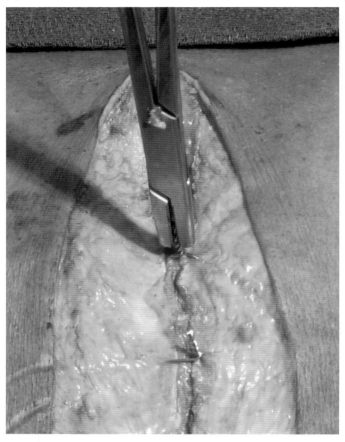

Fig. 14.7(a),(b). *(cont.)*

Anterolateral thoracotomy

- This is the incision of choice for resuscitative thoracotomy, suspected injuries to the lung or the posterior heart, and cross-clamping of the aorta for resuscitation; it provides poor exposure of the anterior mediastinal vessels.
- Mark the incision with a marking pen prior to skin incision.
- The incision is made through the fourth to fifth intercostal space (below the nipple in males, infra-mammary fold in females), starting from the parasternal border and extending to the posterior axillary line, aiming towards the axilla.
- The pectoralis major and pectoralis minor are encountered and divided in the anterior part of the incision.
- The serratus anterior muscle is encountered and divided in the posterior part of the incision.
- The intercostal muscles are then divided close to the superior border of the rib in order to avoid the neurovascular bundle, and the pleural cavity is entered with the use of scissors, taking care to avoid injuring the underlying inflated lung.
  - Withholding ventilation during entry into the pleural cavity reduces the risk of iatrogenic lung injury.
- A Finochietto retractor is then placed and the ribs are spread slowly to avoid rib fractures.

(a)

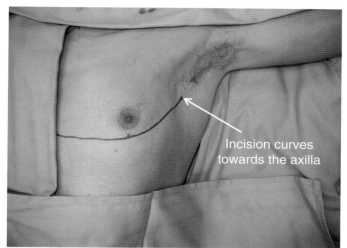

(a)

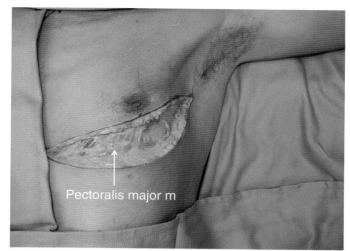

(b)

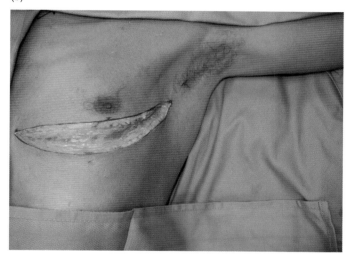

(b)

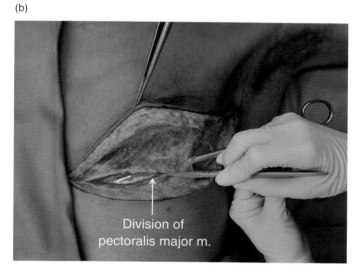

Fig. 14.8(a),(b). The incision for an anterolateral thoracotomy is placed through the fourth to fifth intercostal space, starting from the parasternal border and extending to the posterior axillary line, aiming towards the axilla.

Fig. 14.9(a)–(e). Anterolateral thoracotomy: the pectoralis major muscle is encountered in the anterior part of the incision and is divided (a), (b). The lower part of the pectoralis major is encountered under the pectoralis major and divided (c). The serratus anterior muscle is encountered and divided in the lateral part of the incision. The intercostal muscles are then divided with the use of scissors, close to the superior border of the rib (d). A Finochietto retractor is then placed and the ribs are spread slowly to avoid rib fractures (e).

(c)

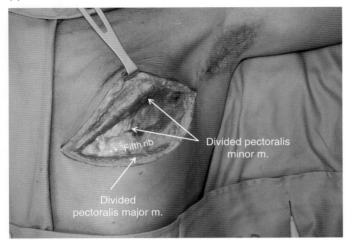

(e)

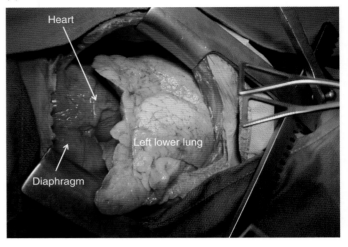

Fig. 14.9(a)–(e). *(cont.)*

(d)

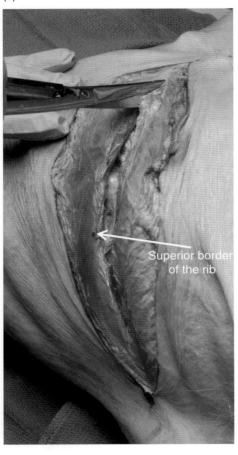

Fig. 14.9(a)–(e). *(cont.)*

Closure of anterolateral thoracotomy incision

- Insert a thoracostomy tube at the mid axillary line.
- Close the chest wall in layers, reapproximating the divided muscles with heavy figure-of-eight absorbable sutures.

Clamshell incision

- It is usually performed as an extension of a standard anterolateral thoracotomy to the opposite side, for suspected bilateral lung injuries, superior mediastinal vascular injuries or cardiac resuscitation and aortic cross-clamping.
- It provides good exposure of the anterior aspect of the heart, the superior mediastinal vessels (aortic arch and branches, superior vena cava and innominate veins), and both lungs.
- The incision is made through the fourth to fifth intercostal spaces bilaterally with transverse division of the sternum, using bone cutters or heavy scissors.
- During division of the sternum, both internal mammary arteries are transected and identification and ligation of the proximal and distal ends should be performed.

(a)

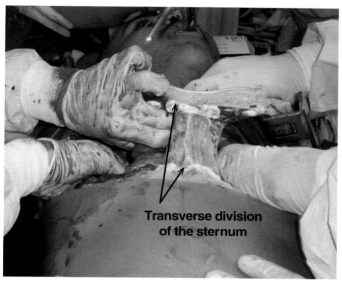

Transverse division of the sternum

(b)

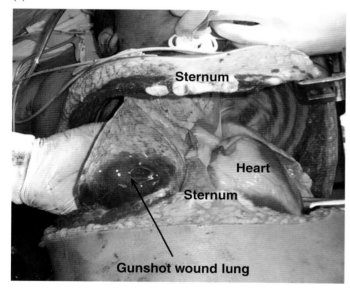

Sternum

Heart

Sternum

Gunshot wound lung

Fig. 14.10(a),(b). The clamshell incision is made through the fourth to fifth intercostal space bilaterally, with transverse division of the sternum. It provides good exposure of the anterior aspect of the heart, the superior mediastinal vessels, and both lungs.

Closure of clamshell incision

- The divided sternum is reapproximated with steel wires and the thoracotomy incisions are closed as described above.

Posterolateral thoracotomy

- This approach requires special patient positioning. It is usually indicated for injuries to the descending aorta, thoracic esophagus, distal trachea, and mainstem bronchi.
- For optimal exposure of the upper portion of the thoracic cavity, the chest is entered through the fourth or fifth intercostal space.
  - A thoracotomy through the fifth intercostal space allows good access to the pulmonary hilum and is considered the approach of choice for major pulmonary resections.
- A low left posterolateral thoracotomy through the sixth or seventh intercostal space provides good exposure to the distal third of the thoracic esophagus, and a high right thoracotomy through the fourth intercostal space provides good access to the upper and middle esophagus.
- A curvilinear skin incision is made, extending from the anterior axillary line, coursing approximately one to two finger breadths below the tip of the scapula, and extending posteriorly and cephalad midway between the spine and the medial border of the scapula (the tip of the scapula is usually over the sixth or seventh intercostal space).
- The latissimus dorsi is identified and divided in line with the incision using electrocautery.
- The serratus anterior muscle is then divided as low as possible to minimize the amount of denervated muscle.
- In the same plane posteriorly, the trapezius muscle (or more superiorly the rhomboid muscles) may need to be divided for additional exposure.
- The scapula is elevated using a scapula retractor, the appropriate intercostal space is selected and the pleural cavity is entered at the superior border of the rib, in order to avoid injuring the neurovascular bundle.
- Resection of a 3 cm to 4 cm portion of the fifth or sixth rib posteriorly improves exposure and prevents iatrogenic fracturing of the ribs.

Closure of posterolateral thoracotomy

- Approximation of the divided muscles and the subcutaneous tissue as described in the anterolateral thoracotomy.

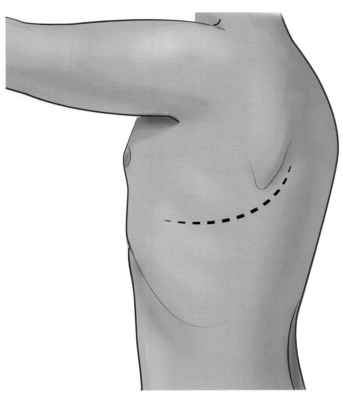

Fig. 14.11. The skin incision for a posterolateral thoracotomy extends from the anterior axillary line, coursing about 1–2 finger breadths below the tip of the scapula, and extends posteriorly and cephalad midway between the spine and the medial border of the scapula.

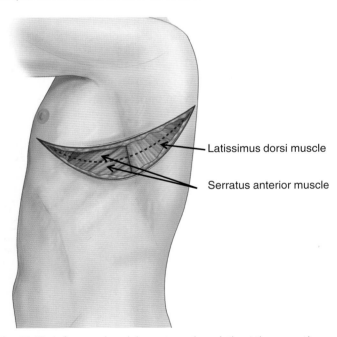

Latissimus dorsi muscle

Serratus anterior muscle

Fig. 14.12. Left posterolateral thoracotomy through the sixth or seventh intercostal space. The latissimus dorsi and the serratus anterior muscles are divided. More posteriorly, the trapezius muscle (or more superiorly the rhomboid muscles) may need to be divided for additional exposure.

Tips and pitfalls

- **Sternotomy incision**
  - Failure to divide the interclavicular ligament at the suprasternal notch and clear its attachments to the sternum causes malfunction of the pneumatic saw, as the pneumatic saw does not work in the presence of soft tissues.
  - The median sternotomy goes off midline, through the costal cartilages. This complicates the closure and increases the risk of sternal dehiscence. To avoid this problem, score the sternum in the midline with electrocautery to guide the saw or the Lebsche knife.
  - The sternal retractor is placed in the lower part of the sternotomy. This is the weakest part of the sternum and increases the risk of sternal fracture. Place the retractor in the upper part of the median sternotomy.
- **Anterolateral thoracotomy**
  - The incision does not follow the intercostal space, making entry into the chest cavity difficult and messy! The incision should curve upward, directed towards the axilla.
  - Excessive spreading of the rib retractor may cause rib fractures and increase postoperative pain.
  - Failure to inspect for injury to the left internal mammary artery after removal of the retractor. The blades of the retractor may obscure an injury to the artery with subsequent bleeding.
  - Failure to approximate the divided muscles in layers may result in functional and aesthetic problems.
- **Clamshell incision**
  - Failure to identify and ligate all four ends of the two divided internal mammary arteries.
  - Failure to approximate the divided muscles in layers may result in functional and aesthetic problems.
- **Posterolateral thoracotomy**
  - The incision is too low or too high resulting in poor exposure.
  - Making the skin incision over the scapula results in poor aesthetic results. The incision should be one to two finger breadths below the tip of the scapula.
  - Failure to approximate the divided muscles in layers may result in functional and aesthetic problems.

Cardiac injuries

Demetrios Demetriades and Scott Zakaluzny

Surgical anatomy

- The pericardium envelops the heart and attaches to the roots of the great vessels. This includes the ascending aorta, pulmonary artery, pulmonary veins, the last 2 cm to 4 cm of superior vena cava, and inferior vena cava.
- The phrenic nerves descend on the lateral surfaces of the pericardium.
- Acute accumulation of as little as 200 mL of fluid in the pericardial sac may result in fatal cardiac tamponade.
- The right atrium is paper thin, approximately 2 mm. The left atrium is slightly thicker at approximately 3 mm.
- The right ventricle is approximately 4 mm thick and the left ventricular wall thickness is approximately 12 mm.
- The two main coronary arteries, left main and right coronary arteries, originate at the root of the aorta, as it exits the left ventricle. The left main coronary artery divides into the left anterior descending artery (LAD) and the circumflex artery, and provides blood supply to the left heart. The right coronary artery divides into the right posterior descending and acute marginal arteries, supplying blood to the right heart as well as to the sinoatrial and atrioventricular nodes, responsible for regulating cardiac rhythm.

General principles

- Cardiac injuries are highly lethal and most victims die at the scene. In those who survive to the emergency department, immediate diagnosis and surgical intervention remain the cornerstones of survival. The diagnosis is based on clinical examination and the Focused Assessment Sonography for Trauma (FAST) exam. There is no role for diagnostic pericardiocentesis in a hospital environment. Most patients have no signs of life or have severe hypotension on arrival. If there is a short prehospital time or small cardiac injury, the patient may arrive with normal initial vital signs.

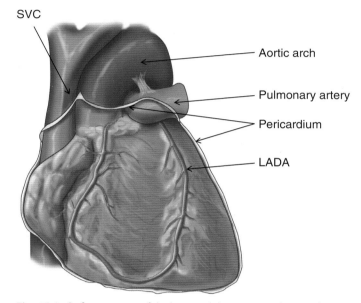

SVC

Aortic arch

Pulmonary artery

Pericardium

LADA

Fig. 15.1. Surface anatomy of the heart and the great vessels. Note the attachment of the pericardium to the roots of the major vessels.

- The majority of cardiac injuries are due to penetrating trauma from stab wounds or gunshot wounds. Stab wounds usually involve the right ventricle and gunshot wounds often damage multiple chambers or internal cardiac structures. Cardiac rupture due to blunt trauma is usually fatal and the victims die before reaching medical care.
- Patients with no vital signs or imminent cardiac arrest on arrival should be managed with a resuscitative emergency room thoracotomy (see Chapter 4).
- Cardiac bypass is almost never required during the initial operation for cardiac repair. The use of temporary intra-aortic balloon pump augmentation may be considered.
- Injuries to the low-pressure cardiac chambers may be complicated by air embolism. Look for air bubbles in the coronary veins. If seen, aspirate the right ventricle.

Atlas of Surgical Techniques in Trauma, ed. Demetrios Demetriades, Kenji Inaba, and George Velmahos. Published by Cambridge University Press. © Cambridge University Press 2015.

Special surgical instruments

- The emergency room thoracotomy tray should be kept simple, with only the absolutely necessary instruments (scalpel, Finochietto retractor, two Duval lung forceps, two vascular clamps, one long Russian forceps, four hemostats, one bone cutter, one pair of long scissors, one pair of suture scissors). In addition, good lighting, working suction, and an internal defibrillator should be immediately available.
- In the operating room, the thoracotomy trauma tray should include a power sternal saw, Lebsche knife with hammer, and bone cutter. The surgeon should wear a headlamp for optimal lighting in anatomically difficult areas.

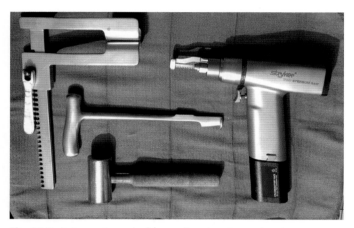

Fig. 15.2. Instruments required for median sternotomy: sternal power saw, Lebsche knife, hammer, Finochietto retractor.

Patient positioning

- For an emergency room left thoracotomy, the patient remains supine on the gurney, with the left arm abducted or elevated above the head. Antiseptic solution is applied on the skin over the anterior chest and both hemithoraces. There is no time for draping or meticulous antiseptic precautions.
- In the operating room the patient is placed in the supine position with both arms abducted at 90 degrees to allow anesthesia access to the extremities. The left arm may be elevated further above the head if a left anterolateral thoracotomy is to be performed. The skin preparation and draping should include the anterior chest and both hemithoraces. The abdomen should be included if there are suspected associated intra-abdominal injuries.

Incisions

- The choice of incision depends on the clinical condition of the patient, the location of the operation (emergency room or operating room), the need for thoracic aortic cross-clamping, and the suspected anatomical site of cardiac injury.
- Patients transported to the emergency room with no vital signs or in imminent cardiac arrest should undergo an immediate left antero-lateral thoracotomy on the gurney.

This incision is fast, does not need power instruments, and allows cross-clamping of the thoracic aorta for resuscitation purposes (see Chapter 4).

- In most patients undergoing an operation in the operating room, a median sternotomy is the incision of choice. It provides good exposure to the heart and both lungs, it is relatively bloodless and is associated with less postoperative pain and fewer complications. However, the exposure of the posterior heart or cross-clamping of the aorta may be difficult.
- A left thoracotomy in the operating room is preferable to sternotomy in patients who might need cross-clamping of the aorta or in suspected cases of injury to the posterior wall of the heart.
- Extension of the left thoracotomy into the right chest to create a clamshell incision may be required in patients with bilateral chest trauma (see Chapter 14).

Media sternotomy incision

- The incision is made over the center of the sternum, extending from the suprasternal notch to the xiphoid. The incision is carried through the sternocostal radiate ligaments, down to the sternum. The interclavicular ligament, at the suprasternal notch, is cleared from its attachment to the sternum, using a combination of cautery and blunt dissection with a right angle. Confirm the clearance of the posterior wall of the suprasternal notch by passing the index finger behind the manubrium. The pneumatic saw does not work in the presence of soft tissues! Score the sternum in the midline with electrocautery to direct the saw or the Lebsche knife to stay in the middle during the sternal division.

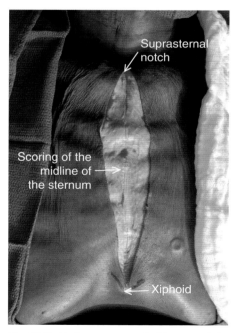

Fig. 15.3. Median sternotomy incision extends from the suprasternal notch superiorly to the xiphoid process inferiorly, and is carried down to the sternum. The sternum is scored in the midline to guide the sternal saw.

(a)

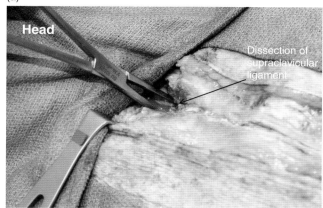

(b)

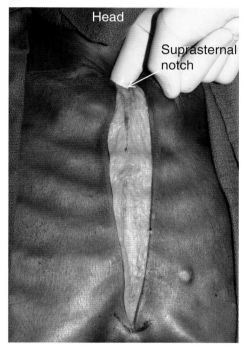

Fig. 15.4(a),(b). The interclavicular ligament is divided, using a combination of cautery and blunt dissection with an angled forceps, prior to division of the sternum with the saw or Lebsche knife. Palpation with a finger of the posterior surface of the sternal notch confirms that soft tissues have been dissected free prior to dividing the sternum.

- Place the hook of the pneumatic saw or the Lebsche knife under the suprasternal notch and lift upward on the sternum. Ask anesthesia to hold ventilation temporarily and divide the sternum, maintaining an upwards traction and always staying in the midline.
- Place the Finochietto retractor in the upper part of the sternum and spread open. The anterior pericardium is now exposed.

(a)

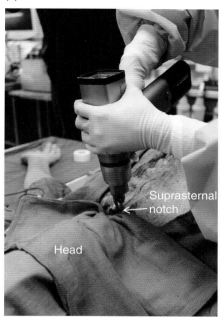

(b)

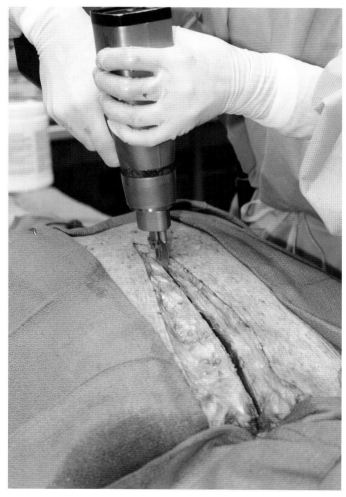

Fig. 15.5(a),(b). The hook of the saw or Lebsche knife is placed under the suprasternal notch and the sternum is lifted slightly upward. The sternum is divided with constant upward traction, always keeping in the scored midline.

117

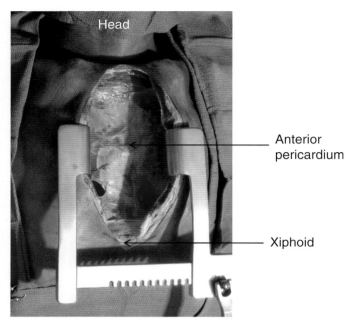

Fig. 15.6. The sternum is spread open with a Finochietto retractor and the pericardium is exposed.

Left thoracotomy incision

- The incision is made through the left fourth to fifth intercostal space (below the nipple in males, in the inframammary fold in females), starting from the left of the parasternal border and extending to the posterior axillary line. Follow the curve of the ribs by aiming towards the axilla (see Chapter 14).
- The pectoralis major and pectoralis minor are encountered and divided in the anterior part of the incision. The serratus anterior muscle is encountered and divided in the posterior part of the incision (see Chapter 14).
- The intercostal muscles are then divided close to the superior border of the rib, in order to avoid the neurovascular bundle, and the pleural cavity is entered with the use of scissors taking precautions to avoid injury to the underlying inflated lung (see Chapter 14).
- Right-stem intubation or withholding ventilation during entry into the pleural cavity reduce the risk of iatrogenic lung injury.
- A Finochietto retractor is then applied and the ribs are spread (see Chapter 14).

Tips and pitfalls

- During sternotomy, failure to divide the interclavicular ligament at the suprasternal notch and clear its attachment to the sternum. The pneumatic saw does not work in the presence of soft tissues!

- The median sternotomy goes off midline, through the costal cartilages. To avoid this problem, score the sternum in the midline with electrocautery to direct the saw or the Lebsche knife and stay in the middle.
- Placement of the Finochietto retractor in the lower part of the sternum may cause transverse fracture of the sternum. The retractor should be placed in the upper part where the sternum is thicker and stronger.
- During left thoracotomy: (a) The incision is made too low. This risks injury to an elevated diaphragm and poor exposure of the upper part of the heart. Do not go below the fourth to fifth intercostal space. (b) The incision does not follow the intercostal space, making entry into the chest difficult and messy! The incision should curve with a direction towards the axilla.
- Failure to inspect for injury to the left internal mammary artery after removal of the retractor. The blades of the retractor may obscure any injury to the artery and subsequent bleeding.

Pericardiotomy

In the absence of tense cardiac tamponade, the pericardium is grasped in the midline with two hemostats and a small pericardiotomy incision is made. In the presence of a tense tamponade it is difficult to apply the hemostats on the pericardium. In these cases a small pericardiotomy is performed with a scalpel and the pericardium is then opened longitudinally with scissors. If a median sternotomy is performed, the pericardiotomy is performed in the midline. With a left thoracotomy, the left phrenic nerve is seen along the lateral surface of the pericardium and the pericardiotomy is performed superiorly and parallel to the phrenic nerve.

(a)

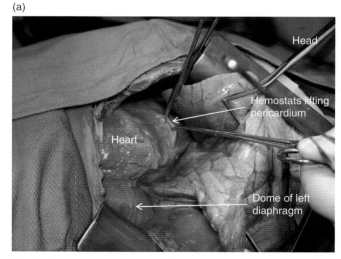

Fig. 15.7(a). The non-tense pericardium can be grasped and elevated with hemostats in order to safely make a pericardiotomy without injuring the underlying heart.

(b)

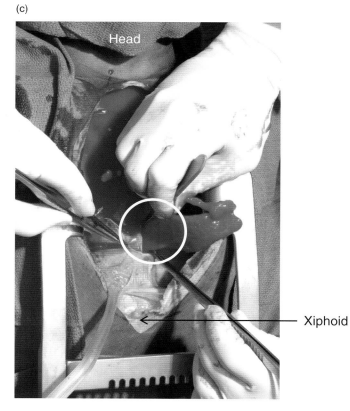

(d)

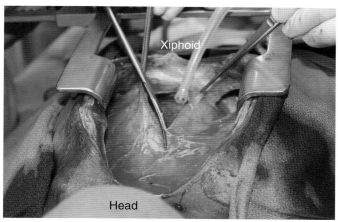

Fig. 15.7(d). Tense cardiac tamponade is released through the pericardiotomy.

(a)

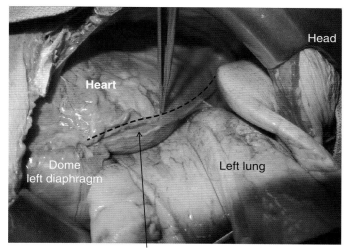

Fig. 15.8(a). The pericardiotomy through a left thoracotomy should be performed in front of the left phrenic nerve. The tip of the forceps shows the site of the pericardiotomy, in front of the nerve.

(b)

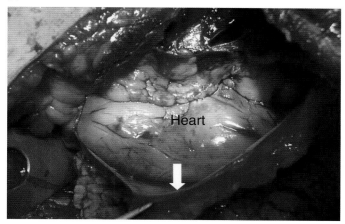

(c)

Fig. 15.7(b),(c). In the presence of a tense cardiac tamponade, the pericardium is entered with a scalpel and opened longitudinally with scissors.

Fig. 15.8(b). The pericardium is opened and the heart exposed.

Tips and pitfalls

- In patients with a tense pericardium, it may be difficult to grasp the pericardium. Make a small pericardiotomy with a scalpel to facilitate entry. Locate and avoid cutting the phrenic nerve.

Bleeding control and cardiac repair

- After the pericardiotomy and release of the tamponade, any direct cardiac bleeding is controlled by finger compression. For larger atrial injuries, a vascular clamp may be used, taking care not to worsen the injury. For emergency room thoracotomies where a small cardiac injury is found, temporary bleeding control may be achieved by inserting and inflating a Foley catheter.
- The cardiac wound is repaired with figure-of-eight, horizontal mattress or running sutures, using non-absorbable 2/0 or 3/0 suture on a large tapered needle. Routine use of pledgets is time consuming and unnecessary in the majority of cases and should be reserved for cases where the myocardium tears during tying the sutures.
- Injuries close to a major coronary vessel should be repaired with horizontal mattress sutures under the vessel.

(a)

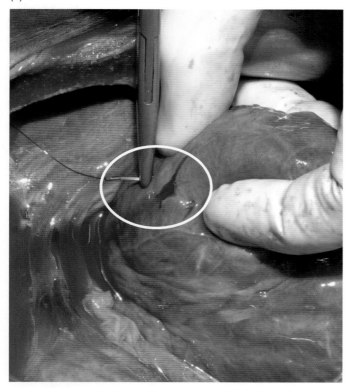

Fig. 15.9(a). Digital compression between the thumb and index finger is used initially to control bleeding from the cardiac wound and allow suturing.

(b)

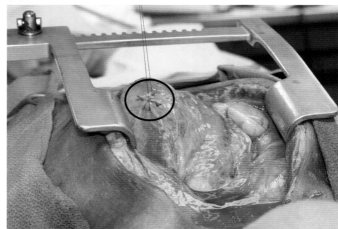

Fig. 15.9(b). Most cardiac wounds can be repaired with figure-of-eight stitches of non-absorbable 2/0 or 3/0 suture on a tapered needle.

(c)

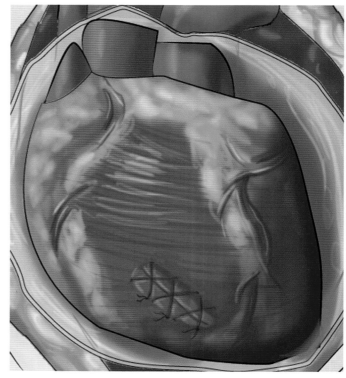

Fig. 15.9(c). Repair of a right ventricular wound with figure-of-eight sutures.

(a)

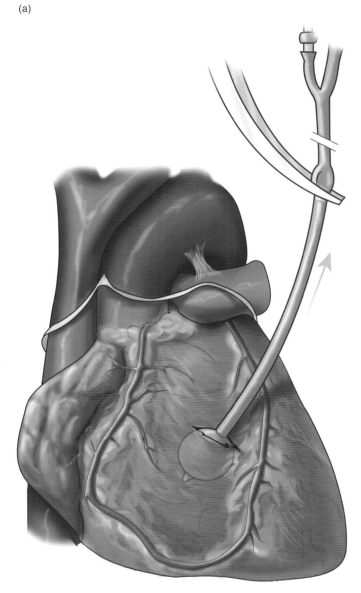

(b)

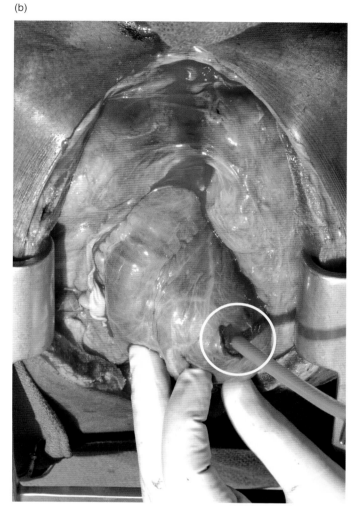

Fig. 15.10(a),(b). (*cont.*)

Fig. 15.10(a),(b). A Foley balloon can be used to temporarily control the bleeding from a cardiac wound. Exert gentle traction on the catheter to achieve tamponade of the wound. Avoid excessive traction to prevent pulling the balloon through the defect and creating a larger wound.

- Skin staples may be used temporarily for cardiac wound closure in the emergency room, and are primarily effective for stab wounds. This does not work well in patients who have sustained gunshot wounds associated with cardiac tissue loss. The staples should be replaced by sutures in the operating room.

- Partial transection of a major coronary artery can be repaired with interrupted sutures under magnification, while the heart is beating. If this is not technically possible, ligation is performed and the cardiac activity is observed. Distal injuries are usually tolerated well. If no arrhythmia develops, then nothing further is

required. If arrhythmia occurs, the suture is removed and gentle finger pressure is applied, while a cardiac team with cardiopulmonary bypass capabilities is mobilized.

- Cardiopulmonary bypass is largely unnecessary during the acute operation. The surgical goal is to save the patient's life. Any non-life-threatening intracardiac defects should be repaired electively under optimal conditions at a later stage.

- Inspection and repair of injuries to the posterior cardiac wall can be difficult, as lifting of the heart often causes arrhythmia or cardiac arrest. These injuries can be exposed and repaired by grasping the apex of the heart with a Duval clamp and applying mild traction and elevation. Another option is to place a figure-of-eight 2–0 suture on a tapered needle through the apex of the heart for traction and elevation. This option should be performed cautiously because the myocardium may tear during traction. An alternative approach is to slowly elevate the heart by placing sequential laparotomy pads, one at a time, under the heart to allow adaptation to the change in position. Inflow occlusion of the superior and inferior vena cava, in order to induce cardiac arrest and facilitate repair of the wound, is not advisable, because it is unlikely that the already compromised heart will tolerate normothermic cardiac arrest, even for brief periods of time.

- In cases of persistent arrhythmias or cardiac arrest, use epicardial pacing (see Chapter 4).

(a)

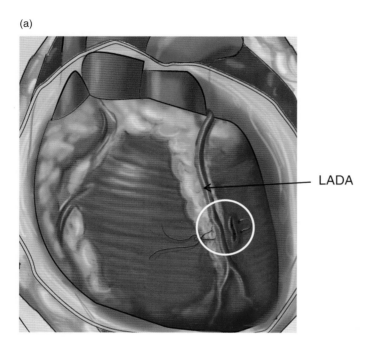

LADA

(b)

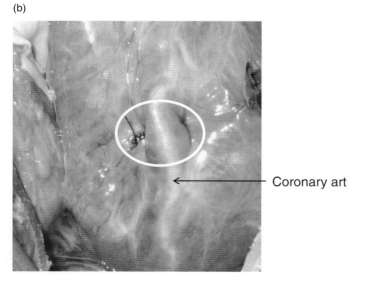

Coronary art

Fig. 15.11(a),(b). Injuries near coronary vessels should be repaired with a horizontal mattress suture, placed under the vessel.

(a)

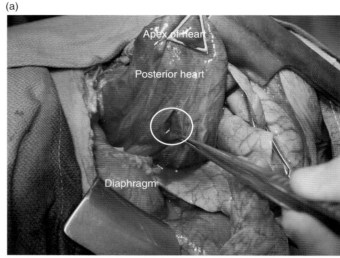

Fig. 15.12(a),(b). The posterior aspect of the heart can be exposed and repaired by grasping the apex with a Duval clamp and gently elevating the heart.

(b)

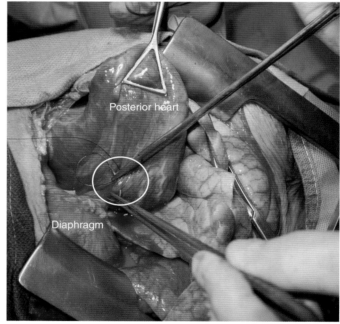

Fig. 15.12(a),(b). (*cont.*)

Pericardial closure

Following cardiac repair and stabilization of the patient, the pericardium is closed with continuous 2–0 sutures, leaving an opening near the base of the pericardium to avoid tamponade in case of a rebleed. In patients with acute cardiac enlargement due to cardiac failure or massive fluid resuscitation, the pericardium should be left open to prevent arrhythmias.

Tips and pitfalls

- Closure of the pericardium under tension may precipitate an arrhythmia and cardiac arrest.

Closure of median sternotomy

- Ensure hemostasis of the sternal edge with cautery or bone wax application.

Check for bleeding from the internal mammary arteries, under the sternum, after removal of the sternal retractor.

- Place at least one water-sealed chest drain under the sternum.
- Close the sternum with steel wires, using the heavy needle driver.
- Close the presternal fascia with heavy absorbable sutures.

(a)

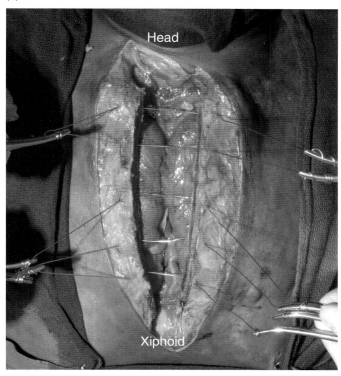

(b)

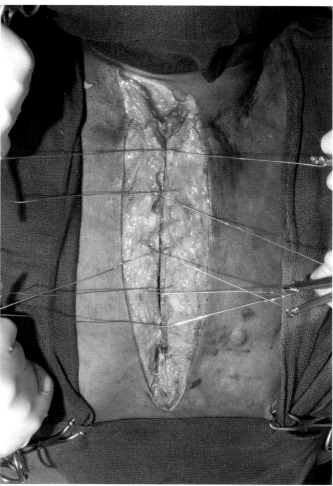

Fig. 15.13(a)–(d). (*cont.*)

Fig. 15.13(a)–(d). Closure of the sternotomy in layers. The sternum is closed with wires and the fascia with heavy, continuous absorbable suture.

(c)

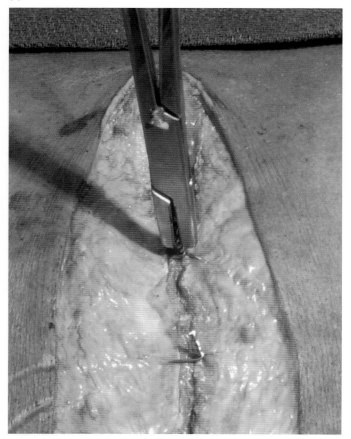

Fig. 15.13(a)–(d). *(cont.)*

(d)

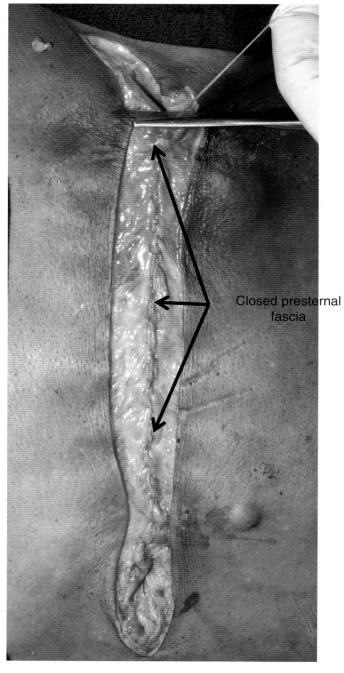

Closed presternal fascia

Fig. 15.13(a)–(d). *(cont.)*

Tips and pitfalls

- Failure to inspect the integrity of the inferior mammary artery after the removal of the sternal retractor can result in significant and persistent postoperative bleeding.

Postoperative evaluation

All survivors should undergo routine early and late echocardiographic evaluation to rule out significant intracardiac injuries, which include septal defects, valvular or papillary muscle dysfunction, myocardial dyskinesia, and late pericardial effusion.

Thoracic vessels

16

Demetrios Demetriades and Stephen Varga

Surgical anatomy

- The upper mediastinum contains the aortic arch with the origins of its major branches. These include the innominate artery, proximal left common carotid, and proximal left subclavian arteries. The left and right innominate veins join to become the superior vena cava (SVC).
- The thymic remnant and surrounding mediastinal fat are the first tissues encountered when entering the upper mediastinum. These tissues lie over the left innominate (brachiocephalic) vein and the aortic arch.
- The left innominate vein is approximately 6–7 cm long, transverses the upper mediastinum under the manubrium sterni and over the superior border of the aortic arch. It joins the right innominate vein, at the level of the first to second intercostal space on the right parasternally, to form the SVC.

- The right innominate (brachiocephalic) vein is approximately 3 cm in length, courses vertically downward and joins the left innominate vein at a 90 degree angle, to form the SVC.
- The SVC is approximately 6–7 cm in length and is located lateral and parallel to the ascending aorta. A small segment is enclosed within the pericardium.
- The ascending aorta is contained within the pericardium. The aortic arch begins at the superior attachment of the pericardium. The first branch of the aortic arch is the innominate (brachiocephalic) artery, which branches into the right subclavian and right common carotid arteries. The next branch of the arch is the left common carotid artery, followed by the left subclavian artery. The innominate artery and the left common carotid originate relatively anteriorly, while the left subclavian artery originates more posteriorly. Anatomical variants include a common origin for the left common carotid artery and innominate artery as well as a common origin for the left subclavian and left common carotid artery.

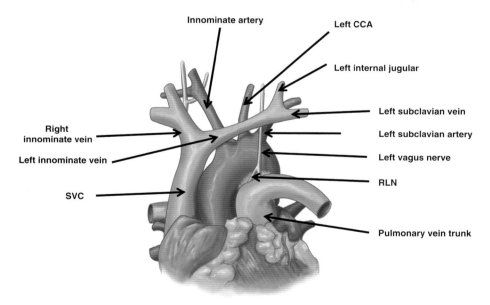

Fig. 16.1. Anatomy of the vessels of the superior mediastinum. Note the left innominate vein transversing over the superior border of the aortic arch and its major branches (SVC = superior vena cava, RLN = recurrent laryngeal nerve, CCA = common carotid artery.)

Innominate artery

Left CCA

Left internal jugular

Left subclavian vein

Right innominate vein

Left subclavian artery

Left innominate vein

Left vagus nerve

RLN

SVC

Pulmonary vein trunk

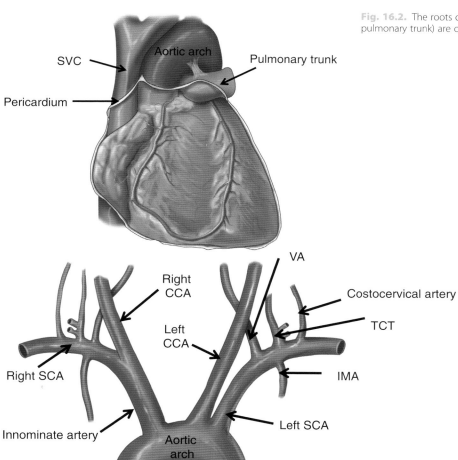

Fig. 16.2. The roots of the major vessels (aorta, superior vena cava, and pulmonary trunk) are covered by the pericardium.

SVC

Aortic arch

Pulmonary trunk

Pericardium

VA

Right CCA

Costocervical artery

Left CCA

TCT

Right SCA

IMA

Innominate artery

Left SCA

Aortic arch

Fig. 16.3. The major vessels of the aortic arch (innominate artery, left common carotid, left subclavian artery). The left common carotid originates directly from the aorta, while the right common carotid branches from the innominate artery. (SCA = subclavian artery, CCA = common carotid artery, VA = vertebral artery, IMA = internal mammary artery, TCT = thyrocervical trunk.)

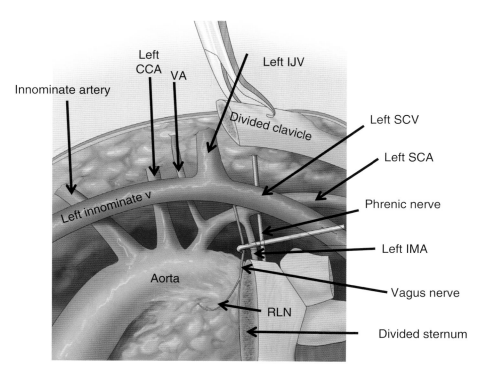

Fig. 16.4. Anatomy of the aortic arch and its major trunks; note the anatomical relationship with the left innominate vein, the left vagus, and left phrenic nerves. The vagus nerve is medial and the phrenic nerve lateral to the internal mammary artery. (SCA = subclavian artery, SCV = subclavian vein, CCA = common carotid artery, VA = vertebral artery, IMA = internal mammary artery, RLN = recurrent laryngeal nerve.)

Left CCA

VA

Left IJV

Innominate artery

Divided clavicle

Left SCV

Left SCA

Phrenic nerve

Left innominate v

Left IMA

Aorta

Vagus nerve

RLN

Divided sternum

- The left vagus nerve travels between the left common carotid and subclavian arteries just anterior to the arch and branches off into the recurrent laryngeal nerve, which loops around the aortic arch and ascends along the tracheoesophageal groove.
- The right vagus nerve crosses over the right subclavian artery, immediately gives off the recurrent laryngeal nerve, which

loops behind the subclavian artery and ascends behind the common carotid artery along the tracheoesophageal groove.

- The thoracic or descending aorta begins at the fourth thoracic vertebra on the left side of the vertebral column. Below the root of the lung, it courses to a position anterior to the vertebral column as it passes into the abdominal cavity through the aortic hiatus in the diaphragm at the twelfth thoracic vertebra.
- The esophagus lies on the right side of the aorta proximally. Distally, as it enters the diaphragm, it courses in front of the aorta.
- The aorta has nine pairs of aortic intercostal arteries that arise from the posterior of the aorta and travel to the associated intercostal spaces. The bronchial and esophageal arteries are additional branches of the aorta as it descends in the thorax.

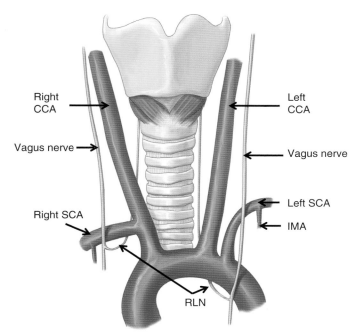

Fig. 16.5. Anatomical relationship between the vagus nerves and the major vessels. They cross in front of the proximal subclavian artery. The recurrent laryngeal nerve loops around the subclavian on the right side and around the aortic arch on the left side. (SCA = subclavian artery, CCA = common carotid artery, IMA = internal mammary artery, RLN = recurrent laryngeal nerve.)

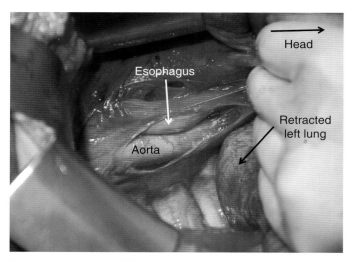

Fig. 16.7. Anatomical relationship between the esophagus and the thoracic aorta: the esophagus lies on the right side of the aorta. Above the diaphragm, it courses in front of the aorta.

Fig. 16.6. The left vagus nerve crosses over the proximal left subclavian artery and the aortic arch. At the inferior border of the arch it gives the left recurrent laryngeal nerve. (SCA = subclavian artery, RLN = recurrent laryngeal nerve).

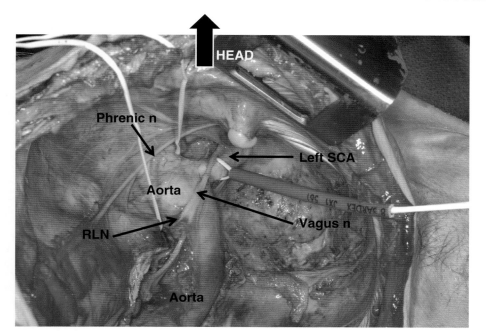

General principles

- Greater than 90% of thoracic great vessel injuries are due to penetrating trauma. Most patients with penetrating trauma to the major mediastinal vessels die at the scene and never reach hospital care.
- For those who survive to present to a hospital, most patients arrive with hemodynamic instability and require emergency operation without any diagnostic studies.
- Patients with no vital signs or imminent cardiac arrest on arrival should be managed with a resuscitative emergency room thoracotomy (see Chapter 4).
- In hemodynamically stable patients with suspected injuries to the mediastinal vessels, CT arteriography is the most effective screening diagnostic investigation.
- Thoracic great vessel injuries can present with external or internal hemorrhage, vascular thrombosis from intimal flaps, or pseudoaneurysms. Consequently, the absence of a significant amount of bleeding does not rule out a vascular injury.

Special surgical instruments

- In the operating room, the thoracotomy trauma tray should include vascular instruments, a power sternal saw, Lebsche knife with hammer, and bone cutter. The surgeon should wear a headlight for optimal lighting in anatomically difficult areas.

Patient positioning

Positioning for upper mediastinal vascular injuries

- The patient is placed in the supine position with both arms abducted at 90 degrees to allow anesthesia access to the extremities.
- Skin preparation and draping should include the neck, anterior chest, and hemithoraces. As for all acute trauma operations, the abdomen and groin should be prepared as well in case of an unexpected missile trajectory or the need for saphenous vein conduit.

Positioning for exposure of the descending thoracic aorta

- Place patient in right lateral decubitus position (see Chapter 14).
- If possible use a double-lumen endotracheal tube and have the left lung deflated once the pleura has been entered.

Incisions

Median sternotomy

- A median sternotomy provides excellent exposure of the upper mediastinal vessels. In addition, it provides good exposure to the heart and to both lungs.

- The median sternotomy incision can also be extended into the neck with a sternocleidomastoid incision or a clavicular extension to allow more distal exposure of the common carotid or the subclavian vessels.

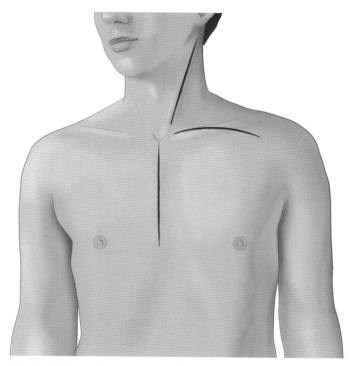

Fig. 16.8. The median sternotomy incision may be extended into the neck with a sternocleidomastoid incision for improved exposure of the common carotids or a clavicular incision to allow more distal exposure of the subclavian vessels.

Clamshell incision

- The clamshell incision provides good exposure of the anterior aspect of the heart, the superior mediastinal vessels, and both lungs. It is usually performed as an extension of a standard anterolateral thoracotomy to the opposite side.
- The incision is made through the fourth to fifth intercostal space bilaterally with transverse division of the sternum, using a bone cutter or heavy scissors.
- During the division of the sternum, both internal mammary arteries are transected, and identification and ligation of the proximal and distal ends should be performed.

(a)

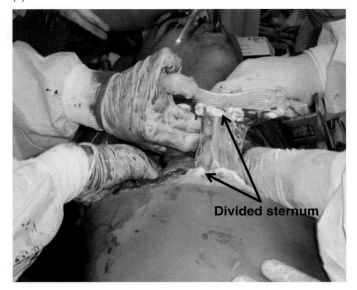

(b)

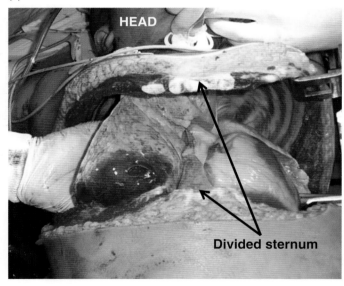

Fig. 16.9(a),(b). The clamshell incision is made through the fourth to fifth intercostal space bilaterally with transverse division of the sternum. It provides a good exposure of the anterior aspect of the heart, the superior mediastinal vessels, and both lungs.

Posterolateral thoracotomy

- This is the optimal incision for the management of injuries to the descending thoracic aorta. However, in the majority of penetrating trauma cases, due to severe hemodynamic instability, the patient is placed in the supine position and an extended anterolateral incision is performed.
- If possible, use a double-lumen endotracheal tube and have the left lung deflated once the pleura has been entered.

- Perform a generous left posterior lateral thoracotomy in the fourth or fifth intercostal space just below the left nipple all the way up between the scapula and the spine, making sure to divide the latissimus dorsi and the serratus anterior.

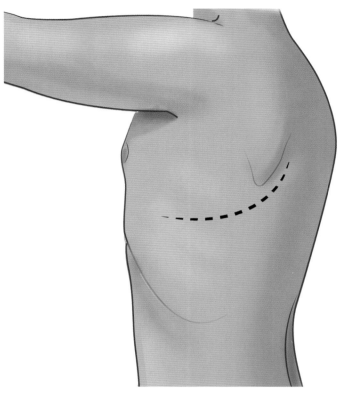

Fig. 16.10. Positioning and incision for the exposure of the descending thoracic aorta.

Exposures
Exposure of the upper mediastinal vessels

- Following median sternotomy or clamshell incision, the first step is to open the pericardium to rule out injury to the heart or the intrapericardial segment of the great vessels.
- All mediastinal hematomas due to penetrating trauma should be explored, if possible after proximal and distal control.
- The first tissues encountered under the sternum in the upper mediastinum are the thymus remnant with surrounding fat pad, which lies directly over the left innominate vein and the aortic arch. These tissues are grasped with an Allis forceps and lifted towards the patient's head. Careful blunt dissection exposes the left innominate vein.
- Vessel loops are placed around the left innominate vein. Dissection of the vessel allows identification of its near perpendicular junction with the right innominate vein, where the SVC begins. The SVC lies parallel and to the right of the ascending aorta.

(a)

(b)

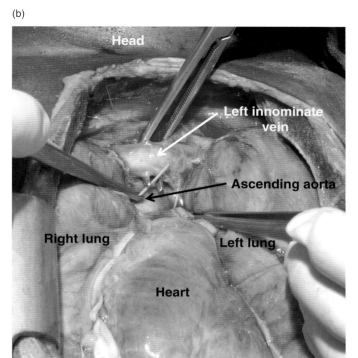

Fig. 16.11(a),(b). Mobilization of the thymus and upper mediastinal fat pad. The first tissues encountered under the sternum in the upper mediastinum are the thymus remnant with the surrounding fat pad, which lie directly over the left innominate vein and the aortic arch. Mobilization of these tissues exposes the left innominate vein, which is encircled with a vessel loop.

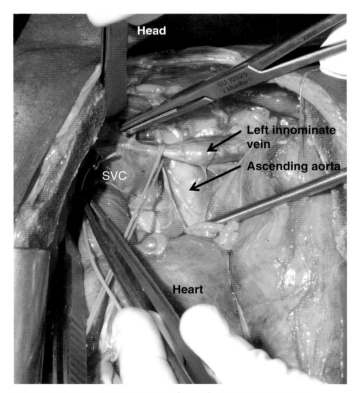

Fig. 16.12. Complete mobilization of the left innominate vein and exposure of the superior vena cava.

- Exposure of the aortic arch and the origins of the major vessels requires retraction of the left innominate vein, which lies directly over the upper border of the arch. On rare occasions, the left innominate vein may need to be ligated to provide better exposure of the transverse aorta and its branches.
- The innominate and left carotid arteries originate from the anterosuperior aspect of the aortic arch and are easy to identify and control with vessel loops. However, the left subclavian artery is more posterior and more difficult to isolate.
- Mobilization and isolation of the distal innominate artery may be difficult through a median sternotomy. In these cases the incision may be extended to the right neck through a standard sternocleidomastoid incision, to improve the exposure.
- Mobilization and isolation of the left subclavian artery may require a combination of a median sternotomy with a left clavicular incision.
- Identify and protect the left vagus nerve as it descends into the mediastinum between the left carotid and the left subclavian arteries, over the aortic arch.

(a)

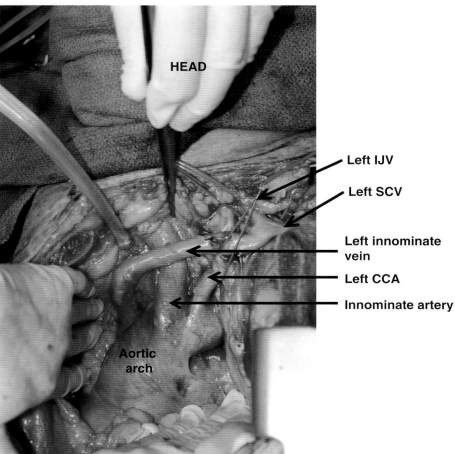

HEAD

Left IJV

Left SCV

Left innominate vein

Left CCA

Innominate artery

Aortic arch

Fig. 16.13(a)–(c). The proximal innominate artery and left common carotid artery lie directly under the left innominate vein (a). The left subclavian artery is lateral and more posterior and needs further dissection for exposure (b). Complete exposure of the left innominate vein (formed by the left internal jugular and left subclavian veins) and the trunks of the aortic arch. (SCA = subclavian artery, CCA = common carotid artery, IJV = internal jugular vein, SCV = subclavian vein.)

(b)

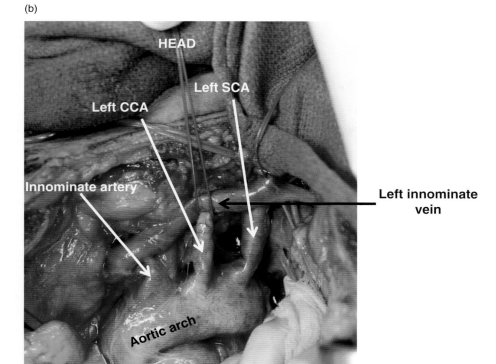

HEAD

Left SCA

Left CCA

Innominate artery

Left innominate vein

Aortic arch

(c)

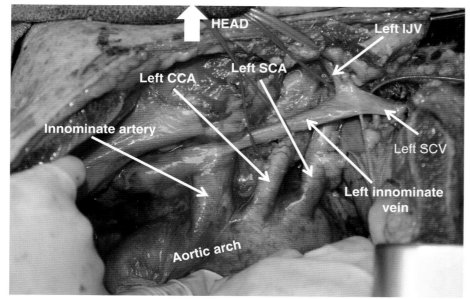

Fig. 16.13(a)–(c). (cont.)

(a)

(b)

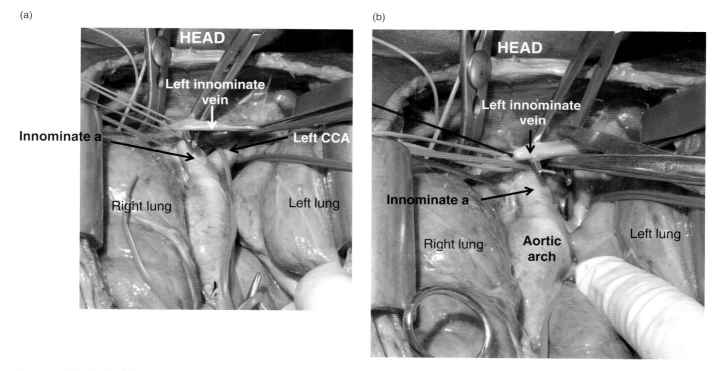

Fig. 16.14(a)–(c). The left innominate vein may be ligated and divided to allow for greater exposure to the transverse aorta and proximal innominate artery.

(c)

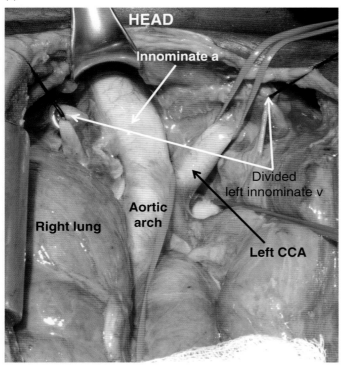

Fig. 16.14(a)–(c). (*cont.*)

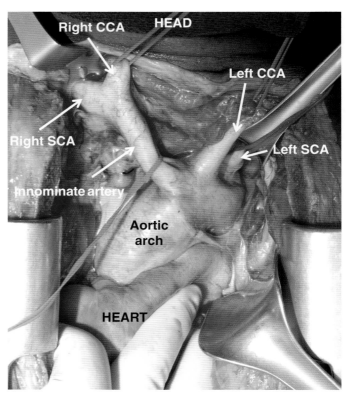

Fig. 16.15. The aortic arch after division of the left innominate vein. The innominate artery, with the origins of the right common carotid and right subclavian arteries are identified. Note the limited exposure of the left subclavian artery due to its posterior position. (SCA = subclavian artery, CCA = common carotid artery.)

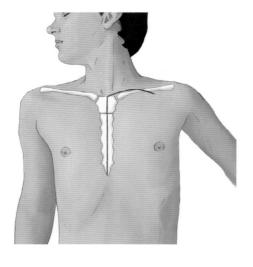

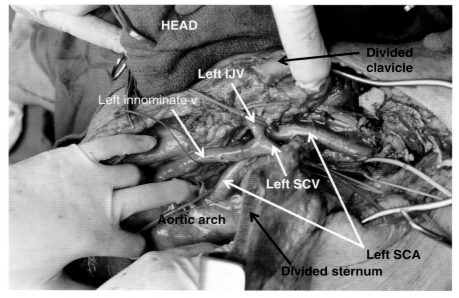

Fig. 16.16. Satisfactory exposure of the left subclavian artery may require a combination of a median sternotomy with a left clavicular incision (inset). Note the junction of the left internal jugular and left subclavian vein to form the left innominate vein. (IJV = internal jugular vein, SCV = subclavian vein.)

Exposure of the descending thoracic aorta

- Optimal exposure is achieved through a generous left posterolateral incision through the fourth intercostal space.
- During dissection and isolation of the aorta, the esophagus should be identified and protected. It lies on the right side of the aorta, but as it enters the diaphragm it courses in front of the aorta.
- The left vagus nerve courses over the aortic arch, between the subclavian and left common carotid arteries. In proximal dissections it should be isolated and protected.

Management of mediastinal venous injuries

- Ligation of the innominate vein is usually well tolerated. Transient arm edema is the most common complication. Repair of the vein should be considered only if it can be done with lateral venorrhaphy and without stricture formation. For an acute injury, especially in the hemodynamically compromised patient, complex reconstruction with synthetic grafts should not be performed.
- Ligation of the SVC is not compatible with life because of the development of massive brain edema. Repair or reconstruction should always be attempted.
- Intraoperative air embolism is a common and potentially lethal complication because of the negative venous pressures in the severely hypovolemic patient. Early occlusion of the venous tear by compression or application of a vascular clamp helps to prevent this complication.

Management of mediastinal arterial injuries

Many patients with injuries to the major mediastinal arteries arrive in extremis. However, ligation of these vessels is not advisable because it may not be compatible with life and is associated with a high incidence of limb loss. Simple suture repair is the preferred choice whenever possible, and is often the case with stab wounds. For more complex injuries with tissue loss, usually due to gunshot wounds or blunt trauma, a more complex reconstruction with prosthetic conduit may be required. Damage control procedures, using a temporary intravascular shunt, is ideal for all injuries involving the branches of the aortic arch. However, for injuries involving the aorta, shunting is not technically possible. In these cases, temporary bleeding control and cardiopulmonary bypass may be the only options.

Innominate artery or proximal right carotid artery

- Identify the origins of the right subclavian and right common carotid arteries and isolate with vessel loops and vascular clamps for control. Extension of the sternotomy into a right sternocleidomastoid incision is often necessary in order to achieve good exposure of the right carotid artery.

- Identify and protect the right vagus nerve, as it crosses over the subclavian artery.
- In selected patients with small partial tears in the vessel, primary repair is often possible. Use a 4–0 polypropylene suture for a lateral arteriorrhaphy.
- In most cases with gunshot wounds or blunt injury to the innominate artery, repair using the bypass exclusion technique is required.
  - Gently palpate the aortic arch to determine suitability for clamping. A side biting clamp is applied just proximal to the innominate take off. Resect the injured artery and examine the intima in the proximal end. If the intimal disruption extends into the aortic arch, this area is not suitable for proximal graft placement.
  - If unable to use the proximal end of the innominate artery, place the clamp on the proximal intrapericardial ascending aorta using a side-biting C clamp. Make an aortotomy with an 11-blade.
  - Select an 8–10 mm low-porosity knitted polyester graft and bevel it appropriately to avoid an acute right angle at its origin. This graft is then placed from the ascending aorta to the distal innominate artery immediately proximal to the bifurcation of the

(a)

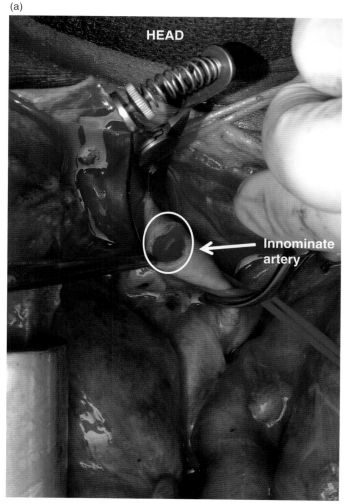

Fig. 16.17(a),(b). Repair of a simple injury (circle) of the innominate artery with continuous suture.

(b)

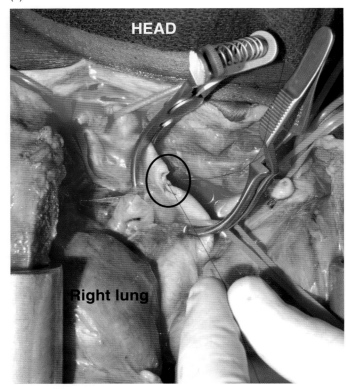

Fig. 16.17(a),(b). *(cont.)*

(a)

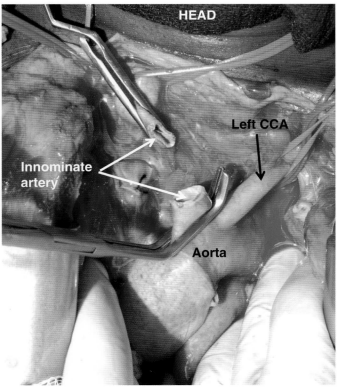

Fig. 16.18(a),(b),(c). Repair of complex injury of the innominate artery with a synthetic graft. A vascular clamp is applied on the proximal innominate artery, at its junction with the aortic arch (a). An interposition size 8 synthetic graft is placed (b),(c).

(b)

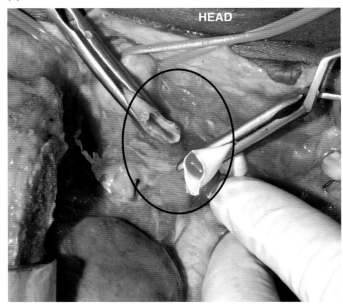

(c)

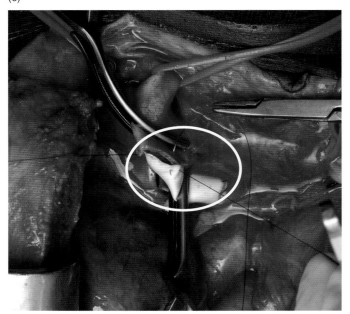

Fig. 16.18(a),(b),(c)

subclavian and right carotid arteries. The anastomosis should be performed using a running 4–0 polypropylene suture.

o Restore flow first to the subclavian artery, then to the carotid artery.

o Once the bypass is complete, oversew the proximal innominate artery stump with a 4–0 polypropylene suture.

Proximal left carotid artery

- Proximal exposure is excellent through a median sternotomy. However, a standard left sternocleidomastoid incision may be necessary for adequate distal control.
- Damage control with a temporary arterial shunt is a good option for patients in extremis. This approach may not be technically feasible for very proximal injuries.
- Primary repair is possible for most stab wounds.
- Reconstruction with saphenous vein or synthetic graft is required in most cases after gunshot wounds or blunt trauma. In any complex reconstruction, temporary shunting should be utilized to reduce the risk of ischemic stroke.

Proximal subclavian artery

- Exposure and repair of the proximal right and left subclavian arteries require combined sternotomy and clavicular incisions.
- Damage control with a temporary arterial shunt is a good option in patients in extremis. This approach may not be technically feasible for very proximal injuries.
- Ligation of the subclavian artery should not be considered as an acceptable method of damage control because of the high incidence of limb ischemia and compartment syndrome.
- Primary repair is possible for most stab wounds. However, reconstruction with a size 6–8 mm PTFE graft is required in most gunshot wounds or blunt injuries (see chapter 9).

Descending thoracic aorta

- Placement of a double-lumen tube and deflation of the left lung upon entering the chest cavity improve the exposure of the thoracic aorta.
- The lung is retracted and the posterior mediastinal structures come into view.
- The first step is to obtain proximal control. This is facilitated by first palpating and isolating the left subclavian artery, and tracing it back to the aortic arch. Identify and protect the left vagus nerve during the dissection.
- Once the proximal aorta is identified, place a finger carefully between the left carotid and left subclavian artery, around the aorta to create a proximal clamping site. Place umbilical tape around the aorta to facilitate clamp placement.
- Once the proximal dissection is complete, obtain distal control. Locate the aorta distal to the hematoma or the bleeding site and incise the pleura over it. Encircle the aorta with finger dissection followed by an umbilical tape. The dissection of the aorta should be limited to avoid avulsion of the intercostal vessels.
- When everything is ready to complete the repair, apply the vascular clamps. Start with the proximal aortic clamp, followed by the distal aortic clamp, then secure the subclavian artery with a vascular clamp or Rummel tourniquet.

(a)

Fig. 16.19(a)–(c). Proximal and distal control of the descending thoracic aorta. Proximal dissection and identification of the origin of the left subclavian artery, which is encircled with a vessel loop (white loop). Identify and protect the left vagus nerve (yellow loop) (a). The pleura over the distal thoracic aorta is dissected and the aorta is encircled (b).

(b)

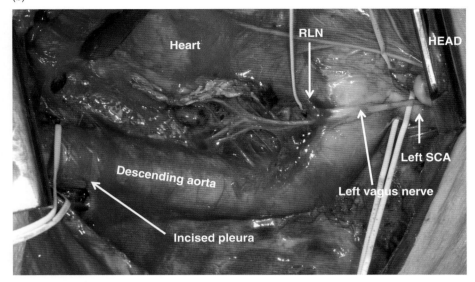

Fig. 16.19(a)–(c). (cont.)

(c)

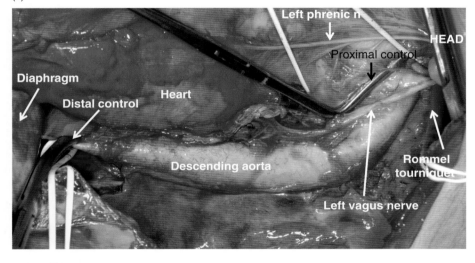

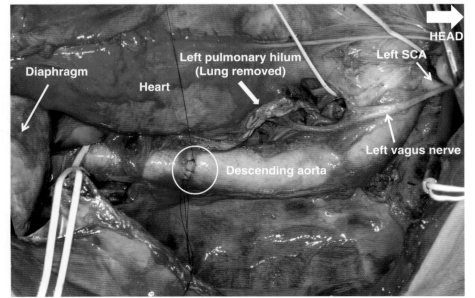

Fig. 16.20. Repair of a simple laceration of the descending aorta with a transverse continuous suture, after proximal and distal control (circle).

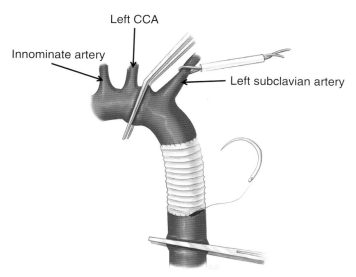

Left CCA

Innominate artery

Left subclavian artery

Fig. 16.21. Repair of the descending aorta with an interposition graft, after proximal and distal control.

- After the proximal and distal dissections are complete, the area of the aortic injury is dissected and the extent of the damage assessed. Small penetrating injuries may be repaired with primary repair (4–0 or 5–0 polypropylene sutures).
- Complex injuries or injuries with extensive intimal involvement will require an interposition graft. Identify the ends of the aorta and excise to healthy tissue. Look for bleeding from the intercostals; if identified, oversew with 4–0 polypropylene sutures.
- Sew proximal graft in first using a double-armed 4–0 polypropylene running suture without pledgets. Once the proximal anastomosis is completed, stretch and cut the graft to an appropriate length and perform the distal anastomosis. Just prior to completion of the distal anastomosis, release the distal clamp to check hemostasis and to de-air the aorta. Complete the distal anastomosis and remove the proximal clamp.
- Once hemostasis is achieved, cover the graft by closing the mediastinal pleura with absorbable sutures to exclude the graft from the lung.
- Place chest tubes and close the thoracotomy incision.

Tips and pitfalls

- The most serious and common error is performing the operation without excellent knowledge of the local anatomy.
- Using a double-lumen tube is not mandatory, but will facilitate exposure and repair of the injury.
- Perform the posterolateral thoracotomy through the fourth intercostal space. Choosing the wrong space makes exposure difficult. If exposure using the fourth intercostal space is still inadequate, cut a rib above or below the initial incision.
- After a clamshell incision, both internal mammary arteries are transected. Identify and ligate all four arterial ends.
- There is a significant risk of air embolism in venous injuries. In a hypovolemic patient it may take only a few seconds. Control the venous injury by compression or clamping as soon as possible.
- The left innominate vein lies under the thymus remnant and surrounding fat. There is a risk of accidental injury to the vein during the exploration of the upper mediastinum.
- There is a risk of iatrogenic injury to the left vagus nerve, as it crosses over the aortic arch, between the left carotid and left subclavian artery, during dissection for proximal aortic control.
- During innominate artery reconstruction, restoring blood flow to the carotid artery prior to the subclavian artery could potentially send debris or air to the brain rather than to the arm.
- Attempting to obtain proximal aortic control distal to the subclavian artery may make the repair difficult, with a very short proximal aorta on which to sew the graft. Obtaining control distal to the left carotid and proximal to the left subclavian provides extra room for repair.
- Be careful while dissecting the distal aorta away from the vertebral column. Stay between the intercostal vessels and minimize superior and inferior dissection to prevent bleeding and avulsion of the intercostal vessels.
- When dissecting out the distal aorta, be sure to palpate and protect the esophagus to prevent injury and avoid including the esophagus in the distal aortic clamp.

Lung injuries

Demetrios Demetriades and Jennifer Smith

Surgical anatomy

- The trachea divides into the right and left main bronchi at the level of the sternal angle. The right bronchus is wider, shorter, and more vertical compared to the left. The right bronchus divides into three lobar bronchi, supplying the right upper, middle, and lower lung lobes, respectively. The left bronchus divides into two lobar bronchi, supplying the left upper and lower lobes.
- The lung has a unique dual blood supply. The pulmonary arteries originate from the right ventricle. The right pulmonary artery passes posterior to the aorta and superior vena cava. The left pulmonary artery courses anterior to the left mainstem bronchus. The pulmonary arteries supply deoxygenated blood from the systemic circulation directly to alveoli where gas exchange occurs. These vessels are large in diameter, but supply blood in a low pressure system.
- The bronchial arteries arise directly from the thoracic aorta. These vessels are smaller in diameter, and supply the trachea, bronchial tree, and visceral pleura.
- The venous drainage of the lungs occurs via the pulmonary veins. They originate at the level of the alveoli. There are two pulmonary veins on the right and two on the left. These four veins join at or near their junction with the left atrium, usually within the pericardium. These veins carry oxygenated blood back to the heart for distribution to the systemic circulation.
- The lung is covered superiorly, anteriorly, and posteriorly by pleura. At its inferior border, the investing layers come into contact forming the inferior pulmonary ligament that connects the lower lobe of the lung, from the inferior pulmonary vein to the mediastinum and the medial part of the diaphragm. It serves to retain the lower lung lobe in position.

(a)

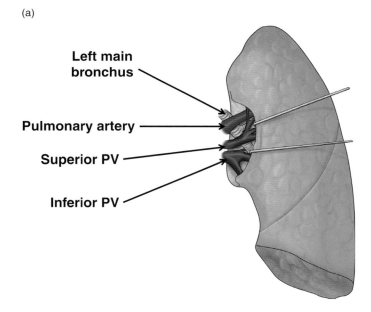

Left main bronchus

Pulmonary artery

Superior PV

Inferior PV

(b)

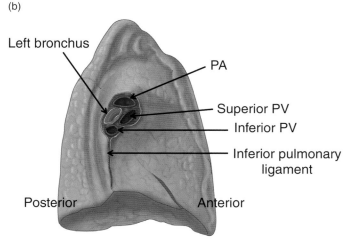

Left bronchus

PA

Superior PV

Inferior PV

Inferior pulmonary ligament

Posterior   Anterior

Fig. 17.1(a)–(d). Anatomy of the left hilum. The pulmonary artery is the superior most structure within the pulmonary hilum. Note the close relationship between the inferior pulmonary vein and inferior pulmonary ligament. Caution should be taken to avoid injury to the vein during division of the ligament.

Fig. 17.1(a)–(d). (*cont.*)

Atlas of Surgical Techniques in Trauma, ed. Demetrios Demetriades, Kenji Inaba, and George Velmahos. Published by Cambridge University Press. © Cambridge University Press 2015.

(c)

Fig. 17.1(a)–(d). (cont.)

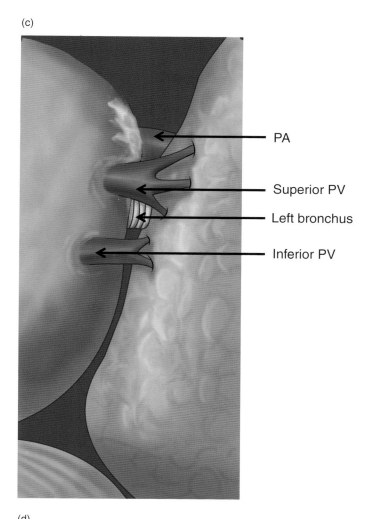

PA

Superior PV

Left bronchus

Inferior PV

(d)

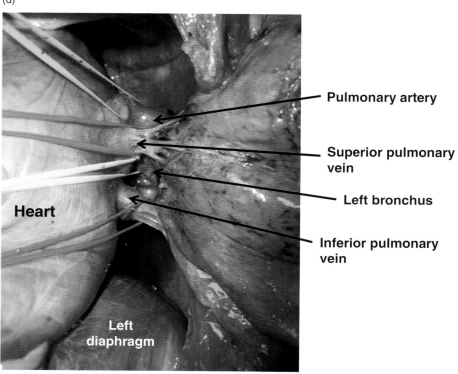

Pulmonary artery

Superior pulmonary vein

Left bronchus

Inferior pulmonary vein

Heart

Left diaphragm

(a)

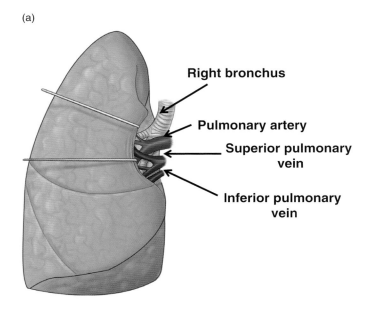

(a)

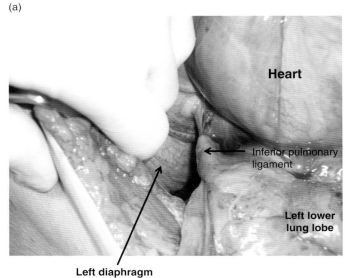

(b)

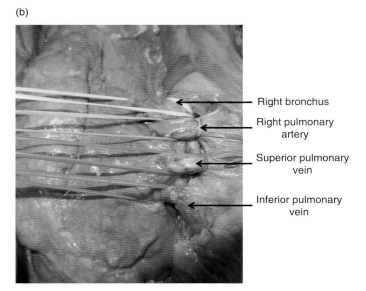

Fig. 17.2(a),(b). Anatomy of the right hilum. There are two structures located anteriorly; the pulmonary artery superiorly, and the superior pulmonary vein inferiorly. The posterior most structure is the right main stem bronchus. The inferior-most structure is the inferior pulmonary vein.

(b)

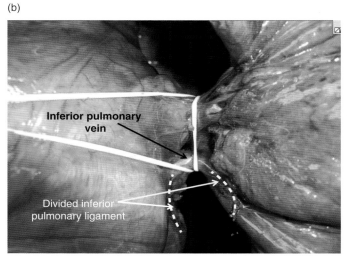

Fig. 17.3(a),(b). The inferior pulmonary ligament (a) connects the lower lobe of the lung, from the inferior pulmonary vein to the mediastinum and the medial part of the diaphragm. During division of the ligament, accidental injury to the vein may occur (b).

General principles

- Lungs have high blood flow, but are part of a low pressure system. In addition, the lung tissue is rich in tissue thromboplastin. This combination results in spontaneous hemostasis from the lung parenchyma in the majority of cases. Hilar or central lung injuries are the most common cause of massive lung hemorrhage requiring operative management.
- About 80%–85% of penetrating and more than 90% of blunt trauma to the lungs can safely be managed with thoracotomy tube drainage and supportive measures alone.
- Lung-sparing non-anatomical lung resections are preferable to more extensive anatomical resections after injury.
- Pneumonectomy after trauma is associated with very high mortality.

Special surgical instruments

The surgeon should have readily available a standard vascular tray, Finochietto retractor, Duval clamps, Allison lung retractor, and a sternal saw or Lebsche knife.

Anesthesia considerations

- If the hemodynamic condition of the patient allows, insert a double-lumen tube.
- Maintain low tidal volumes to reduce the risk of air embolism.

Positioning

The patient is placed supine on the operating room table with both arms abducted to 90 degrees. Skin preparation should include the neck, anterior and bilateral lateral chest walls, and the abdomen down to the groin.

Incisions

Median sternotomy

It is the incision of choice in penetrating injuries to the anterior chest with suspected cardiac or anterior mediastinal vascular injuries. It provides good exposure of the heart, the anterior mediastinal vessels, both of the lungs, the middle and distal trachea, and left mainstem bronchus. It is quick to perform, relatively bloodless, and causes less postoperative pain and fewer respiratory complications than a thoracotomy. However, it does not allow for good exposure of the posterior mediastinal structures and does not provide adequate access for cross-clamping of the thoracic aorta for resuscitation purposes. The technique is described in Chapter 14.

Anterolateral thoracotomy

It is the preferred incision in cases with lung injuries. The technique is described in Chapter 14.

Clamshell thoracotomy

It is usually performed as an extension of a standard antero-lateral thoracotomy to the opposite side, for suspected bilateral lung injuries, superior mediastinal vascular injuries or cardiac resuscitation, and for aortic cross-clamping purposes. The technique is described in Chapter 14.

Operative techniques

- The type of lung operation is determined by the site and severity of lung injury, the shape and direction of the lung wound, the hemodynamic condition of the patient, and the experience of the surgeon. The operative techniques may include suturing of the bleeding lung, lung tractotomy, wedge resection, lobectomy, and total pneumonectomy.
- There is a stepwise increase in both mortality and complications with more extensive resections. This is independent of injury severity and the presence of associated

injuries. In trauma, non-anatomical lung-sparing resections are preferred over extensive anatomical resections.

Pneumonorrhaphy

- This technique is used to repair small, superficial lung injuries. Following careful individual suture ligation of any major bleeders and air leaks, the laceration is repaired with figure-of-eight absorbable sutures, on a large tapered needle. Application of tissue glue prior to approximation of the edges of the laceration may improve hemostasis and control minor air leaks.
- In cases with bleeding and air leaks from deep penetrating lung injuries, suturing of the entry and exit wounds should be avoided because of the risk of air embolism, intrapulmonary hematoma, and hemorrhagic flooding of

(a)

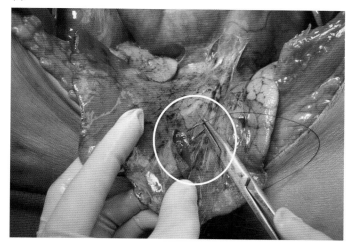

(b)

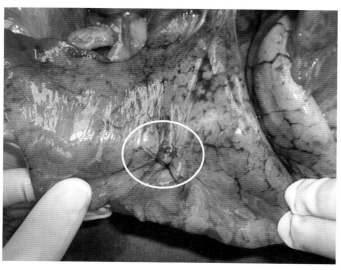

Fig. 17.4(a),(b). Peripheral stab wound to the lung, amenable to primary repair. Pneumonorrhaphy with figure-of-eight repair.

the bronchial tree, including the contralateral lung. These cases should be managed with lung tractotomy or segmental resection.

Lung tractotomy

- This is the procedure of choice in cases with bleeding and/or major air leaks from deep, penetrating injuries. Tractotomy is not indicated in suspected hilar injuries. These injuries usually require lobectomy or total pneumonectomy.
- The wound tract is opened with a GIA stapler with a 2.5 mm white load. Any significant bleeders or air leaks are

suture ligated under direct visualization. Application of tissue glue may be helpful in decreasing any diffuse bleeding and minor air leaks. The tract may be closed with figure-of-eight absorbable sutures on a large tapered needle.

- On rare occasions, tractotomy may devascularize segments of the lung, resulting in subsequent ischemic necrosis and lung abscess. The tractotomy should be performed parallel to the vascular supply whenever possible. The lung adjacent to the tractotomy should always be assessed for viability and any questionable tissue should be resected.

(a)

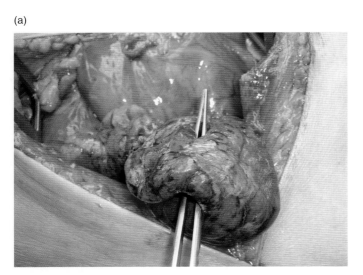

(b)

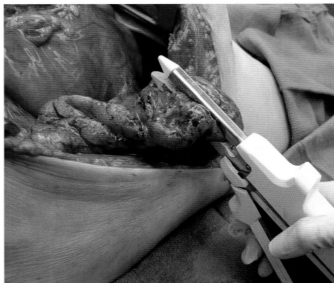

(c)

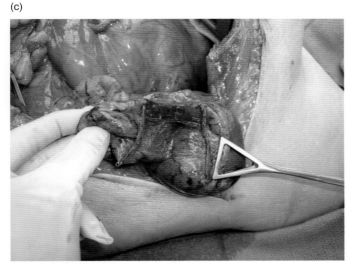

(d)

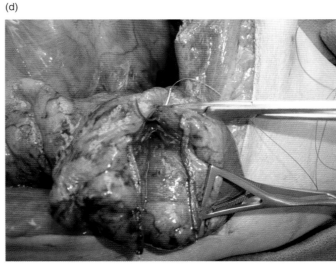

Fig. 17.5(a)–(d). Technique of stapled tractotomy in a through-and-through penetrating injury to the lung (a). Placement of a GIA stapler through the wound (b). Opened tract after tractotomy (c). Oversewing of bleeders and areas of air leak in the tract (d).

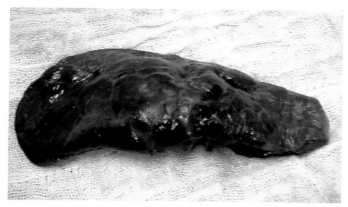

Fig. 17.6. Devascularized and dead lung tissue after tractotomy. To prevent this complication, the tractotomy should be parallel to the vessels.

Wedge resection

For larger peripheral injuries, the injured lung may be resected non-anatomically. Using a GIA stapler with a 2.5 mm white load, "wedge out" the injured tissue. Any persisting bleeding or air leaks can be managed with additional sutures and/or tissue glue. Alternatively, if a stapling device is not available, the injured tissue may be placed between clamps and the tissue "cut out." The edges are then oversewn using a running technique.

Non-anatomic lobe resection

- After temporary bleeding control with digital compression or application of a vascular clamp around the hilar structures, the hilar vessels are dissected free and the injury is identified. Depending on the anatomical location of the injury, the need for a lobectomy or pneumonectomy is determined.
- Anatomic lobe resection is rarely used in trauma and has been replaced by non-anatomical resection, preserving as much normal lung parenchyma as possible.
- During lower lobe resections, the inferior pulmonary ligament should be divided.
- The resection is best accomplished using a TA stapling device. Before release of the stapler, two stay sutures or Allis forceps are applied to the stump in order to prevent retraction. Once the stapler is released, the suture line can be held using the stay suture to inspect for, and control, any bleeding or air leaks.
- During the procedure, care should be taken to avoid devascularization of the remaining normal lung parenchyma.
- After resection of the lower lobe, avoid torsion of the remaining upper lobe. Failure to recognize this problem results in ischemic necrosis of the normal lobe. The remaining lung parenchyma can be tacked into place using superficially placed 3–0 sutures on a tapered needle.

(a)

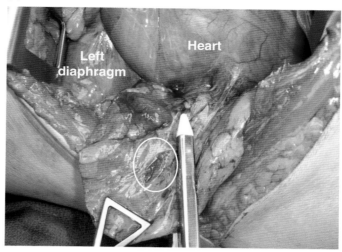

(b)

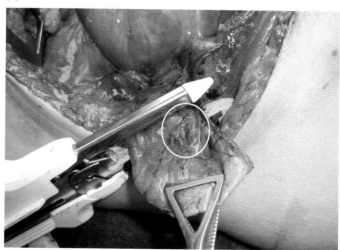

(c)

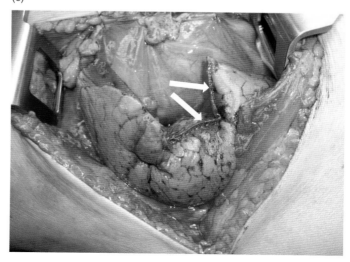

Fig. 17.7(a)–(c). Wedge resection of lung parenchyma using a GIA stapler after a peripheral stab wound.

(a)

(b)

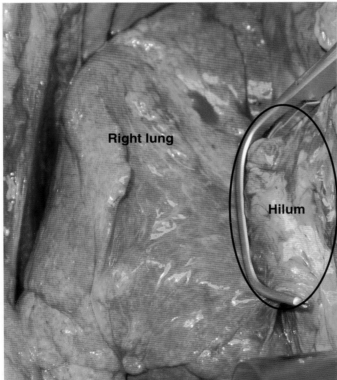

Fig. 17.8(a),(b). Temporary bleeding control with digital compression of the right lung hilum (a). Application of vascular clamp around the left hilum (b).

(a)

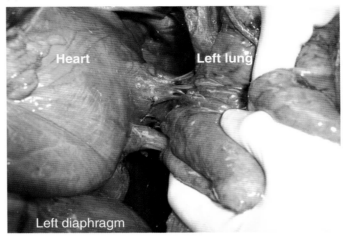

(b)

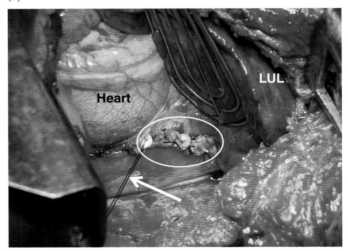

(c)

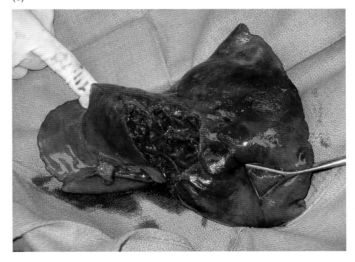

Fig. 17.9(a)–(c). Dissection of the left hilar vessels to determine the need for lobectomy or total pneumonectomy (a). En-masse stapled left lower lobectomy. If necessary, additional sutures may be placed for better hemostasis (circle shows the stump, arrow shows the stay suture to prevent retraction of the stump and check for hemostasis or air leaks). Stapled left lower lobectomy specimen (c).

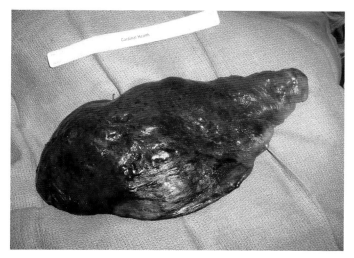

Fig. 17.10. Torsion and ischemic necrosis of the normal upper lobe following lower lobectomy.

Pneumonectomy

- A total pneumonectomy may be necessary in severe hilar injuries not amenable to repair or lobectomy.
- In hilar vascular injuries the patient is usually hemodynamically unstable and there is severe active bleeding. The fastest way to achieve temporary bleeding control is digital compression of the hilum and subsequent application of a vascular clamp, as described above. This maneuver is critical for effective bleeding control, and prevention of air embolism and hemorrhagic flooding of the normal bronchial tree. Acute occlusion may aggravate the hemodynamic condition of the patient because of acute right-sided cardiac strain. An alternative to clamping the hilum is to perform a "hilar twist" after release of the inferior pulmonary ligament. The whole lung is twisted 180° around the hilum.
- Pneumonectomy normally involves individual isolation, ligation, and division of the hilar structures. However, this approach is time-consuming and requires significant technical skills and experience. In the decompensated trauma patient, an acceptable alternative to the anatomical pneumonectomy is the en-masse stapled pneumonectomy.
- The en-masse pneumonectomy can be rapidly performed using a TA stapler.
  - The main bronchus should be divided as close to the carina as possible to avoid pooling of secretions and to reduce the risk of breakdown of the stump.
  - Following division of the inferior pulmonary ligament, the hilum is isolated and the index finger is placed around it.
  - After application and firing of the TA stapler around all hilar structures, the vessels and bronchus are divided approximately 0.5 cm above the instrument.
  - Two figure-of-eight stay sutures or two Allis forceps are placed at the two corners of the stump, before the

(a)

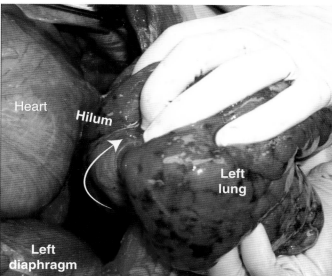

(b)

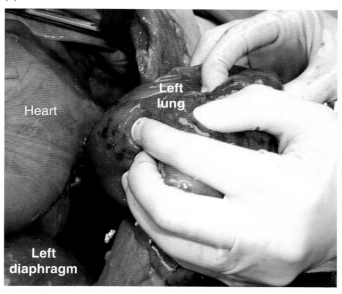

Fig. 17.11(a),(b). Hilar twist for temporary control of hilar bleeding. After division of the inferior pulmonary ligament to free the lung, the lung is grasped in its entirety and rotated 180° in a clockwise direction.

stapler is released. This prevents retraction of the stump after the removal of the stapler and facilitates identification and control of any bleeding or air leaks.
  - Buttressing of the stump with adjacent tissues, such as the pericardial fat pad, parietal pleura, or intercostal muscle flap may be used.
- Total pneumonectomy is associated with a very high mortality, usually due to hemorrhage or acute right cardiac failure.

(a)

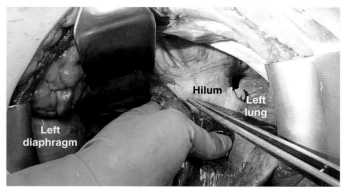

(b)

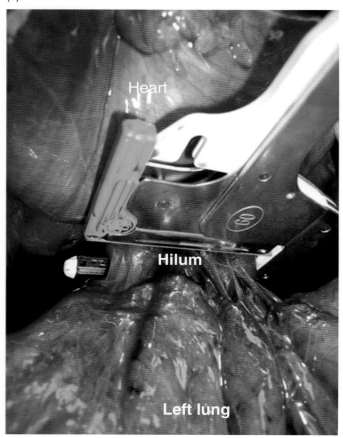

(c)

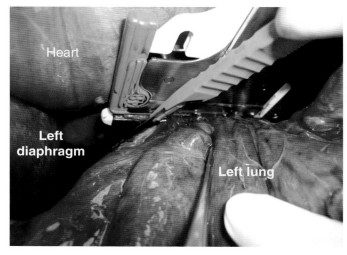

(d)

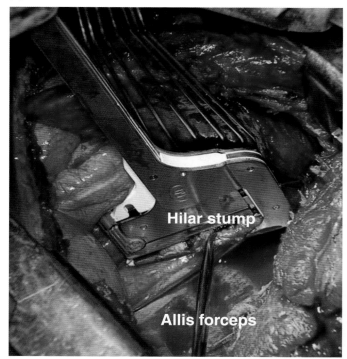

Fig. 17.12(a)–(e). Technique of *en-masse* stapled left total pneumonectomy. The hilum is isolated and the index finger is placed around it (a). A TA stapler is placed around all the structures of the pulmonary hilum (b). Division of all hilar structures with scalpel, about 0.5 cm above the stapler (c). Placement of two stay sutures or Allis forceps on the stump before removal of the stapling device to prevent retraction of the stump (d). Any bleeding or air leaks can be controlled with additional figure-of-eight absorbable sutures (e).

Fig. 17.12(a)–(e). (*cont.*)

(e)

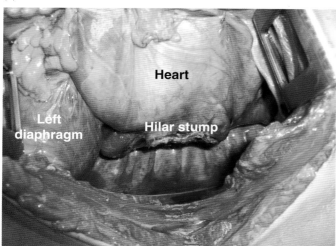

Fig. 17.12(a)–(e). (*cont.*)

Closure

The techniques of sternotomy or thoracotomy closure are described in Chapter 14.

Complications

Air embolism

- This is a potentially lethal complication and may occur in deep penetrating or hilar injuries involving both the bronchial tree and the pulmonary veins.
- Suturing of the entry and exit wounds of a deep tract creates the ideal conditions for air embolism and should never be done. The appropriate procedure is a tractotomy or a resection.
- Air embolism should be suspected when the patient develops arrhythmias or cardiac arrest. Sometimes, air bubbles may be seen in the coronary veins.
- In suspected air embolism the patient is placed in the Trendelenberg position, the apex of the heart is elevated and both ventricles are aspirated.

Right heart failure

- This occurs when a large volume of lung parenchyma is removed acutely. The volume of blood is now distributed over a smaller volume of parenchyma. This complication requires careful fluid status titration and cardiac output support with the use of inotropes.

Tips and pitfalls

- Suturing of the entry and exit wounds of a deep tract creates the ideal conditions for air embolism and should never be done. The appropriate procedure is a tractotomy or a resection.

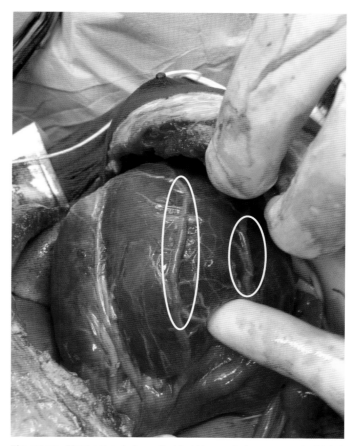

Fig. 17.13. Massive air embolism with air bubbles seen in the coronary veins (circles).

- During lung tractotomy or non-anatomic resection, portions of the residual lung may become ischemic and necrotic. Orient the tractotomy or resection lines parallel to the vessels and check the residual lung for viability.
- During stapled lobectomy or total pneumonectomy, the hilar stump retracts and can make identification of any persistent bleeding difficult. This may be life threatening if the stapler misfires. Never release the stapling device before placement of two stay sutures or Allis forceps on the stump.
- Anatomic lung resections have limited or no role in trauma. Perform non-anatomic, lung-preserving resections.
- During division of the inferior pulmonary ligament, there is a risk of injury to the inferior pulmonary vein. Proceed cautiously and divide only the semi-transparent part of the ligament.
- After major lung resections it is essential to reduce the tidal volume accordingly. Also, restrict fluid administration because many patients develop acute right cardiac failure. This is a common cause of postoperative death.
- After major lung operations, perform a bronchoscopy routinely to aspirate any blood from the remaining and contralateral bronchial tree.
- The main bronchus should be divided as close to the carina as possible to avoid pooling of secretions and reduce the risk of breakdown of the stump.

Chest

Thoracic esophagus

18

Daniel Oh and Jennifer Smith

Surgical anatomy

- The esophagus is approximately 25 cm in length and begins at the level of the C6 vertebra. The external landmark is the cricoid cartilage. It terminates 2–3 cm below the diaphragmatic hiatus, which corresponds to the T11 vertebra.
- The esophagus is divided into three parts: cervical, thoracic, and intra-abdominal. The cervical esophagus begins approximately 15 cm from the upper incisors and is approximately 6–8 cm long. The thoracic esophagus begins approximately 23 cm from the incisors and is approximately 15 cm in length. The intra-abdominal esophagus begins approximately 38 cm from the incisors at the diaphragmatic hiatus and extends for 2–3 cm distally before becoming the gastric cardia.
- The thoracic esophagus rests on the thoracic spine and the longus colli muscles. It passes posterior to the trachea, the tracheal bifurcation, the left main stem bronchus, and the left atrium. It descends to the right of the thoracic aorta and moves anterior to the aorta, just above the diaphragm.
- The azygos vein lies in front of the bodies of the lower thoracic vertebrae and to the right of the esophagus. At the level of the bifurcation of the trachea, it arches anteriorly to drain into the superior vena cava, just before it enters the pericardium.
- The hemiazygos vein passes from the left side of the spine to the right, after crossing the spine and traveling in front of the aorta and behind the esophagus and thoracic duct, to drain into the azygos vein.

- The thoracic duct lies between the esophagus, the aorta and the azygos vein before crossing over, just below the level of the tracheal bifurcation, to the left hemithorax where it drains into the left subclavian vein.
- The esophagus does not have a serosal layer.
- The arterial and venous blood supply and drainage of the esophagus are segmental. The cervical esophagus is supplied by branches of the inferior thyroid artery. The upper thoracic esophagus is supplied by the inferior thyroid artery and an anterior esophagotracheal branch directly from the aorta. The middle and lower esophagus receives its arterial supply directly from the aorta via a bronchoesophageal branch. The lower esophagus and intraabdominal esophagus portions are supplied by small branches from the left gastric artery and the left inferior phrenic artery.
- The parasympathetic innervation of the esophagus is through the vagal nerves. The right and left recurrent laryngeal nerves travel in the tracheoesophageal groove, giving off branches to both the trachea and the cervical and upper esophagus. The vagal nerves join with the fibers of the sympathetic chain to form the esophageal plexus. Together with the esophagus, the vagi pass through the diaphragm and continue along the lesser curvature of the stomach.
- The sympathetic innervation comes from the cervical and thoracic sympathetic chains.

Atlas of Surgical Techniques in Trauma, ed. Demetrios Demetriades, Kenji Inaba, and George Velmahos. Published by Cambridge University Press. © Cambridge University Press 2015.

(a)

(b)

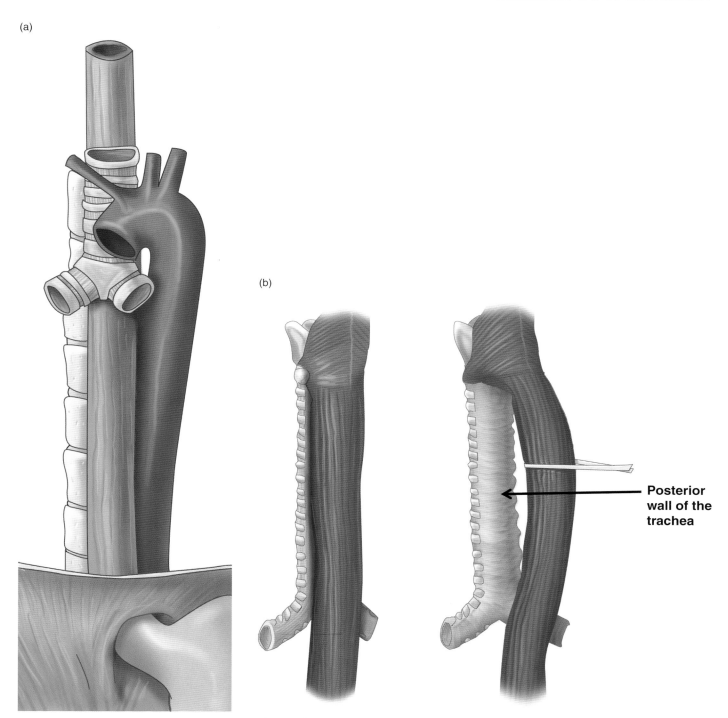

Posterior wall of the trachea

Fig. 18.1(a). Anatomy of the esophagus and its relationship with the spine, trachea, and thoracic aorta.

Fig. 18.1(b). Anatomical relationship between the cervical and upper thoracic esophagus and the larynx and trachea.

General principles

- Most esophageal injuries can be repaired with suturing or a limited resection and primary anastomosis. In rare cases with extensive soft tissue loss or delayed diagnosis it may be necessary to perform resection and reconstruction with gastric pull up or colon interposition. These complex procedures will not be discussed in this chapter.
- Primarily repair the mucosa with absorbable interrupted sutures.
- The primary repair or anastomosis should be tension-free and the edges viable and adequately perfused. Important technical principles for primary repair include the following.
  - Debride all injured, ischemic, and necrotic or infected tissue.
  - Incise the muscular layer longitudinally superiorly and inferiorly to the injury to expose the entire extent of the mucosal injury. Primarily repair the mucosa with absorbable interrupted sutures.
  - Repair the muscularis layer with interrupted non-absorbable sutures.
  - Avoid narrowing the esophageal lumen.
  - Reinforce the primary repair with well-vascularized adjacent tissue flaps.

- Place drains adjacent to the repair.
- Consider placement of a draining gastrostomy tube and a jejunostomy tube for nutritional support.

Special surgical instruments

- General thoracic tray (Allison lung retractor, Bethune rib shears, Duval lung forcep, Davidson scapula retractor, Finochietto retractor)
- 1″ Penrose drain, thoracotomy tubes
- Head light

Anesthesia considerations

- Single lung ventilation is critical for exposure of the thoracic esophagus.

Patient positioning

- Upper and middle thoracic esophageal injuries: left lateral decubitus (right side up)
- Lower thoracic esophageal injuries: right lateral decubitus (left side up)

- Supine for patients undergoing a laparotomy for intra-abdominal esophageal injuries.
- For lateral decubitus positioning, ensure the following:
  - An axillary roll is placed in the axilla.
  - Penis and testes are not compressed.
  - Padding is placed between the knees.

(a)

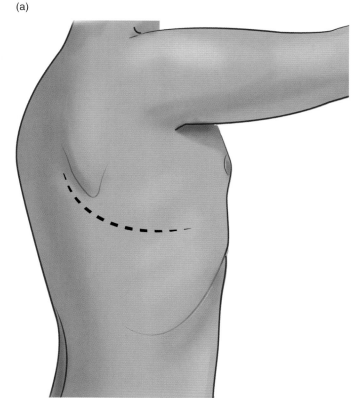

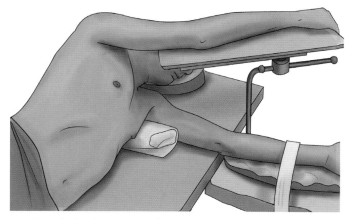

Fig. 18.2. Positioning of patient for a right posterolateral thoracotomy.

Incisions

- Choice of incision depends on the location of the injury.
- Cervical esophagus: standard left neck incision along the sternocleidomastoid muscle (see Chapter 7).
- Upper and middle thoracic esophagus: right posterolateral thoracotomy in the fifth or sixth intercostal space.
- Lower thoracic esophagus: left posterolateral thoracotomy in the seventh or eighth intercostal space.
- Intra-abdominal esophagus: laparotomy.

Standard posterolateral thoracotomy

- Identify the scapula border and mark the skin.
- The skin incision for a posterolateral thoracotomy extends from the anterior axillary line, coursing about 1–2 finger breadths below the tip of the scapula, and extends posteriorly and cephalad midway between the spine and the medial border of the scapula.

Fig. 18.3(a),(b). The skin incision for a posterolateral thoracotomy extends from the anterior axillary line, coursing about one to two finger breadths below the tip of the scapula, and extends posteriorly and cephalad midway between the spine and the medial border of the scapula.

- Divide the subcutaneous tissue. Identify and divide the latissimus dorsi muscle, but can preserve the rhomboid muscle posteriorly. This muscle can be avoided by locating the "empty triangle" between the two muscle groups.
- Use the scapula retractor and palpate the number of rib spaces.
- Divide the intercostal muscle from its insertion site on the superior border of the sixth rib to avoid the neurovascular bundle coursing along the inferior rib border.
- Remove a 2 cm segment of rib using the Bethune rib shears in order to prevent rib fracture during Finochietto retractor placement. If further exposure is needed, a subtotal rib resection may be done.
- Place the Finochietto retractor.

(b)

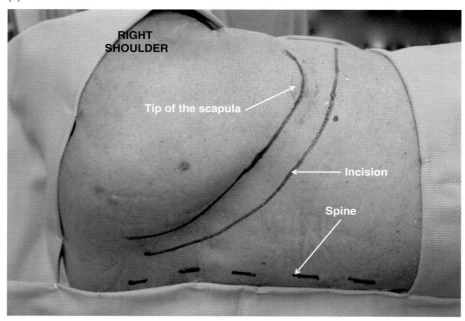

Fig. 18.3(a),(b). (*cont.*)

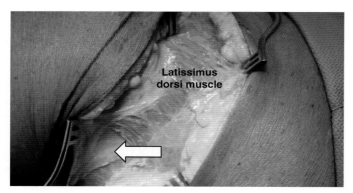

Fig. 18.4. Exposure of the latissimus dorsi muscle. Note the "empty triangle" (arrow), which separates the latissimus from the more posterior rhomboid muscle.

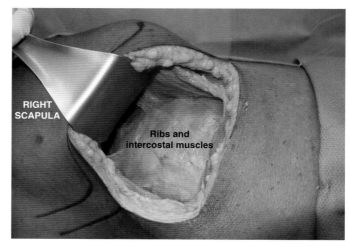

Fig. 18.5. Cephalad retraction of the scapula exposes the underlying ribs and intercostal spaces (the tip of the scapula is usually over the sixth or seventh intercostal space).

(a)

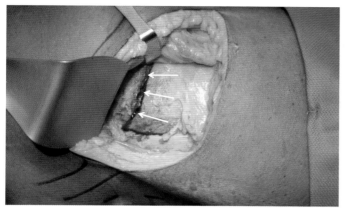

Fig. 18.6(a). Division of the intercostal muscle at its insertion on the superior border of the rib (arrows) to avoid the neurovascular bundle, which is located at the inferior border of the rib.

(c)

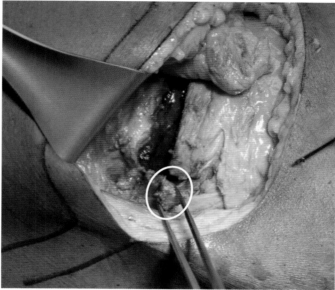

Fig. 18.6(c). Removal of 2 cm segment of the rib (circle) in order to prevent rib fracture during Finochietto retractor placement.

(b)

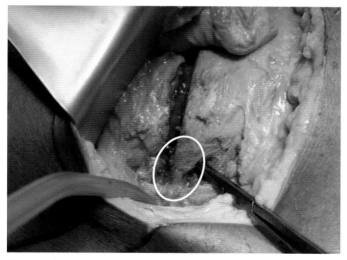

Fig. 18.6(b). Limited mobilization of the sixth rib to prepare for excision (circle).

Exposure of the thoracic esophagus

- The upper and middle thoracic esophagus is exposed through a right posterolateral thoracotomy, as described above.
  - Divide the inferior pulmonary ligament and retract the right lung anteriorly.
  - Visualize the mediastinal pleura and inspect for violation or injury. Evacuate debris and devitalized tissue.
  - The azygos vein will be seen coursing across the esophagus toward the superior vena cava.
  - Open the posterior mediastinal pleura overlying the esophagus, along the length of the azygos vein.
  - If necessary for exposure, ligate and divide the azygos vein as it crosses the esophagus.
  - Mobilize the esophagus and place a Penrose drain around it.

(a)

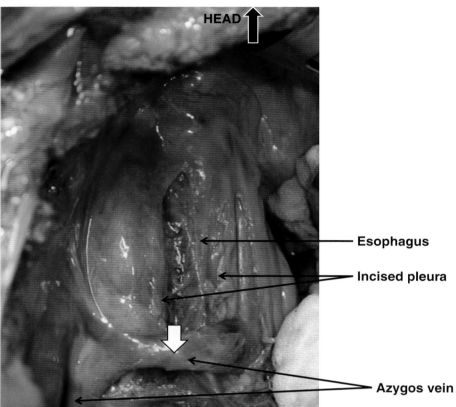

HEAD

Esophagus

Incised pleura

Azygos vein

Fig. 18.7(a). Posterior mediastinum with retraction of the right lung anteriorly. The azygos vein is seen coursing over the esophagus (white arrow), toward the superior vena cava (SVC). The posterior mediastinal pleura overlying the esophagus is incised.

(b)

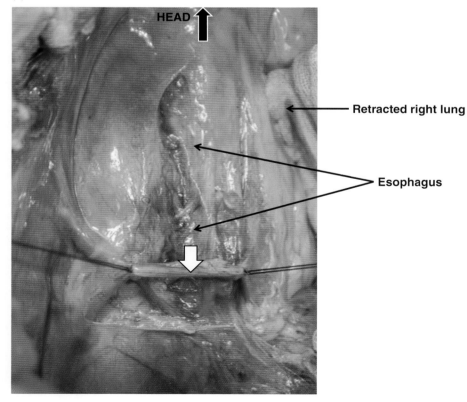

HEAD

Retracted right lung

Esophagus

Fig. 18.7(b). Ligation and division of the azygos vein (white arrow), improves the exposure of the underlying esophagus.

(c)

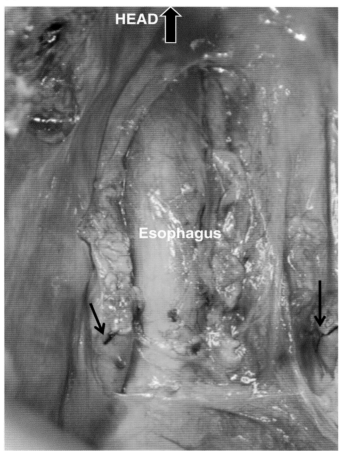

Fig. 18.7(c). Exposure of the esophagus after division of the azygos vein (arrows show the divided ends of the azygos).

- The lower third of the esophagus is exposed through a left posterolateral thoracotomy, as described above.
  - o Divide the inferior pulmonary ligament and retract the left lung anteriorly.
  - o The esophagus is located to the right of the thoracic aorta and can easily be palpated after placement of a nasogastric tube.
  - o Incise the pleura over the esophagus, mobilize, and place a Penrose drain around it.

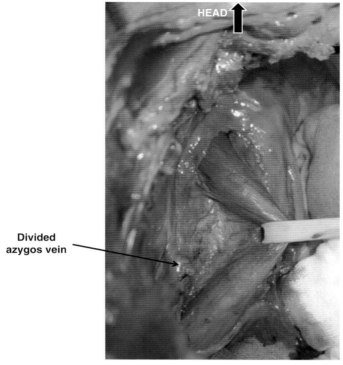

Fig. 18.8. A Penrose drain is placed around the esophagus for retraction.

Repair of the esophagus

- Identify the injury and mobilize the esophagus above and below. Take care not to devitalize the esophagus during mobilization. Open the muscle fibers longitudinally to fully expose the extent of the mucosal injury.
- Repair the mucosa with interrupted absorbable sutures.
- Repair the muscle layer with interrupted non-absorbable sutures.
- Create a flap from the parietal pleura on the chest wall and secure it over the esophageal repair.
- Additionally or in lieu of the pleura, an intercostal muscle flap with its neurovascular bundle may be mobilized from an adjacent interspace and brought over the esophageal repair for additional coverage. Alternatively, a pericardial fat-pad flap can be used.
- The wound is copiously irrigated and drained using standard chest tubes.
- If not placed previously, a nasogastric tube is guided past the site of repair and into the stomach, taking care to avoid damaging the repair site.
- A jejunostomy feeding tube can be inserted through a mini-laparotomy at the time of the esophageal repair.

(a)

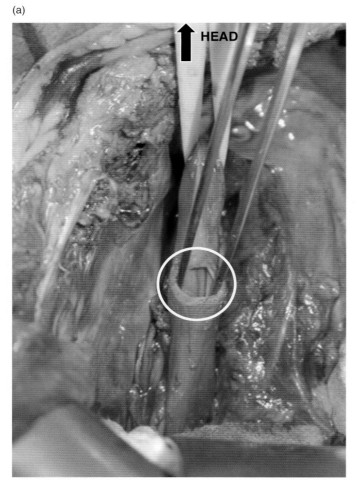

Fig. 18.9(a). Identification of the esophageal perforation (circle).

(b)

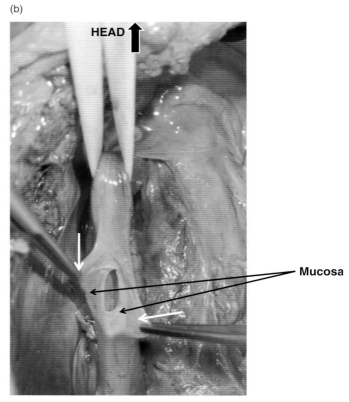

Fig. 18.9(b). The esophageal muscle fibers (white arrows) are opened longitudinally to fully expose the extent of the mucosal injury (black arrows).

(a)

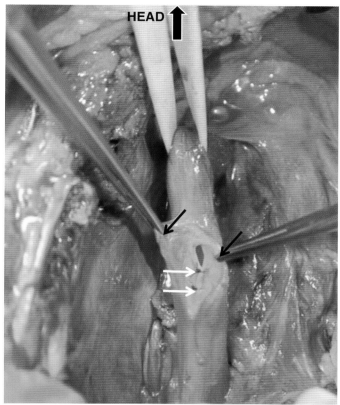

Fig. 18.10(a). The mucosa is repaired with an interrupted absorbable suture (white arrows). Muscularis layers are retracted by forceps (black arrows).

(b)

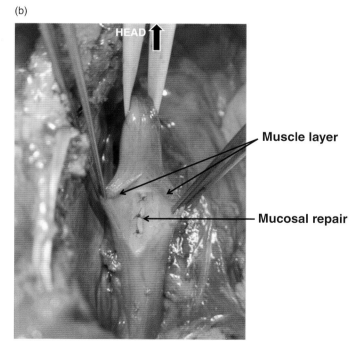

Muscle layer

Mucosal repair

Fig. 18.10(b). Completed mucosal repair.

(c)

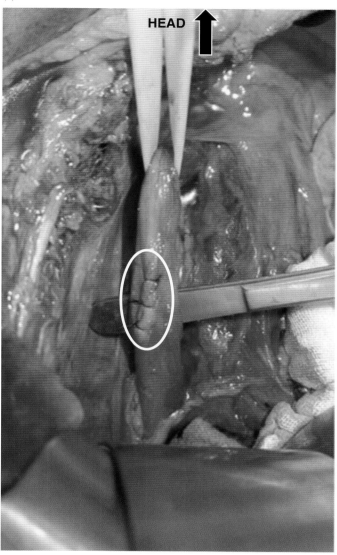

Fig. 18.10(c). The muscle layer is repaired with an interrupted non-absorbable suture (circle).

(a)

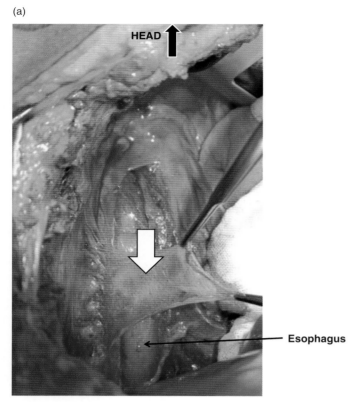

Fig. 18.11(a). A flap (white arrow) from the parietal pleura is created and brought over the esophageal repair.

(b)

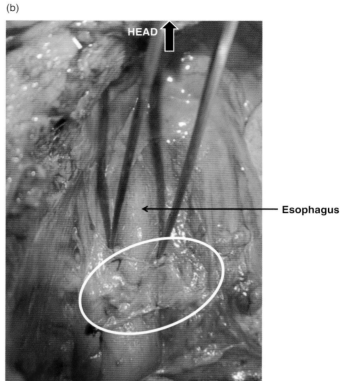

Fig. 18.11(b). The pleural flap is sutured over the esophageal repair (circle).

(a)

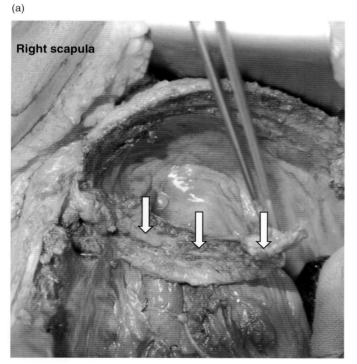

Fig. 18.12(a). Creation of an intercostal muscle flap (white arrows) with its neurovascular bundle from an adjacent intercostal space.

(b)

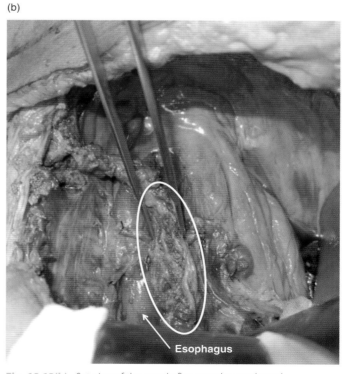

Fig. 18.12(b). Suturing of the muscle flap over the esophageal repair (circle).

Exposure and repair of the intra-abdominal esophagus

- A laparotomy is the approach used to repair an injury to the intra-abdominal esophagus.
- The left triangular ligament is divided and the liver is retracted. This exposes the esophageal hiatus.
- The short gastric vessels can be divided to aid with mobilization of the gastroesophageal junction for improved exposure of the injury.
- Following primary repair, the hiatus is closed with interrupted non-absorbable sutures to recreate an opening that only accommodates the esophagus and one fingertip.
- A feeding jejunostomy tube is placed for postoperative alimentation.
- For destructive injuries, a circular stapled anastomosis placed through a gastrotomy is an acceptable alternative.

Tissue reinforcement options

- Pleural flap, intercostal muscle flap, pericardial fat-pad flap.

Tips and pitfalls

- Delayed recognition and repair of the esophagus is associated with a high incidence of infectious complications and death.
- Cervical esophageal leaks usually cause an abscess or an esophageal fistula and are rarely life threatening. However, thoracic esophageal leaks can cause severe mediastinitis and are often life threatening.
- Any repair or anastomosis should be tension free and well perfused.
- Routine wide drainage of all esophageal repairs is critical.
- Use tissue flaps to reinforce the esophageal repair. This is particularly important in the presence of associated tracheal injuries due to the risk of tracheoesophageal fistula or vascular injuries due to the risk of arterioesophageal fistula.

19

Diaphragm injury

Lydia Lam and Matthew D. Tadlock

Surgical anatomy

- The diaphragm consists of a peripheral muscular segment and a central aponeurotic segment. It is attached to the lower sternum, the lower six ribs, and the lumbar spine. During expiration, it reaches the level of the nipples. The central tendon of the diaphragm is fused to the base of the pericardium.
- It has three major openings, which include the aortic foramen which allows passage of the aorta, the azygos vein, and the thoracic duct, the esophageal foramen for the esophagus and the vagus nerves and finally the vena cava foramen, which contains the inferior vena cava.
- The arterial supply stems from the phrenic arteries that are direct branches off the aorta as it exits the hiatus, while the venous drainage is directly into the inferior vena cava.
- The diaphragm is innervated by the phrenic nerve, which originates from the C3–C5 nerve roots, courses over the anterior scalene muscle, continues into the mediastinum along the pericardium, and terminates in the diaphragm.

General principles

- The diagnosis of an isolated, uncomplicated diaphragmatic injury can be challenging because such injuries are often asymptomatic and the radiological findings may be subtle. Untreated diaphragmatic injuries will result in a diaphragmatic hernia, which can manifest long after the injury. This complication usually occurs on the left diaphragm, although both sides are at risk.
- Any asymptomatic penetrating injury to the left thoracoabdominal area, between the nipple superiorly and the costal margin inferiorly, should be evaluated laparoscopically to rule out diaphragmatic injury.
- Repair of isolated diaphragmatic injuries can be performed laparoscopically or through a laparotomy.

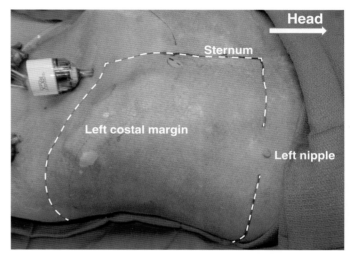

Fig. 19.1. Any asymptomatic penetrating injury in the left thoracoabdominal area, between the nipple superiorly and the costal margin inferiorly, should be evaluated laparoscopically to rule out diaphragmatic injury.

Special instruments

- Equipment for the open operation would include a major laparotomy tray. A Bookwalter retractor improves the exposure of posterior diaphragmatic injuries.

Laparoscopic repair

Positioning

- The patient should be placed in the supine position.
- Once the laparoscope is inserted, the patient should be placed in reverse Trendelenberg and right decubitus to improve visualization of the left diaphragm.

Incisions

- Trocar placement should adhere to general laparoscopy principles of triangulation to allow access to likely areas of injury on the diaphragm. To begin, a standard supra-umbilical trochar can be used to insert a camera for

---

Atlas of Surgical Techniques in Trauma, ed. Demetrios Demetriades, Kenji Inaba, and George Velmahos. Published by Cambridge University Press. © Cambridge University Press 2015.

diagnostic confirmation of the injury. Once the injury is localized, additional ports can be inserted to maximize access to the injury.

(a)

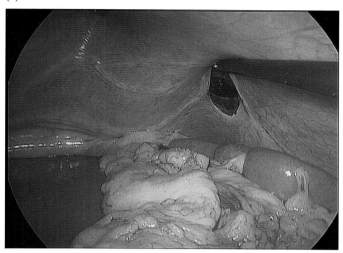

(b)

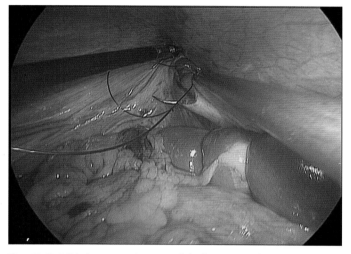

Fig. 19.4(a),(b). Laparoscopic repair of diaphragm with figure-of-eight with non-absorbable suture. It is important to grasp the diaphragm and pull toward the camera for a good suture bite.

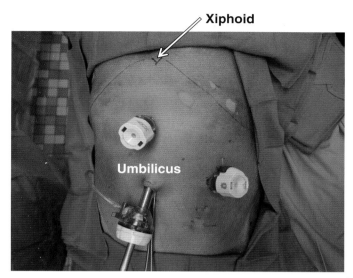

Fig. 19.2. Trocar placement for diagnostic laparoscopy for diaphragm evaluation.

(a)

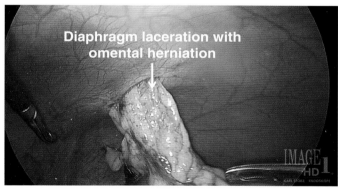

(b)

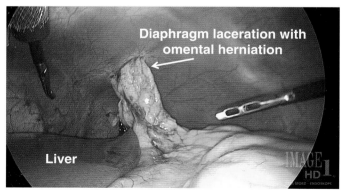

Fig. 19.3(a),(b). Diagnostic laparoscopy view of diaphragm injury with omental herniation.

Repair

- Lacerations should be repaired with interrupted non-absorbable sutures. Alternatively, laparoscopic hernia staples may be used.

Open repair

Positioning

- Patient should be placed in the supine position with both arms abducted.
- A standard trauma preparation from the chin to the knees is used as access to the chest may be necessary.

Incision

- A standard midline laparotomy incision should be used for repair of the diaphragm to enable a complete investigation of the remaining abdomen. For chronic injuries, a thoracic approach may be considered.

Exposure

- Superior cephalad retraction of the costal margins is key to adequate exposure of the diaphragm. The use of a fixed retractor such as the Bookwalter retractor is strongly recommended.
- The diaphragmatic wound edges are grasped with Allis clamps and pulled anteriorly, to improve exposure and repair. Clamps can be placed at the apices to line up the edges of the laceration and facilitate suturing. This is particularly important for posterior injuries, which are difficult to access.
- If there is a diaphragmatic hernia, reduce the contents with gentle traction. If necessary, enlarge the diaphragmatic defect to reduce incarcerated contents. Inspect contents for any ischemic necrosis.

Repair

The diaphragmatic defect can be repaired with interrupted figure-of-eight sutures, using number 0 or 1 monofilament, non-absorbable sutures. Alternatively, for larger injuries, a running suture can be used.

- High-energy deceleration injuries can result in avulsion of the diaphragm from its chest wall attachments. In these instances, the diaphragm will need to be secured to the chest wall. It may be necessary to perform an ipsilateral thoracotomy to allow horizontal mattress sutures to be placed around the ribs to secure the diaphragm in its typical position. The use of synthetic meshes typically is not necessary in the acute setting, as tissue loss and domain loss have not had time to occur.
- Prior to definitive closure, perform transdiaphragmatic irrigation of the pleural cavity to minimize contamination, especially in the presence of concomitant hollow viscus injuries.
- A tube thoracotomy should always be placed after the diaphragm repair.

Tips and pitfalls

- In the presence of a diaphragmatic defect, there is a risk of tension pneumothorax during abdominal insufflation for laparoscopy. Monitor closely the hemodynamic and oxygenation status and peak inspiratory pressures. If any sign of tension pneumothorax develops, release abdominal insufflation and insert a chest drain.
- In some cases laparoscopic repair may be difficult because of the loss of pressure through the diaphragmatic defect and into the chest drain. Grasping the edge of the wound with a forceps and partially twisting it can occlude the defect and allow repair.

(a)

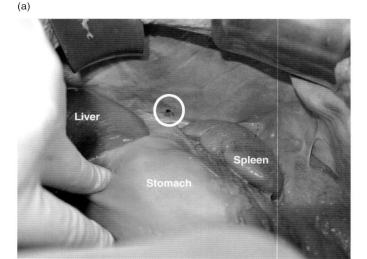

(b)

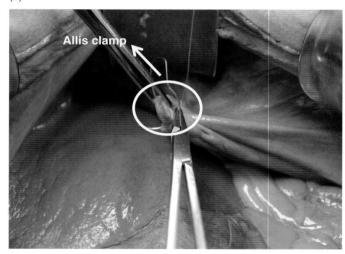

Fig. 19.5(a),(b). Posterior diaphragm laceration (circle) at laparotomy. Repair may be difficult because of the deep location and poor exposure of the wound (a). The exposure can improve significantly by grasping the diaphragm injury with a forceps and pulling it toward the umbilicus (arrow) (b).

- Repair of posterior diaphragmatic wounds during laparotomy is difficult due to poor exposure. Improve exposure by grasping the edges of the wound and pulling the diaphragm towards the laparotomy incision.
- In the presence of peritoneal intestinal content contamination there is an increased risk of empyema. Wash out the pleural cavity through the diaphragmatic defect and remove any gross contamination.
- Although rare, during repair of the diaphragm below the pericardium, place the sutures under direct visualization to avoid inadvertent injury to the myocardium.
- After diaphragmatic repair, always place a thoracotomy tube for postoperative drainage.

Chapter

20

General principles of abdominal operations for trauma

Heidi L. Frankel and Lisa L. Schlitzkus

Surgical anatomy

- The anterior abdominal wall has four muscles: the external oblique, the internal oblique, the transversalis, and the rectus muscles. The aponeuroses of the first three muscles form the rectus sheath, which encloses the rectus abdominis muscle.
- The linea alba is a midline aponeurosis which runs from the xiphoid process to the pubic symphysis and separates the left and right rectus abdominis muscles. It is widest just above the umbilicus, facilitating entry into the peritoneal cavity.
- For vascular trauma purposes, the retroperitoneum is conventionally divided into four anatomic areas:

  o *Zone I.* Extends from the aortic hiatus to the sacral promontory. This zone is subdivided into the supramesocolic and inframesocolic areas. The supramesocolic area contains the suprarenal aorta and its major branches (celiac axis, superior mesenteric artery (SMA), and renal arteries), the supramesocolic inferior vena cava (IVC) with its major branches, and the superior mesenteric vein (SMV). The inframesocolic area contains the infrarenal aorta and IVC.

  o *Zone II.* Includes the kidneys, paracolic gutters, and renal vessels.

  o *Zone III.* Includes the pelvic retroperitoneum and contains the iliac vessels.

  o *Zone IV.* Includes the perihepatic area, with the hepatic artery, the portal vein, the retrohepatic IVC, and hepatic veins.

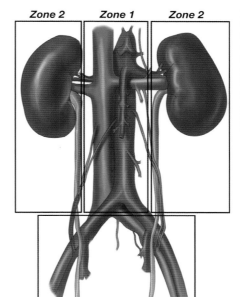

Fig. 20.1. Retroperitoneal vascular zones: *Zone I* includes the midline vessels from the aortic hiatus to the sacral promontory; *Zone II* includes the kidneys with the renal vessels; and *Zone III* includes the pelvic retroperitoneum, with the iliac vessels.

General technical principles

- A laparotomy for bleeding is different from a laparotomy for peritonitis.
- The top priority of the surgeon is to stop the bleeding! This should be followed by a methodical exploration of all structures to identify and repair other non-life-threatening injuries.
- Consider damage control early before major physiological deterioration (coagulopathy, hypothermia, acidosis) occurs. In determining the need for damage control, take into account the nature of the injury, associated injuries, the physiological condition of the patient, the hospital capabilities, and the skillset of the surgeon.
- Removal versus repair for organs such as the spleen and kidney should be determined by the injury severity and

Atlas of Surgical Techniques in Trauma, ed. Demetrios Demetriades, Kenji Inaba, and George Velmahos. Published by Cambridge University Press. © Cambridge University Press 2015.

physiologic condition of the patient. Splenectomy or nephrectomy should be considered even in moderate severity injuries if the patient is unstable.

- If damage control packing does not stop the bleeding, do not terminate the operation. Re-explore and look for surgical bleeding.

- In damage control procedures the abdomen should always be left open using temporary closure techniques in order to prevent intra-abdominal hypertension or abdominal compartment syndrome.

Positioning of patient and skin preparation

- The patient should be placed in the supine position with the arms abducted to 90 degrees.

- If there is concern for rectal or anal canal injury, the patient may be placed in lithotomy.

- The bed rails should be free and exposed for fixed surgical retractor placement.

- The patient should undergo a standard trauma preparation from chin to knees and laterally to the bed. Inclusion of the groins in the field is important because of the possibility of the need of saphenous vein graft.

(a)

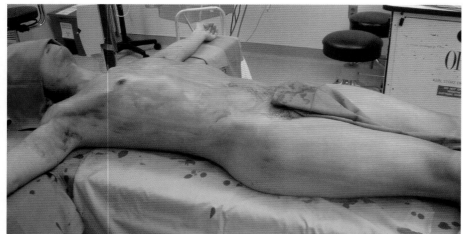

Fig. 20.2(a),(b). Position and skin preparation for trauma laparotomy. The patient should be prepped from chin to knees and laterally to the bed (posterior axillary lines).

(b)

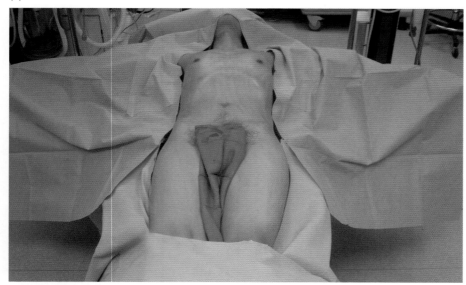

Special instruments

- A trauma laparotomy set should include basic vascular instruments.
- A Bookwalter retractor or other fixed surgical retractor will facilitate surgical exposure, especially in anatomically difficult areas.

(a)

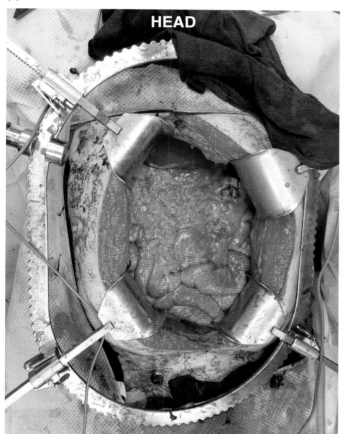

(b)

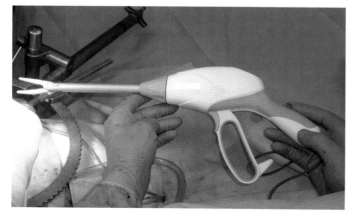

Fig. 20.3(a). Bookwalter retractor in place. (b) Electrothermal bipolar vessel sealing system device (LigaSure device).

- Head lights are strongly recommended.
- An electrothermal bipolar vessel sealing system device (LigaSure device) may be useful. It expedites division of the mesentery in cases requiring bowel resection. It is also a useful instrument for liver resections and splenectomy.

Incisions

- A full midline laparotomy is the standard incision in trauma. The extent of the incision is determined by the location of any penetrating injury and the condition of the patient. The incision should be long enough to provide comfortable exposure and allow a complete exploration of the abdomen. A xiphoid to pubic symphysis incision should be considered in hemodynamically unstable patients with penetrating trauma and unknown missile trajectories. The concept of routine xiphoid to pubic symphysis incision in all trauma laparotomies is not advisable.
- In a hypotensive patient, the abdomen should be entered quickly, without wasting time for local hemostasis. The skin, subcutaneous tissue, and the linea alba are incised sharply. The best place to incise the linea alba is 2–3 cm above the umbilicus, where the aponeurosis is at its widest part and where there is a reduced risk of entering the rectus sheath. The preperitoneal fat is then swept away, and the peritoneum is identified and entered. A finger can be used to enter the peritoneal cavity just superior to the umbilicus at the thinnest point.

(a)

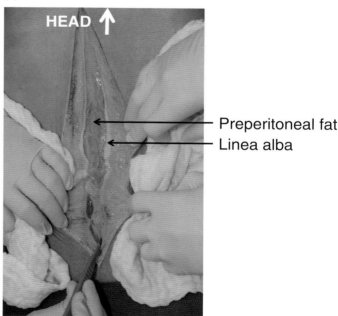

Fig. 20.4(a),(b). The skin, subcutaneous tissue, and the linea alba are incised. The preperitoneal fat is then swept away and the peritoneum is identified and entered.

(b)

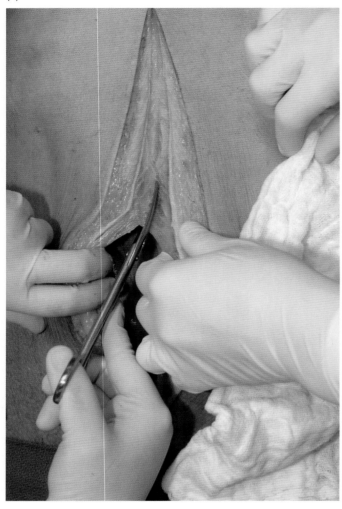

Fig. 20.4(a),(b). *(cont.)*

- In some cases with complex posterior liver or retrohepatic major venous injuries, the exposure can be improved by adding a right subcostal incision to the standard midline laparotomy. The standard subcostal incision is made one to two finger breadths below the costal margin. Avoid an acute angle between the two incisions to prevent ischemic necrosis of the skin. The rectus abdominis, external oblique, internal oblique, and transversalis muscles are divided.

(a)

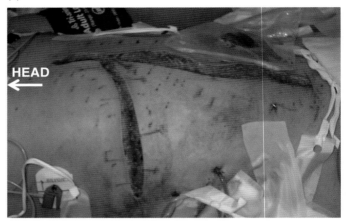

(b)

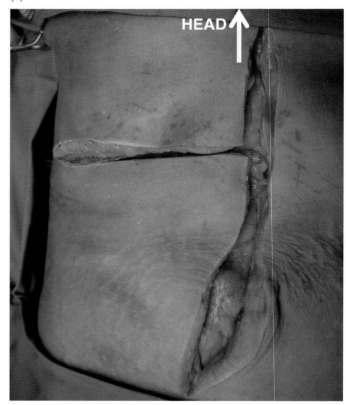

Fig. 20.5(a),(b). Addition of a right subcostal incision to the standard midline laparotomy, for improved exposure of the liver. The subcostal incision is made one to two finger breadths below the costal margin. Avoid an acute angle between the two incisions to prevent ischemic necrosis of the skin.

- Extension of the midline laparotomy into a median sternotomy can be useful in cases with severe liver injuries requiring atriocaval shunting or total liver vascular isolation. The technique of median sternotomy is described in Chapter 14.

(a)

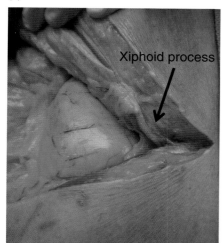

Xiphoid process

Fig. 20.6(a) Cranial extension of the midline to either side of the xiphoid can provide several more centimeters of exposure.

(b)

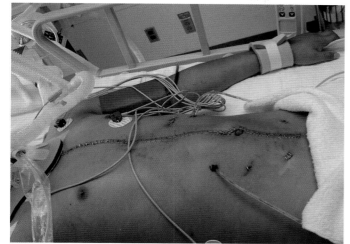

Fig. 20.6(b). Extension of the midline laparotomy into a median sternotomy in cases with associated intrathoracic injuries or severe liver injuries requiring atriocaval shunt or total liver vascular isolation.

Abdominal exploration

- Upon entering the abdomen, the top priority is the temporary control of all significant bleeding. This can be achieved by a combination of packing and direct compression.
- Blind four-quadrant packing is not as effective as directed packing! There is no point in packing all quadrants in a patient with an isolated stab wound to the left upper quadrant.

- In severe bleeding, which is not compressible, consider temporary aortic compression below the diaphragm. Clamping of the infradiaphragmatic aorta can be facilitated by dividing the left crux of the diaphragm at 2 o'clock. At this site there are no vessels. However, if there is a supramesocolic hematoma or bleeding, infradiaphragmatic aortic clamping may not be possible. In these cases a left thoracotomy with supradiaphragmatic cross-clamping of the aorta may be needed. Another alternative is placement of an endovascular aortic occlusion balloon, insufflated above the diaphragm.
- The exposure and exploration are facilitated by complete evisceration of the small bowel. Keep the eviscerated bowel covered with warm and moist towels.
- All hematomas due to penetrating trauma should be explored! The only exception is a stable retrohepatic hematoma, because it is a difficult and potentially dangerous maneuver.
- Stable hematomas due to blunt trauma should not be explored. However, exploration should be considered for all paraduodenal hematomas and for large, expanding, or leaking hematomas.
- After bleeding control, the abdominal cavity should be explored systematically to identify and treat other injuries.
  - The intestine should be examined from the ligament of Treitz to the rectum. Grasp the transverse colon with two hands and retract towards the patient's chest. The ligament of Treitz is at the center and base of the transverse mesocolon. Ensure that both sides of the small bowel and mesenteric border are carefully examined so as to not miss an injury. This is

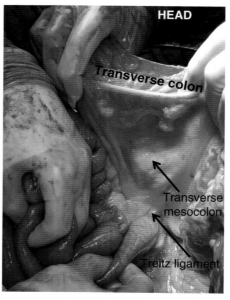

HEAD

Transverse colon

Transverse mesocolon

Treitz ligament

Fig. 20.7. Identification of the beginning of the small bowel at the Treitz ligament. Grasp the transverse colon with two hands and retract towards the patient's chest. The Treitz ligament is at the middle and base of the transverse mesocolon.

particularly germane to penetrating injuries, especially shotgun wounds.

o Evisceration of the small bowel to the left or right allows careful evaluation of the right and left colon. Hematomas in the fat surrounding the

colon wall should be explored to exclude an underlying injury.

o The anterior wall of the stomach and the proximal duodenum can be exposed and inspected by retracting the transverse colon toward the patient's pelvis.

(a)

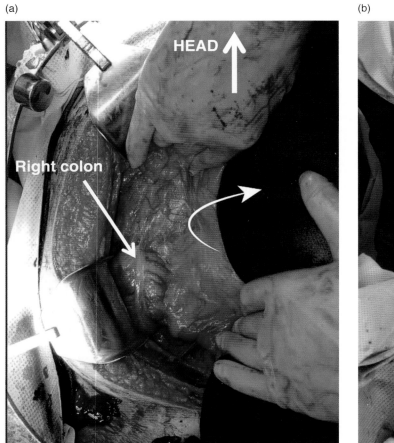

(b)

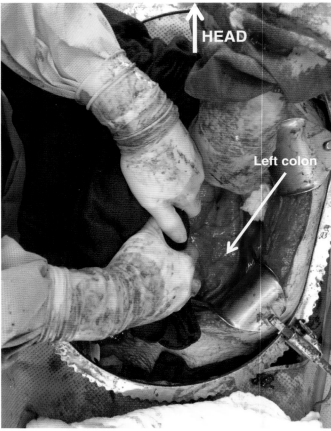

Fig. 20.8(a),(b). Evisceration of the small bowel to the left allows good exposure and visualization of the right colon (a). Evisceration to the right allows exposure of the left colon (b). Note the small bowel retracted under the dark blue towel.

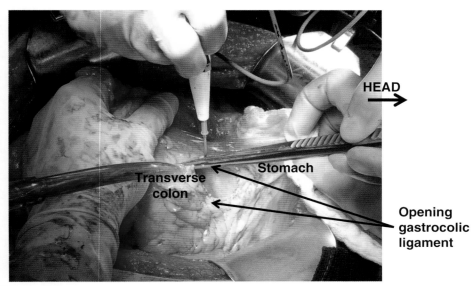

Fig. 20.9. Opening of the lesser sac. The stomach is retracted anteriorly and toward the head and the transverse colon towards the pelvis. The tense gastrocolic ligament is opened at its thinnest part and the sac is entered.

- The posterior wall of the stomach and the pancreas can be inspected by dividing the gastrocolic ligament and entering the lesser sac.
- The liver and spleen should be palpated and visually inspected for injuries. The inspection may be improved by placing laparotomy pads behind the liver or spleen.
- All hollow viscus subserosal hematomas should be unroofed and examined for underlying perforations.
- The diaphragm should always be palpated and inspected for injuries.
- Both kidneys should be palpated for their presence and normal size. This step is important if a nephrectomy is considered. If the patient can tolerate it, preserve kidney mass whenever possible.

Intestinal anastomosis

- In trauma, the outcomes are similar for hand-sewn versus stapled anastomoses or one-layer versus two-layer anastomosis, and continuous versus interrupted sutures. In pediatric cases a one-layer anastomosis is recommended to avoid anastomotic stenosis.

Abdominal closure

- Closed drains are recommended in selected cases, such as complex liver or pancreatic injuries. There is no role for routine drainage.
- Fascial closure should be attempted whenever possible. However, for patients at risk of abdominal compartment syndrome or intra-abdominal hypertension, temporary closure is acceptable. In all patients, close postoperative monitoring of intra-abdominal pressures is warranted (see Chapter 21).
- The skin should be left open in cases where there was intra-operative contamination.

Tips and pitfalls

- Ongoing communication with the anesthesia team is critical during the operation.
- In penetrating abdominal injuries with hemodynamic instability, avoid venous access in the lower extremities, because of the possibility of iliac vein or inferior vena cava injuries.
- The surgeon should consider using a head light, especially for injuries located in difficult anatomical areas.
- Open the linea alba 2–3 cm above the umbilicus, where the aponeurosis is widest to reduce the risk of entering the rectus sheath.
- All hematomas due to penetrating trauma, irrespective of size, should be explored. The only exception is a stable retrohepatic hematoma.
- In multiple small bowel perforations, identify all perforations before starting repairs. Resecting one segment with a single anastomosis may be safer than multiple intestinal repairs in close proximity.
- In complex abdominal trauma where the abdominal wall is closed at the index operation, monitor bladder pressures postoperatively for the development of intra-abdominal hypertension.

21

Damage control surgery

Mark Kaplan and Demetrios Demetriades

General principles of damage control surgery

- Damage control (DC) surgery initially referred to surgical techniques used in the operating room. This concept has now been expanded to include damage control resuscitation, which includes permissive hypotension, early empiric blood component therapy, and the prevention and treatment of hypothermia and acidosis.
- DC techniques can be applied to most anatomical areas and structures, including the neck, chest, abdomen, vessels, and fractures.
- DC surgery is an abbreviated procedure with the goal of rapidly controlling bleeding and contamination so that the initial procedure can be terminated, decreasing surgical stress and allowing a focus on resuscitation. This should be considered in patients with progressive physiologic exhaustion who are at risk of irreversible shock and death. After physiologic resuscitation, the patient is returned to the operating room for definitive reconstruction and eventual definitive closure of the involved cavity.
- The standard indications for DC include:
    o Patients "in extremis," with coagulopathy, hypothermia < 35 °C, acidosis (base deficit >15 mmol/L)
    o Bleeding from difficult to control injuries (complex liver injuries, retroperitoneum, mediastinum, neck, and complex vascular)
    o In suboptimal environments, such as the rural or battlefield setting or with inexperienced surgeons without the adequate skillset to definitively manage the injury.
- For maximum benefit, damage control should be considered early, before the patient reaches the in extremis condition! Take into account the nature of the injury, the physiologic condition of the patient, comorbid conditions, the available resources, and the experience of the surgeon. The timing of damage control is critical in determining the outcome.

Damage control in vascular trauma

- The standard technical principles used in elective vascular surgery may not be applicable in trauma, because of the poor physiological condition of the injured patient.
- The surgeon has many damage control technical options, including temporary intraluminal shunting, ligation, balloon catheter occlusion, and extremity amputation. Complex repairs, such as end-to-end anastomosis or graft interposition can be undertaken at a later stage, after resuscitation and correction of coagulopathy, hypothermia, and acidosis.
- Details of vascular damage control techniques are described in other chapters.

Damage control in the chest

- Non-anatomical lung-sparing resections, hilar clamping, hilar twisting, gauze packing of the posterior mediastinum, and temporary chest wall closure are all part of damage control in thoracic trauma.
- Temporary sternotomy or thoracotomy incision closure may be necessary in selected cases requiring packing for persistent bleeding or in patients at high risk for postoperative cardiac arrest during the ICU phase of resuscitation. In these cases immediate access to the heart for cardiac massage may be life-saving.
- Details of damage control operative techniques in the lung are described in Chapter 17.

Damage control in the extremities

- DC techniques include external fixation, vascular shunting, or gauze packing.

Damage control in the abdomen

- In abdominal damage control, the goal of the initial exploration is temporary control of bleeding and spillage from the intestine. The definitive reconstruction is

Atlas of Surgical Techniques in Trauma, ed. Demetrios Demetriades, Kenji Inaba, and George Velmahos. Published by Cambridge University Press. © Cambridge University Press 2015.

performed semi-electively, at a later stage, after physiological stabilization.

- Temporary closure can be obtained by use of a vacuum-assisted closure system.

Temporary control of abdominal bleeding

- Temporary bleeding control can be achieved by tight gauze packing of the source of the bleeding (liver, retroperitoneum, and pelvis), application of local hemostatic agents, balloon tamponade in some cases (i.e., bleeding from a deep penetrating tract in the liver or the retroperitoneum), ligation instead of repair of major

venous injuries, temporary shunting of injured arteries, or any combination of the above (see Chapter 24).

- The technique of liver gauze packing (also see Chapter 24), following ligation of major sites of bleeding and non-anatomical resection of non-viable liver, for damage control with tight packing tamponade should be considered if there is persistent bleeding. The liver is wrapped with absorbable mesh and gauze packing is applied around it. The mesh stays permanently in the abdomen and facilitates the removal of the gauze at the second-look laparotomy, without causing bleeding.
- Local hemostatic agents are usually effective in controlling minor bleeding, but they rarely work in major hemorrhage.

(a) (b) (c) (d)

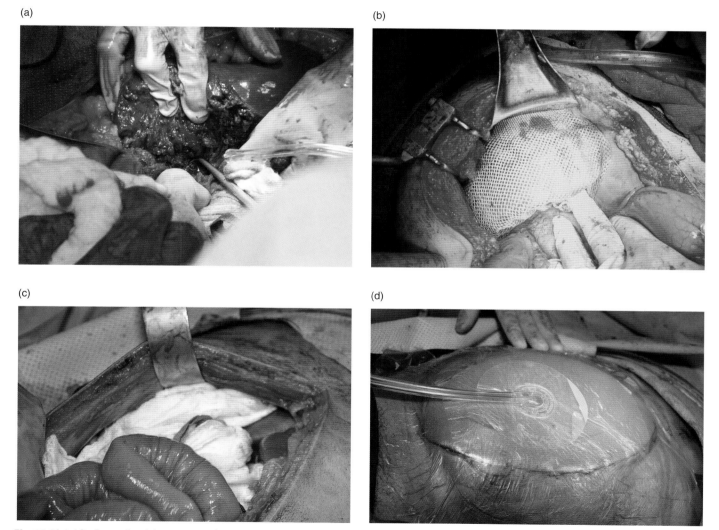

Fig. 21.1(a)–(d). Severe liver injury requiring damage control with packing (a). After ligation of major bleeders and non-anatomical debridement, the liver is tightly wrapped with absorbable mesh (b). Tight gauze packing is applied over the mesh (c). Temporary abdominal wall closure with ABThera negative pressure system.

Control of intestinal spillage

- Ligation or stapling of the injured bowel, without reanastomosis, has been recommended for temporary control of intestinal content spillage. Definitive reconstruction is performed at a later stage, usually about 24–36 hours after the initial operation. Some surgeons do not support this approach because of the concern for creating a closed loop intestinal obstruction, which may promote bacterial and toxin translocation and aggravate bowel ischemia, especially in patients requiring vasopressors. These authors support reconstruction of the bowel or ostomy diversion during the damage control operation whenever possible.

Temporary abdominal wall closure

- Following damage control procedures, the abdominal fascia or skin should never be closed because of the high risk of intra-abdominal hypertension (IAH) or abdominal compartment syndrome (ACS). Temporary abdominal closure (TAC) should always be performed.
- The technique used for temporary abdominal wall closure can influence outcomes, including survival, complications, and success rate as well as time to definitive fascia closure.
- The ideal method of temporary abdominal closure should prevent evisceration, actively remove any infected or toxin-loaded fluid from the peritoneal cavity, minimize the formation of enteroatmospheric fistulas, preserve the facial integrity, minimize abdominal wall retraction, facilitate reoperation, and help achieve early definitive closure.
- Numerous materials and techniques have been used for temporary closure over the last decade. They include the "Bogota bag," the Wittmann patch, absorbable synthetic meshes, and various negative pressure therapy (NPT) techniques. The NPT techniques have the advantage of active removal of contaminated or toxin-rich peritoneal fluid.

1. The "Bogota Bag" can easily be constructed with a 3-liter sterile irrigation bag or a sterile X-ray cassette cover, stapled or sutured to the fascia or to the skin. It prevents evisceration of the abdominal contents while preventing or treating IAH or ACS. It might have limited use in cases with damage control for intra-abdominal bleeding, where definitive abdominal closure is anticipated within the next 24–48 hours. Its major disadvantage is that it does not allow the effective removal of any contaminated or toxin and cytokine-rich intraperitoneal fluid, and it does not prevent the loss of abdominal wall domain.

2. Negative-pressure therapy (NPT) techniques have revolutionized the management of the open abdomen and have improved survival, morbidity and the success rate of primary fascia closure. The three most commonly used NPT techniques are the Barker's vacuum pack technique,

(a)

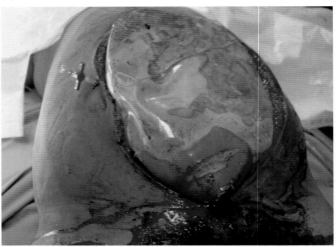

(b)

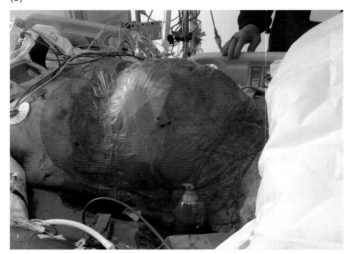

Fig. 21.2(a),(b). Temporary abdominal closure with plastic sheet (Bogota bag). This approach does not allow the effective removal of peritoneal fluid and does not preserve the abdominal domain.

the vacuum-assisted closure (VAC, KCI, San Antonio, Texas), and the ABThera (KCI, San Antonio, Texas).

(a) Barker's vacuum pack technique consists of a fenestrated, non-adherent polyethylene sheet, which is placed over the bowel and under the peritoneum, covered by moist surgical towels or gauze, two large silicone drains placed over the towels, and a transparent adhesive drape over the wound to maintain a closed seal. The drains are connected to continuous wall suction at 100–150 mmHg. The dressing system is changed every 24–48 hours and every time the fascia at the top and bottom of the wound is approximated, if it can be done without tension. Some surgeons use this technique for the first 24–48 hours postoperatively, switching to the VAC therapy afterwards.

(a)

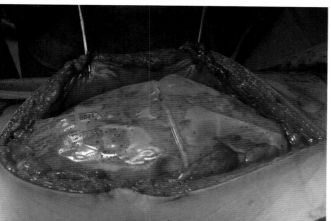

(b)

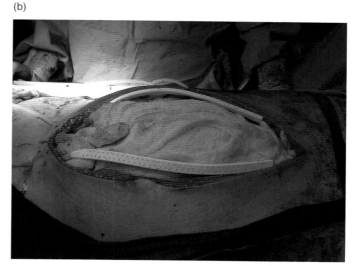

(c)

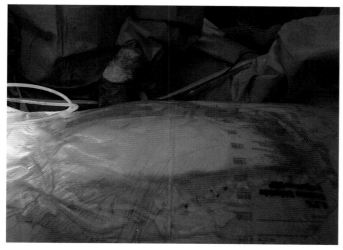

Fig. 21.3(a)–(c). Barker's vacuum pack technique: fenestrated, non-adherent polyethylene sheet is placed over the bowel and under the peritoneum (a), and covered by moist surgical towels or gauze. Two silicone drains are placed over the gauze (b), and a transparent adhesive drape is placed over the wound to maintain a closed seal. The drains are connected to continuous wall suction.

(b) The V.A.C.® Abdominal Dressing System (KCI) is a negative pressure dressing system, which includes polyurethane foam, covered with a protective, fenestrated, non-adherent layer, tubing, a collection canister, and a computerized pump. The system pulls the fascia edges together and prevents adhesions between the bowel and anterior abdominal wall, making subsequent re-exploration of the abdomen and fascia closure easier and safer. In addition, it actively removes any contaminated or inflammatory fluid from the peritoneal cavity.

(c) The ABThera (KCI) is a new NPT device. It consists of a visceral protective layer (VPL), made of a polyurethane foam with six radiating foam extensions enveloped in a polyethylene sheet with small fenestrations. This layer is placed directly over the bowel and tucked under the peritoneum, into the paracolic gutters and pelvis. The VPL does not need to be cut; however, if it is, the foam squares should be divided in the middle, with the residual foam pulled out and discarded. Lateral slits should be made at the level of any ostomies or feeding tubes to allow the VPL to fully extend around them. The second layer consists of fenestrated foam cut into the correct size and shape and placed over the protective foam, under the peritoneum. The third layer consists of a similar foam placed over the previous layer, between the fascia edges. The dressing is then covered with a semi-occlusive adhesive drape. A small piece of the adhesive drape and underlying sponge are excised and an interface pad with a tubing system is applied over this

(a)

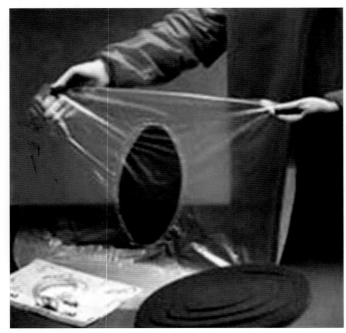

(b)

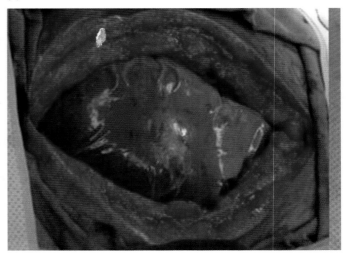

(c)

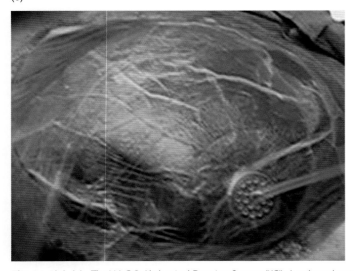

Fig. 21.4(a)–(c). The V.A.C.® Abdominal Dressing System (KCl). A polyurethane foam, covered with a protective, fenestrated, non-adherent layer (a), is placed over the intestine, under the peritoneum (b). A perforated polyurethane foam is placed over the first covered foam, covered with transparent adhesive drapes and connected to a computerized pump (c).

defect and connected to a negative pressure therapy unit. The negative pressure collapses the foam. A pump canister collects and quantifies the fluid evacuated from the abdomen. Dressing changes are usually done every 2 to 3 days.

- The three main NPT modalities (Barker's, V.A.C.® Abdominal Dressing System, ABThera) have different mechanical properties, which may affect outcomes. The most important difference is the distribution pattern of the preset negative pressures, with ABThera having a more even distribution and sustained NPT, promoting a more effective removal of any intraperitoneal fluid.

Caution with NPT

- In cases with incomplete hemostasis, application of high negative pressure may aggravate bleeding. In these cases an initial low negative pressure is advisable. If large amounts of blood are seen in the canister of the vacuum pump, the negative pressure should be immediately discontinued and the patient returned to the operating room for re-exploration and bleeding control.
- IAH may occur in rare cases with temporary abdominal wall closure with NPT dressing. The bladder pressure should be monitored routinely during the first few hours of negative-pressure dressing application.

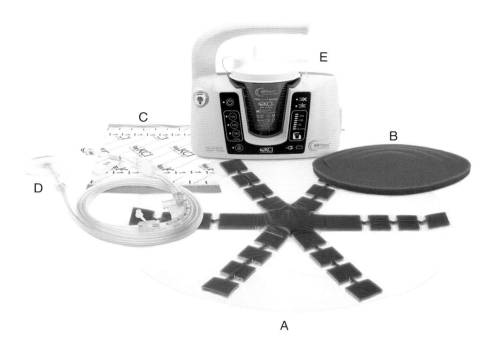

Fig. 21.5. ABThera negative pressure system for temporary abdominal closure: (A) visceral protective layer, (B) fenestrated foam, (C) semi-occlusive adhesive drape, (D) tubing with interface pad, (E) pump.

(a)

(b)

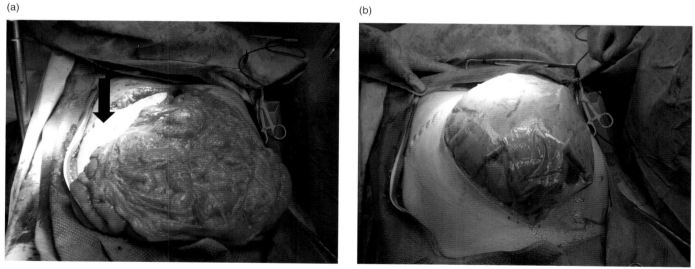

Fig. 21.6(a)–(d). Application of ABThera (KCI) for temporary abdominal closure. (a) Severe liver injury with perihepatic packing (arrow). (b) Application of the visceral protective layer over the intestine and under the peritoneum. (c) Application of two layers of fenestrated foam (one under the peritoneum and one between the edges of the abdominal wound), covered with transparent occlusive adhesive drape. (d) Interface pad and suction tubing.

(c)

(d)

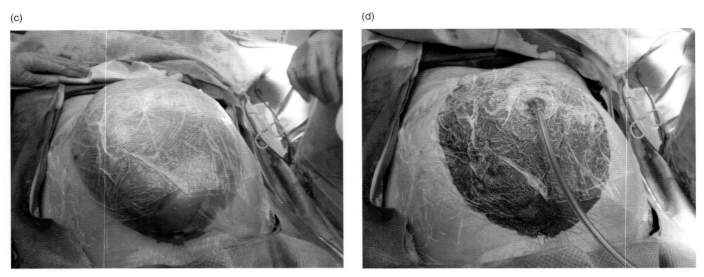

Fig. 21.6(a)–(d). (*cont.*)

(a)

(b)

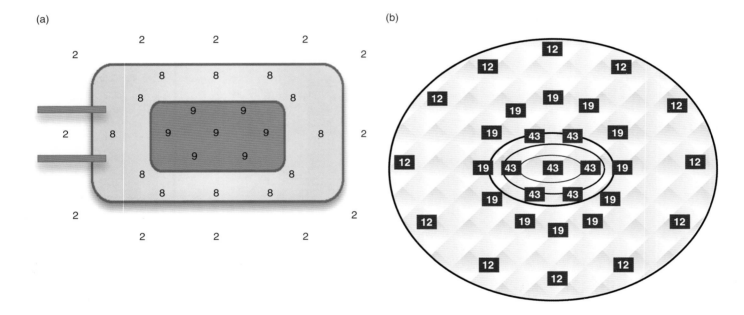

Fig. 21.7. Distribution of negative pressure of −125 mmHg with the Barker's (a), V.A.C.® abdominal dressing system (b), and ABThera system (c). The distribution of negative pressures affects the efficacy of removal of any intraperitoneal fluid (d).

(c)

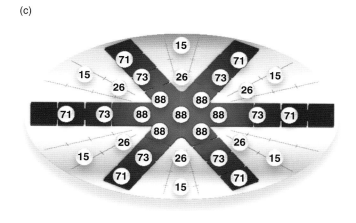

(d)

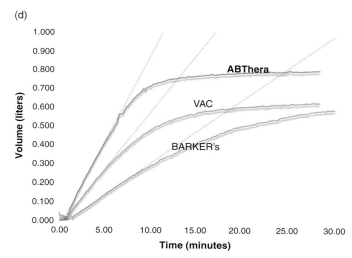

Fig. 21.7. (cont.)

Comparison of NPT techniques for temporary abdominal closure

- There is evidence that the ABThera™ Negative Pressure Therapy System (KCI USA, Inc., San Antonio, TX, USA), is associated with a significantly higher 30-day primary fascia closure rate and a lower mortality rate than the Barker's technique. The superior outcomes with ABThera have been attributed to the more effective removal of toxic lymph and cytokine and toxin-loaded peritoneal fluid.

Definitive fascia closure

- Early, definitive closure of the abdomen reduces the complications associated with the open abdomen. The closure should be achieved without tension or risk of recurrence of IAH.
- Primary fascia closure may be possible in many cases within a few days of the initial operation, and should be considered when all intra-abdominal packing has been removed, any residual infection is cleared, and the bowel edema subsides.
- In some patients early definitive fascial closure may not be possible because of persistent bowel edema or intra-abdominal sepsis. In these cases, progressive closure should be attempted at every return to the operating room for dressing change, by placing a few interrupted sutures at the top and bottom of the fascia defect.

- In patients with persistent large fascial defects, definitive reconstruction should be considered, using synthetic or biological meshes or sheets, or autologous tissue transfer with component separation.

Tips and pitfalls

- Consider early damage control, before the patient becomes in extremis. The timing of damage control is critical in determining the outcome.
- Interventional radiology is an important component of damage control. Consider going to the angiography suite straight from the operating room or utilize a hybrid operating room if available.
- Postoperative continuous bleeding after damage control must be examined in the operating room immediately. Do not assume that it is coagulopathic bleeding!
- The type of negative pressure therapy used for temporary abdominal closure can influence outcomes.
- In the presence of bleeding avoid using high negative pressure therapy.
- In applying ABThera or any other NPT, make sure that the foam does not come into direct contact with the bowel because of the risk of fistula formation.

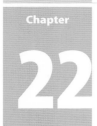

Chapter

22

Gastrointestinal tract

Kenji Inaba and Lisa L. Schlitzkus

Special surgical instruments

- General laparotomy tray
- Bookwalter or other fixed abdominal retractor
- Both TA and GIA stapling devices
- Ostomy supplies
- An electrothermal bipolar vessel sealing system device (LigaSure device)
- Adequate lighting including a headlight.

Positioning

- The patient should be placed in the supine position with the arms abducted to 90 degrees.
- The bed rails should be free and exposed for retractor placement.
- Standard trauma preparation of skin from chin to knees and laterally to the bed.
- If based on pre-operative imaging, there is a possibility of multiple compartment operations including a laparotomy and thoracotomy with one hemithorax involved, the patient can be positioned in a modified taxi-cab hailing position. The patient is placed supine with the injured hemithorax medially rotated 30° anterior to the coronal plane, facilitating further exposure of the chest wall. A beanbag, folded blankets, or a roll may be used to elevate and support the chest. Abduct the arm and slightly flex the elbow. The arm can be prepped into the field if manipulation is required. In general, however, to accommodate any injuries that may be encountered, it is preferable to use the utility supine position.
- In suspected low rectal injuries, the patient may be placed in the lithotomy position to facilitate diagnostic sigmoidoscopy or transanal repair of a rectal injury.

Incisions

- A midline laparotomy incision provides the ideal exposure for all gastrointestinal tract injuries. Adequate visualization and access should not be compromised by the length of the incision. Extension from xiphoid to pubic symphysis may be required, especially in hemodynamically compromised patients.

- Subcostal extensions may be required for cases with complex hepatic or gastroesophageal (GE) junction injuries.
- In a hypotensive patient, the abdomen should be entered using the scalpel in three strokes. First, the skin is incised, followed by the subcuticular tissue, and then the linea alba. A finger can be used to enter the peritoneal cavity just superior to the umbilicus at the thinnest point. Mayo scissors can then be used to extend the peritoneal incision. Cautery electrodissection may be used in hemodynamically stable patients under direct visualization.

Stomach
Surgical anatomy

- The lesser curvature is supplied by the left and right gastric arteries. The origin of the right gastric artery is highly variable, but generally originates from the proper hepatic artery. The left gastric artery arises from the celiac trunk and is encased in the hepatogastric ligament. It gives off the esophageal artery before following the lesser curvature to anastomose with the right gastric artery.
- The greater curvature is supplied by the left and right gastroepiploic arteries. The right gastroepiploic artery is an end branch of the gastroduodenal artery. The left gastroepiploic artery branches off the splenic artery and anastomoses with the right.
- The fundus of the stomach is also supplied by the short gastric arteries that arise from the distal splenic artery.
- The venous drainage parallels the arteries. The gastric veins drain into the portal veins, while the left gastroepiploic and short gastric veins first enter the splenic vein and ultimately the portal vein. The right gastroepiploic vein drains directly into the superior mesenteric vein.
- The angular incisure is the indentation approximately two-thirds of the way along the lesser curvature, and is a landmark for the end of the body and the beginning of the pyloric antrum.
- The upper part of the stomach begins with a physiologic sphincter, the lower esophageal sphincter. The outlet consists of a thickened muscular ring called the pylorus.

Atlas of Surgical Techniques in Trauma, ed. Demetrios Demetriades, Kenji Inaba, and George Velmahos. Published by Cambridge University Press. © Cambridge University Press 2015.

- The spleen is posterolateral to the fundus of the stomach, and the stomach creates an impression on the medial, visceral aspect of the spleen. The short gastric arteries lie within the gastrosplenic ligament.
- The anterior surface of the body of the pancreas is located posterior and inferior to the stomach.
- The left portion of the transverse colon lies posterior and inferior to the stomach. The gastrocolic ligament attaches to the greater curvature of the stomach and to the superior, anterior surface of the transverse colon.

General principles

- Most gastric injuries are secondary to penetrating trauma and are identified during operative exploration.
- The stomach is redundant and can be easily managed with primary suture closure in one or two layers or stapled wedge resection of the injured segment except near the GE junction and pylorus. For these injuries, see description below.
- The anterior and posterior walls of the stomach must be fully visualized to exclude injuries regardless of the mechanism.
- Division of the gastrocolic ligament allows entrance into the lesser sac for exposure of the posterior wall of the

(a)

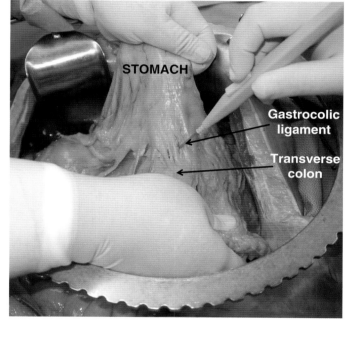

Fig. 22.1(a). One surgeon grasps the stomach with one hand and the opposite transverse colon in the other hand. The second surgeon or assistant enters the avascular plane of the gastrocolic ligament.

(b)

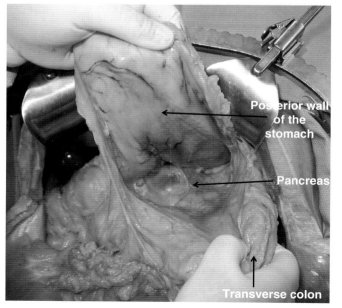

Fig. 22.1(b). After division of the gastrocolic ligament, elevating the stomach with downward traction of the transverse colon provides the critical view of the posterior wall of the stomach and the pancreas.

stomach. Elevation of the stomach with downward retraction of the colon provides the critical view. A wide malleable retractor withdrawn slowly may facilitate viewing the posterior wall of the stomach.

Distal esophageal injuries

- The gastroesophageal junction may be better visualized by placing the patient in the reverse Trendelenberg position. Taking down the triangular ligament and retracting the left lobe of the liver and dividing the gastrohepatic ligament, or the lesser omentum, exposes the medial aspect of the GE junction. To gain access to the lateral aspect, the short gastric

(a)

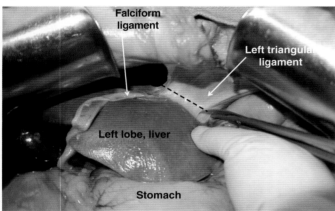

Fig. 22.2(a). Exposure of the gastroesophageal junction can be achieved by adequate mobilization and medial retraction of the left lobe of the liver and division of the gastrohepatic ligament. The falciform and and left triangular ligament are divided; division of the left triangular ligament of the liver (interrupted line).

(b)

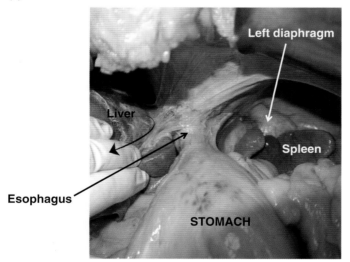

Fig. 22.2(b). Medial rotation of the liver, division of the gastrohepatic ligament and division of the short gastric arteries along the greater curvature exposes the gastroesophageal junction.

(c)

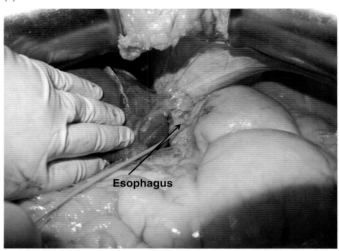

Fig. 22.2(c). Vessel loop around the esophagus and enter downward, caudal retraction on the stomach, exposes the esophagus and gastroesophageal junction.

(d)

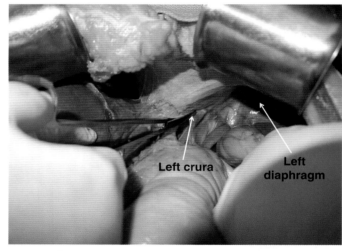

Fig. 22.2(d). Division of the diaphragmatic crura maximizes the exposure of the distal esophagus.

arteries can be divided. A Penrose can be placed around the GE junction to retract it caudally. Use of a Bookwalter or other fixed abdominal retractor and a headlamp can improve the exposure. Division of the diaphragmatic crura provides the maximal exposure cranially.

- Most simple injuries can be primarily repaired with absorbable 3–0 interrupted sutures in one layer. The repair may be buttressed with omentum, pleura, muscle, or stomach.
- Larger injuries may require resection and re-anastomosis, which can be handsewn or stapled utilizing an EEA stapler.

(a)

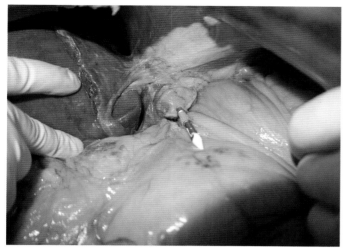

Fig. 22.3(a). Stapled esophago-gastrostomy: the EEA anvil can be placed through the injury site and pushed cranially in the esophagus. The injured GE junction can then be resected, and the anvil brought out the distal healthy end of the esophagus.

(b)

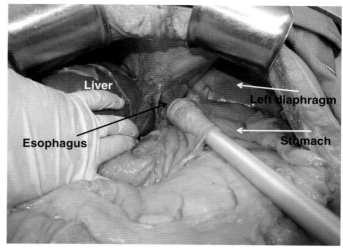

Fig. 22.3(b). A separate gastrotomy can be made to insert the EEA stapler.

(c)

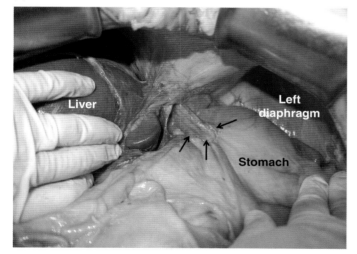

Fig. 22.3(c). The circular stapler creates a neo-gastroesophageal junction (arrows).

(d)

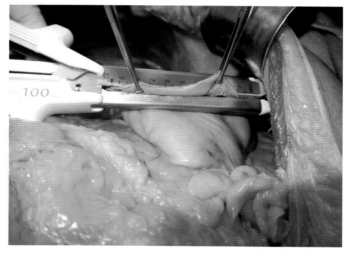

Fig. 22.3(d). The gastrotomy can later be closed with a TA or GIA stapler.

All devitalized tissue should be debrided. An anterior gastrotomy allows insertion of the EEA stapler and this opening can be closed using a GIA or TA stapler.

Pyloric injuries

- This area is prone to stenosis. Simple injuries may be repaired with a pyloroplasty, but destructive injuries may require an antrectomy.
- Options for reconstruction include a Billroth I, Billroth II, or a Roux-en-Y reconstruction.
- The gastrojejunostomy may be stapled or handsewn, antecolic or retrocolic. If the jejunum is brought through the mesocolon, the middle colic vessels should be avoided and the jejunum secured to the mesocolon to prevent an internal hernia.

Tips and pitfalls

- Exposure and good lighting are critical for avoiding missed injuries. All hematomas along the curvatures must be opened and explored for underlying perforations. Injuries to the posterior wall and along the curvatures of the stomach may be easily missed, even in the absence of an anterior injury.
- Excessive tension on the stomach may easily tear the short gastric vessels and cause iatrogenic bleeding.

Small intestine

Surgical anatomy

- The jejunum begins at the ligament of Treitz and the ileum terminates at the ileocecal valve. About two-fifths of the small intestine is jejunum and the remainder is ileum.

183

- The mesentery is the folding of peritoneum over the vascular supply and attaches the small intestine to the posterior abdominal wall. The attachment is about 15 centimeters from the upper left to lower right of the abdomen.
- The jejunum and ileum are supplied by the superior mesenteric artery (SMA) and drainage is by the superior mesenteric vein (SMV). The artery has multiple arcades, and the veins parallel the arteries. The SMV lies slightly anterior and to the right of the SMA within the mesentery and joins the splenic vein to form the portal vein posterior to the neck of the pancreas.

General principles

- Injury should be suspected in any penetrating trauma that enters or traverses the peritoneal cavity. Multiple concurrent injuries may be present along the length of the small bowel.
- Perforation after blunt trauma results from shearing forces or bowel entrapment causing a closed loop obstruction with perforation due to a sudden increase in intraluminal pressure. Traction injuries may occur at points of fixation such as the ligament of Treitz or the ileocecal junction. A bucket handle injury of the mesentery may also occur where the bowel is initially intact and viable, but later necroses due to impaired blood supply from an injured mesentery.

(a)

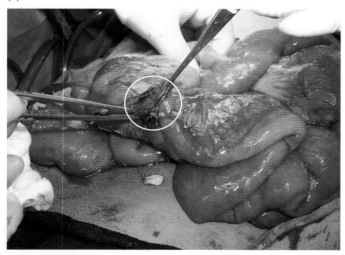

Fig. 22.4(a). Small bowel perforation in blunt abdominal trauma due to increased intraluminal pressure. The perforation usually occurs at the antimesenteric border.

(b)

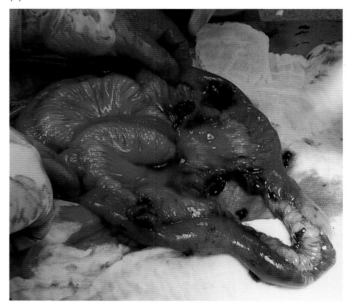

Fig. 22.4(b). Bucket handle injury of the small bowel mesentery due to deceleration injury. Note the ischemic necrosis of the bowel.

- The small intestine must be examined from the ligament of Treitz to the ileocecal valve. The entire circumference of the intestine including the mesenteric border should be visualized. Stay methodical to avoid missing injuries.

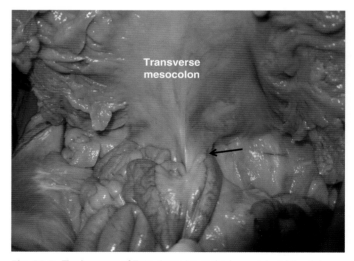

Fig. 22.5. The ligament of Treitz (arrow) is at the base and middle of the transverse mesocolon.

Resection versus repair

- If multiple injuries are identified, consider a single rather than multiple anastomoses.
- All injuries should be closed in a transverse orientation to avoid narrowing the lumen.
- Resection versus primary repair will depend on the extent of the injury.

Intestinal anastomosis

- The outcomes are similar for hand-sewn versus stapled anastomoses for trauma.
- In settings where the bowel is edematous, friable, or where there is a large size mismatch, a hand-sewn anastomosis may be preferred.
- Even in the damage control setting, always attempt to perform the gastrointestinal tract anastomosis at the first operation. If unable, stapling and leaving the patient in discontinuity may be considered.

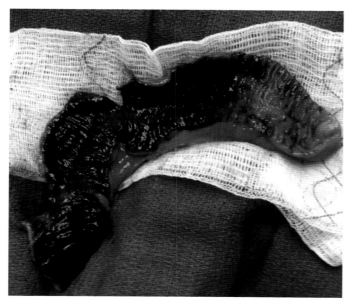

Fig. 22.6. Distended and ischemic segment of bowel proximal to the staple line in a patient who had a damage control procedure with bowel stapled and left in discontinuity.

Tips and pitfalls

- All bowel wall hematomas due to penetrating trauma must be unroofed and explored. A common error is the failure to explore hematomas at the junction of the bowel and the mesentery.
- Perform a complete evaluation of the small bowel before starting any repairs or resections. The presence of other perforations may change the management plan.
- In cases with multiple small bowel perforations, a single resection of a larger segment is preferable to multiple smaller resections.

- In planning major small bowel resections, try to preserve a minimum of 100 cm of small bowel to avoid "short bowel syndrome."
- Consider hand-sewn rather than stapled anastomosis in the presence of bowel edema.
- Bowel left in discontinuity following damage control may be at risk of ischemia; when able, perform the anastomosis at the index operation.

Colon

Surgical anatomy

- The colon is divided into four parts: the ascending, transverse, descending, and sigmoid. Along the length of the colon are three longitudinal muscles called the taenia coli.
- The cecum is the first part of the ascending colon. It has no mesentery, is almost entirely covered by peritoneum, and gives off the appendix. Its vascular supply is the ileocolic artery and vein, an end branch of the SMA and SMV. The appendiceal artery, a branch of the ileocolic, lies within the mesentery of the appendix.
- The remainder of the ascending colon is retroperitoneal and can be freed by taking down the white line of Toldt. It is supplied by the right colic artery, a branch of the SMA, and drains by the right colic vein into the SMV. The ascending colon transitions into the transverse colon at the hepatic flexure located at the inferior edge of the liver.
- The transverse colon is the largest and most mobile part of the colon. It is supplied by the middle colic artery from the SMA with the parallel veins draining into the SMV. The transverse colon ends at the splenic flexure. This turn is more acute, less mobile and more superior than the hepatic flexure. This is also the watershed transition point of the vascular supply from the superior mesenteric vessels to the inferior mesenteric vessels.
- The descending colon mirrors the ascending, but on the left. It is supplied by the left colic artery and vein, which originate from the inferior mesenteric artery (IMA) and inferior mesenteric vein (IMV). As the descending colon becomes more mobile and turns midline to drop down into the pelvis, it becomes the sigmoid colon supplied by the sigmoid artery. The sigmoid and left colic vein drain into the IMV, then the splenic vein to enter the portal vein.

General principles

- Hemorrhage must first be controlled, followed by contamination control. Once all injuries are identified, definitive repair can be undertaken. Contamination control may include placing a Babcock on the injury, oversewing, or stapling the injury.
- Antibiotics to include aerobic and anaerobic coverage should be given preoperatively to all suspected colon

injuries and should not be continued for more than 24 hours postoperatively unless active infection is present.

- Primary repair is advocated in all non-destructive colon injuries. The majority of destructive injuries requiring resection can safely be managed with primary anastomosis. Diversion should be considered in cases with massive wall edema, poor quality colon tissue, or questionable blood supply.

- The risk of intra-abdominal infection following destructive colon injuries requiring resection is high, irrespective of the method of management.

- Hand-sewn anastomoses are favored for edematous bowel, otherwise a stapled anastomosis can be used.

- Given the complications of bowel left in discontinuity during damage control, an attempt at primary anastomosis should be performed whenever possible at the index operation.

- Mobilization is key to evaluating the colon. The right and left colon may be taken down along the white line of Toldt. The splenocolic and hepatocolic ligaments may be divided.

- During mobilization of the splenic flexure, excessive traction on the colon may cause avulsion of the splenic capsule with bleeding.

- During mobilization of the right or left colon, the ureters should be identified and protected.

(a)

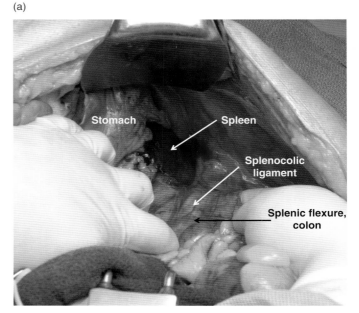

Fig. 22.8(a). During mobilization of the splenic flexure of the colon and division of the splenocolic ligament, avoid excessive traction on the colon to prevent avulsion of the splenic capsule.

(b)

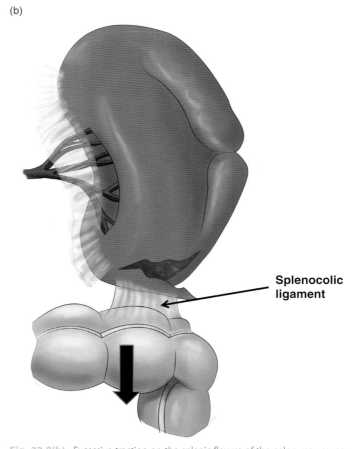

Fig. 22.8(b). Excessive traction on the splenic flexure of the colon may cause avulsion of the splenic capsule and bleeding.

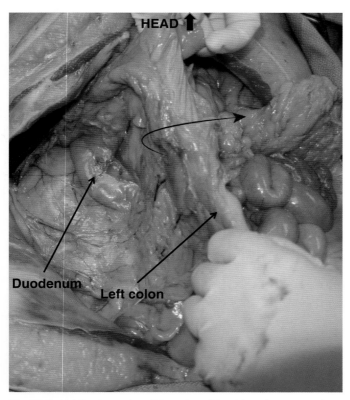

Fig. 22.7. Mobilization and medial rotation of the right colon exposes the C loop of the duodenum.

Resection versus repair

- For penetrating colon injuries, primary repair is recommended. For simple wounds, debridement followed by a one- or two-layer repair is acceptable using a transmural absorbable running or interrupted inner layer. If used, the second layer would consist of interrupted Lembert sutures.
- Resection is required when the injury encompasses >50 percent of the circumference or when it results in a devascularized segment. The anastomosis may be hand-sewn or stapled.
- A common injury pattern is de-serosalization, usually of the sigmoid colon. Separation of the muscular and serosal layers occurs with an intact mucosal tube. To repair, telescope the mucosa back upon itself. Debride the muscular and serosal edges, and then reapproximate them with one layer of interrupted or running suture. The mucosa within will redistribute and does not lead to stenosis or obstruction. Healing occurs without having to open the lumen, avoiding contamination. Extensive defects, especially those with associated mesenteric injury, will require resection and anastomosis.

Wound closure

- The skin should always be left open because of the high incidence of wound infection and fascial dehiscence with primary skin closure. Delayed primary closure can be performed 3–4 days after the initial operation.

Tips and pitfalls

- All paracolic hematomas due to penetrating trauma should be explored.
- Excessive tension on the hepatic and splenic flexures may cause capsular tears and further bleeding.
- Whenever possible, the colon should be transected obliquely, with the mesenteric border left longer than the anti-mesenteric border in order to optimize blood supply to the bowel wall.
- Adequate debridement of all penetrating wounds, especially gunshot wounds, is critical before a repair is performed. In destructive injuries the bowel wall should be resected to well-perfused and healthy edges.
- While the colon is unlikely to become narrowed, all injuries should be closed in a transverse orientation to avoid this complication.
- Injuries to the splenic flexure can be difficult to expose and the flexure should be taken down to allow adequate visualization.

Rectum

Surgical anatomy

- The rectum is approximately 15 centimeters long and is only partially intraperitoneal. The anterior and lateral sides of the upper third and the anterior middle third are covered by peritoneum. The lower third of the rectum is completely extraperitoneal.
- The rectum is highly vascular. The superior rectal artery from the IMA supplies the upper third, the two middle rectal arteries from the internal iliac arteries supply the middle third and the inferior rectal arteries from the internal pudendal arteries supply the lower third, the anorectal junction, and the anal canal. The superior rectal veins drain into the IMV (portal system), whereas the middle and inferior rectal veins drain into the internal iliac and internal pudendal veins (systemic).

General principles

- Injuries to the intraperitoneal rectum are treated like colonic injuries.
- Extraperitoneal rectal injuries are rare after blunt trauma due to the protection afforded by the bony pelvis. They can, however, result from bone fragments secondary to pelvic fracture or from rectal foreign bodies. The majority of extraperitoneal injuries result from transpelvic gunshot wounds. This should be suspected if blood is noted on digital rectal examination or if there is a suspicious missile trajectory seen on CT.
- For these patients, the diagnosis can be confirmed by anoscopy followed by sigmoidoscopy. If an associated intraperitoneal component of the rectal injury is suspected, laparoscopic confirmation or laparotomy can be performed. Isolated small, non-destructive extraperitoneal injuries can be observed or repaired through a trans-anal approach. Routine diversion is not necessary.
- A large destructive extraperitoneal rectal injury may be primarily repaired and protected using a diverting ostomy.
- Some large injuries cannot be repaired due to their anatomical location. Diversion alone has been used with success.
- A properly constructed loop colostomy may achieve complete fecal diversion, thus avoiding the complex reconstruction required after a Hartmann end-colostomy. The Hartmann's procedure should be reserved for patients with extensive destruction of the rectum.
- Routine pre-sacral drainage and distal rectal washout for extraperitoneal rectal injuries are no longer recommended.

Tips and pitfalls

- Patients with suspected extra-peritoneal rectal injuries should be placed on the operating table in the lithotomy position for anoscopy and sigmoidoscopic evaluation with

(a)

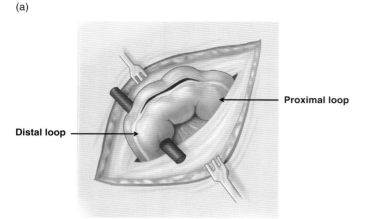

Proximal loop

Distal loop

Fig. 22.9(a). Loop colostomy with complete fecal diversion. A "bridge" is created with a plastic rod placed through the mesocolon close to the distal loop of the colostomy.

(b)

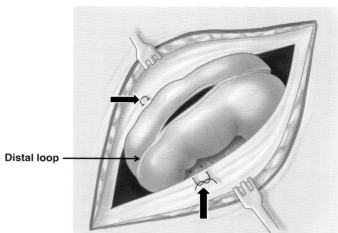

Distal loop

Fig. 22.9(b). Loop colostomy with complete fecal diversion, using a heavy horizontal mattress suture as a temporary bridge (thick arrows), close to the distal loop of the colostomy, through the aponeurosis of the external oblique muscle.

(c)

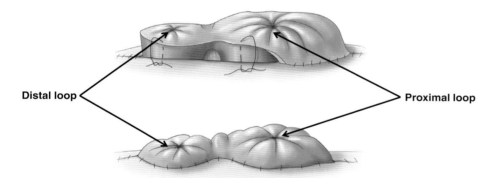

Distal loop

Proximal loop

Fig. 22.9(c) Completion of the diverting loop colostomy. Loop colostomy with complete fecal diversion. A "bridge" is created by a plastic rod placed through the mesocolon close to the distal loop of the colostomy (left). Alternatively, a heavy horizontal mattress suture (silk 1) through the aponeurosis of the external oblique muscle and the mesocolon can be used instead of the plastic rod (right).

possible trans-anal repair. In the hemodynamically unstable patient due to associated intra-abdominal injuries, an exploratory laparotomy for bleeding control precedes the rectal evaluation.

- A properly constructed loop colostomy can provide effective fecal diversion and be the primary treatment for an extraperitoneal rectal injury. Alternatively, a heavy horizontal mattress suture (silk 1) through the aponeurosis of the external oblique muscle and the mesocolon can achieve an excellent fecal diversion.

- Associated bladder or iliac vascular injuries are common. Every effort should be made to separate the repairs with well-vascularized tissue such as omentum, in order to reduce the risk of vascular graft infection or the formation of a rectovesical fistula.

- Complex anorectal injuries after open pelvic fractures should be managed acutely with hemostasis, wound packing, and a sigmoid colostomy.

Duodenum

23

Edward Kwon and Demetrios Demetriades

Surgical anatomy

- The duodenum lies in front of the right kidney and renal vessels, the right psoas muscle, the inferior vena cava, and the aorta.

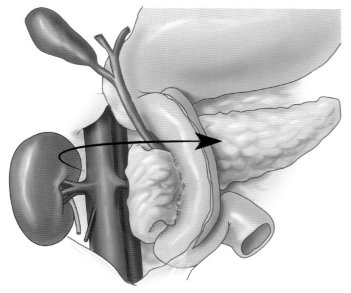

Fig. 23.1. The duodenum lies in front of the right kidney and renal vessels, the inferior vena cava, and the aorta. Exposure after medial rotation of the duodenum and head of the pancreas.

- The duodenum is approximately 25 cm in length. It is the most fixed part of the small intestine and has no mesentery. It is anatomically divided into four parts:
  - The superior or first portion is intraperitoneal along the anterior half of its circumference. Superiorly, the first portion is attached to the hepatoduodenal ligament. The posterior border is associated with the gastroduodenal artery, common bile duct, and the portal vein.
  - The descending or second portion is bordered posteriorly by the medial surface of the right kidney, the right renal vessels, and the inferior vena cava. The transverse colon crosses anteriorly. The common bile duct and main pancreatic duct drain into the medial wall of the descending duodenum.
  - The transverse or third portion is also entirely retroperitoneal. Posteriorly, it is bordered by the inferior vena cava and the aorta. The superior mesenteric vessels cross in front of this portion of the duodenum.
  - The ascending or fourth portion of the duodenum is approximately 2.5 cm in length and primarily retroperitoneal, except for the most distal segment. Posteriorly, it is bordered by the aorta and it ascends to the left of the aorta to join the jejunum at the ligament of Treitz.
- The common bile duct descends within the hepatoduodenal ligament to course posterior to the first portion of the duodenum and pancreatic head, becoming partially invested within the parenchyma of the pancreas. The main pancreatic duct then joins the common bile duct to drain into the ampulla of Vater within the second portion of the duodenum. The ampulla of Vater is located approximately 7 cm from the pylorus. The accessory pancreatic duct drains approximately 2 cm proximal to the ampulla of Vater.
- The vascular supply to the duodenum is intimately associated with the head of the pancreas. The head of the pancreas and the second portion of the duodenum derive their blood supply from the anterior and posterior pancreaticoduodenal arcades. These arcades lie on the surface of the pancreas near the duodenal C loop. Attempts to separate these two organs at this location usually result in ischemia of the duodenum.

Atlas of Surgical Techniques in Trauma, ed. Demetrios Demetriades, Kenji Inaba, and George Velmahos. Published by Cambridge University Press. © Cambridge University Press 2015.

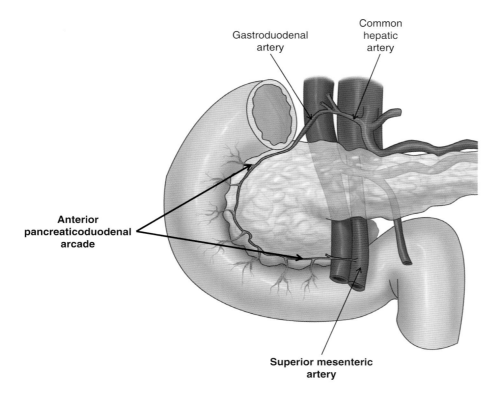

Gastroduodenal artery

Common hepatic artery

Anterior pancreaticoduodenal arcade

Superior mesenteric artery

Fig. 23.2. The head of the pancreas and the second portion of the duodenum derive their blood supply from the anterior and posterior pancreaticoduodenal arcades. Attempts to separate the two organs at this location usually result in ischemia of the duodenum.

General principles

- All periduodenal hematomas secondary to blunt or penetrating trauma found during laparotomy should be explored to rule out underlying perforation.

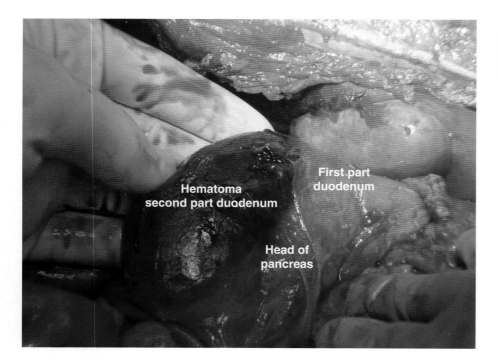

Hematoma second part duodenum

First part duodenum

Head of pancreas

Fig. 23.3. Hematoma of the second part of the duodenum due to blunt trauma. All duodenal hematomas secondary to blunt or penetrating trauma found during laparotomy should be explored to rule out underlying perforation.

- The majority of duodenal lacerations can be managed with debridement and transverse duodenorrhaphy.
- Resection and primary anastomosis of the second portion of the duodenum are tenuous due to the high risk of vascular compromise during mobilization and proximity to the ampulla of Vater.
- Injuries involving the medial aspect of the second portion of the duodenum may be more effectively explored from within the lumen via a lateral duodenotomy. Avoid dissection of the duodenum from the head of the pancreas due to the high risk of devascularization and duodenal necrosis.
- Routine pyloric exclusion should not be performed. Exclusion should be reserved for severe injuries requiring a complex repair or a repair with tenuous blood supply.
- In complex pancreaticoduodenal injuries, consider damage control techniques and delayed reconstruction.
- Wide local drainage with closed suction drains of duodenal repairs should be performed. The drains should not directly overlie the repair.
- Distal feeding access, through a feeding jejunostomy, should routinely be considered in patients with complex duodenal injuries.
- Although rare, severe destructive injuries to the duodenum that include the pancreatic head may require a pancreaticoduodenal resection. These cases should be handled using damage control principles with a staged resection followed by delayed reconstruction.

Special surgical instruments

- Complete trauma laparotomy tray, Bookwalter self-retaining abdominal retractor, surgical headlight, and tube for possible jejunal feeding access.

Positioning

- Standard supine positioning with arms abducted to 90 degrees
- Standard trauma preparation from the nipples to the mid thighs.

Incision

- A standard midline laparotomy incision from the xiphoid process to the pubic symphysis.

Operative technique
Exposure

- A self-retaining abdominal retractor is useful to retract the abdominal wall and the liver cephalad to expose the duodenal–pyloric junction.
- The anterior surface of the first portion of the duodenum is readily visible.

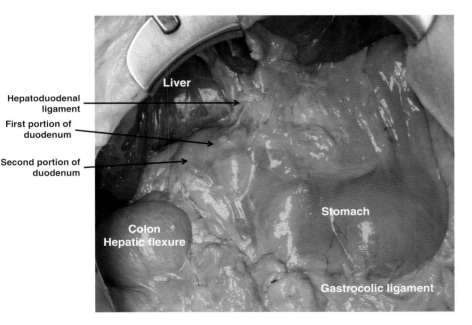

Fig. 23.4. Duodenum in situ. The anterior half of the first portion of the duodenum is intraperitoneal and easily visible. The hepatoduodenal ligament is attached to the superior aspect of the first portion of the duodenum. The proximal aspect of the second portion of the duodenum is also visible, although often the second portion is covered anteriorly by the hepatic flexure of the colon.

- A Kocher maneuver is performed by incising the lateral peritoneal attachments of the first, second, and proximal third portions of the duodenum to the superior mesenteric vein (SMV) exposing their lateral aspects. Avoid injury to the SMV.

  o The C-loop of the duodenum and the pancreatic head are retracted medially to expose their posterior surfaces. Avoid excessive superior traction to prevent superior mesenteric vein injury.

  o Gerota's fascia of the right kidney and the inferior vena cava are visible posteriorly.

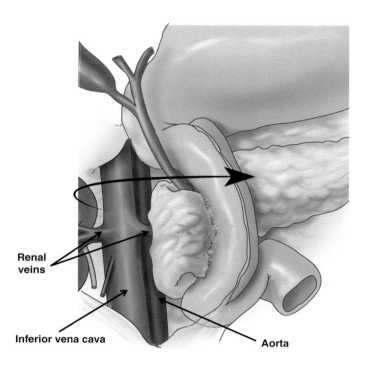

Fig. 23.5. Kocher maneuver: the posterior and lateral aspects of the second portion of the duodenum may be exposed by performing a Kocher maneuver. The lateral peritoneal attachments of the first, second, and proximal third portions of the duodenum are incised and the pancreaticoduodenal complex is retracted medially. Note the exposure of the inferior vena cava and renal veins, deep to the pancreaticoduodenal complex.

(a)

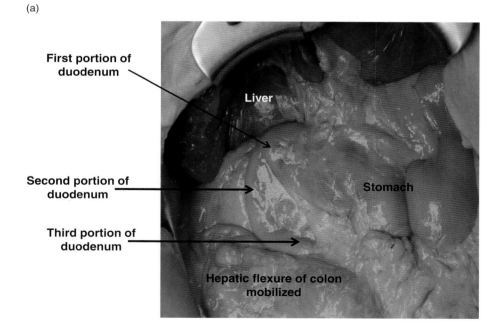

Fig. 23.6(a). Kocher maneuver: the hepatic flexure of the colon is mobilized and retracted toward the pelvis, revealing the underlying anterior and lateral surface of the second and proximal third portion of the duodenum.

(b)

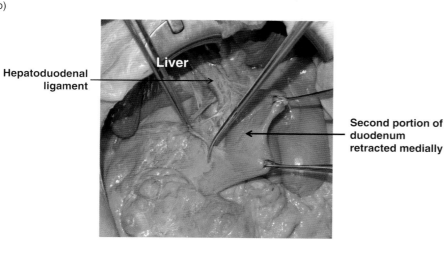

Hepatoduodenal ligament

Liver

Second portion of duodenum retracted medially

Fig. 23.6(b). Kocher maneuver: the lateral attachments of the duodenum are sharply divided, exposing the lateral and posterior surfaces of the second portion of the duodenum.

(c)

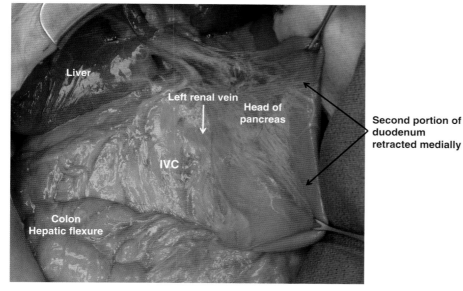

Liver

Left renal vein

Head of pancreas

IVC

Colon Hepatic flexure

Second portion of duodenum retracted medially

Fig. 23.6(c). Kocher maneuver: the duodenum is mobilized medially until the IVC and left renal vein are encountered (IVC = inferior vena cava).

- To increase exposure to the remainder of the third and fourth portions of the duodenum and retroperitoneal vessels, a right medial visceral rotation or Cattell–Braasch maneuver is performed.

  ○ Incise the lateral peritoneal attachments of the right colon from the hepatic flexure to the cecum and retract the colon medially.

  ○ Continue the inferior margin of the lateral peritoneal incision onto the visceral peritoneum, posterior to the small bowel mesentery, in an oblique fashion from the ileocecal junction towards the ligament of Treitz. The right colon and small bowel are retracted cephalad and to the left.

  ○ The superior mesenteric vessels are retracted with the small bowel, towards the patient's head and left side, and are no longer crossing the duodenum. The third and fourth portions are now accessible.

(a)

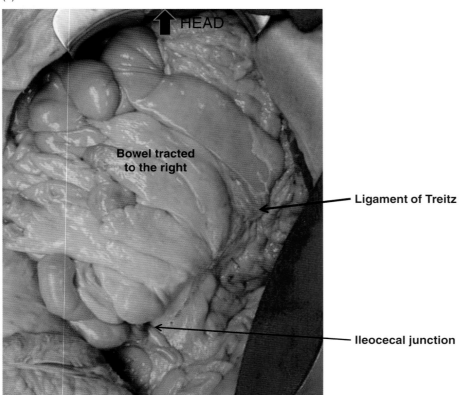

Fig. 23.7(a). Cattell–Braasch maneuver. After mobilization of the right colon, the bowel is retracted to the right. An incision is then made on the visceral retroperitoneum, posterior to the small bowel mesentery (red line), in an oblique fashion from the ileocecal junction towards the ligament of Treitz.

HEAD

Bowel tracted to the right

Ligament of Treitz

Ileocecal junction

(b)

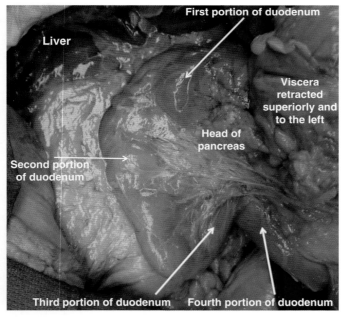

First portion of duodenum

Liver

Viscera retracted superiorly and to the left

Head of pancreas

Second portion of duodenum

Third portion of duodenum   **Fourth portion of duodenum**

Fig. 23.7(b). Complete exposure of all parts of the duodenum after Cattell–Braasch maneuver. The viscera is retracted superiorly and to the left. Note the superior mesenteric vessels are no longer crossing the duodenum.

- The distal fourth portion of the duodenum can also be exposed by incising the ligament of Treitz.
  - The transverse colon is retracted superiorly and the small bowel is gently retracted inferiorly and to the right. The ligament of Treitz is identified at the root of the mesentery where the fourth portion of the

duodenum emerges from the retroperitoneum attached to the superior aspect of the duodenum.

  - The root of the mesentery should be palpated to identify the location of the superior mesenteric vessels to the right of the ligament of Treitz to prevent injury prior to division.

(a)

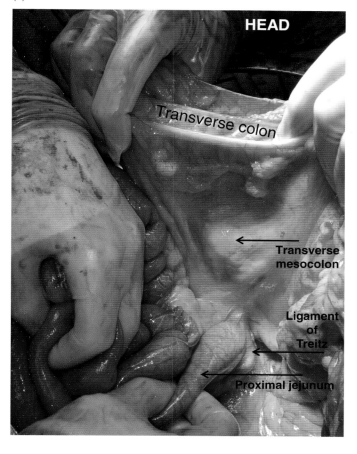

Fig. 23.8(a). The distal most part of the fourth portion of the duodenum is attached to the ligament of Treitz. The Treitz ligament is at the middle and base of the transverse mesocolon.

(b)

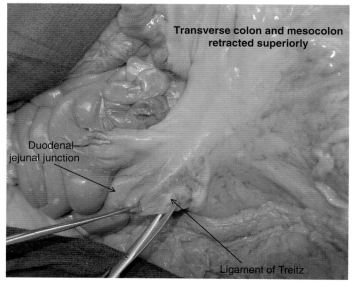

Fig. 23.8(b). Division of the ligament of Treitz to the right of the duodenojejunal junction. The superior mesenteric artery is to the left of the junction.

- Alternatively, the hepatic flexure of the colon can be mobilized inferiorly by serially ligating and dividing the gastrocolic omentum from the mid transverse colon to the hepatic flexure and incising the peritoneal attachments laterally. An electrothermal bipolar vessel sealing system (LigaSure device) may be used as a safe and faster alternative to vessel ligation and division.
- The lesser sac is exposed and the anteromedial surfaces of the second portion of the duodenum and head of the pancreas are visible.

Repair

- All duodenal hematomas identified intraoperatively must be explored to rule out underlying perforation.
  A seromuscular incision is made overlying the hematoma and the hematoma is evacuated. The duodenum should be carefully examined for full thickness injury at the site of the hematoma.
- Most duodenal lacerations can be debrided and repaired primarily. Repairs should be performed transversely in two layers using a full thickness continuous 3–0 absorbable suture as the inner layer and 3–0 seromuscular Lembert sutures as the outer layer.

  o If adequate mobilization is not possible for transverse closure, the injury may be repaired in a longitudinal fashion if there is not significant luminal narrowing. If there is significant stenosis, a gastrojejunostomy should be performed in addition to the repair.
  o Some injuries may not be able to be repaired primarily and require more complex repairs such as jejunal mucosal patch or serosal patch. A serosal patch may also be utilized to buttress a repair.

- Transections and injuries involving >50% of the circumference of the first, third, and fourth portions of the duodenum may require segmental resection and duodenoduodenostomy or duodenojejunostomy.

  o The injured segment is resected and a two-layer end-to-end anastomosis is created using a full thickness continuous 3–0 absorbable suture and seromuscular 3–0 Lembert sutures.
  o If a tension-free anastomosis is unable to be created a Roux-en-y duodenojejunostomy may be required.

- Segmental resection of the second portion is limited by the ampulla of Vater and by the common blood supply with the pancreas, making it particularly susceptible to vascular compromise during mobilization.
- Pyloric exclusion should be used selectively for injuries involving the second portion of the duodenum, combined pancreatic and duodenal injuries, and otherwise tenuous repairs.

  o An anterior gastrotomy is created along the greater curvature of the stomach, near the pylorus.
  o The pylorus is identified and grasped via the gastrotomy with a Babcock clamp and a purse-string suture using a size 0 absorbable suture is placed.
  o An alternative technique involves stapling of the post-pyloric duodenum with a TA 55 4.8 mm stapling device.
  o A gastrojejunostomy is created utilizing the previous gastrotomy.

(a)

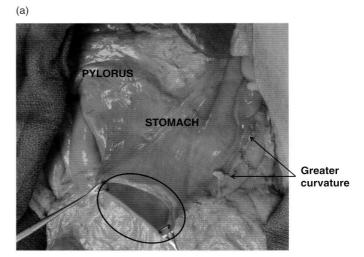

Fig. 23.9(a). Pyloric exclusion: a gastrotomy (circle) is created along the greater curvature, which will also be used to create a gastrojejunostomy.

(b)

Fig. 23.9(b). Pyloric exclusion. The pylorus is grasped with a Babcock clamp via the gastrotomy and delivered.

(c)

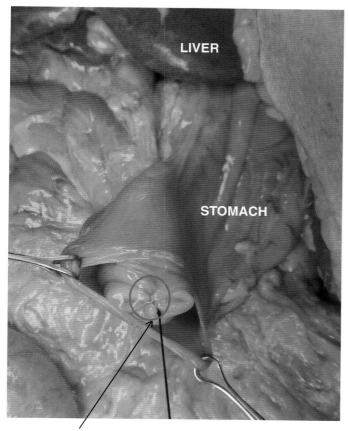

Pylorus sutured closed

Fig. 23.9(c). Pyloric exclusion. A 0 absorbable suture is utilized to close the pylorus (circle). A gastrojejunostomy is then created using the previous gastrotomy.

- Destructive injuries to the pancreatic head and duodenum may require pancreaticoduodenectomy (Whipple procedure).

o These patients are often hemodynamically unstable and these injuries are best managed with completion of the resection and delayed reconstruction as a second planned operation.

o Associated sources of hemorrhage should be considered and include from superficial to deep: (1) duodenum and pancreas, (2) superior mesenteric vessels and portal vein, (3) inferior vena cava, renal vessels and aorta.

- Damage control techniques for duodenal injuries include resection without anastomosis or wide drainage and exteriorization of the injury with lateral duodenostomy and planned delayed reconstruction.

Tips and pitfalls

- The superior mesenteric vein and its branches are easily injured with excessive traction during the Kocher and Cattell–Braasch maneuvers.
- Care should be taken during repairs and anastomoses involving the second portion of the duodenum to identify and preserve the ampulla of Vater.
- Separation of the second portion of the duodenum from the head of the pancreas results in ischemia and necrosis of the duodenum.
- During division of the ligament of Treitz, proceed carefully to avoid injury to the superior mesenteric artery on the right and the inferior mesenteric vein on the left.
- Injuries of the medial aspect of the second portion of the duodenum can be explored from within the lumen, through a lateral duodenotomy.
- In complex injuries, distal feeding access should be considered through a feeding jejunostomy tube.
- Closed suction drains should be placed around, but not directly overlying duodenal repairs.

Abdomen

Liver injuries

Kenji Inaba and Kelly Vogt

Surgical anatomy

- The liver is held in place by the following ligaments:
  - The falciform ligament, which attaches the liver to the anterior diaphragm and the anterior abdominal wall, extending towards the umbilicus.
  - The coronary ligament, which attaches the right lobe of the liver to the diaphragm. The lateral extensions of the coronary ligament form the triangular ligaments, right and left, which are also attached to the diaphragm.
- The anatomical division of the liver into the eight classic Couinaud segments has no practical application in trauma, where the resection planes are dictated by the extent of

injury and are non-anatomical. However, the external anatomical landmarks may be useful in planning operative maneuvers.

  - The plane between the center of the gallbladder and the inferior vena cava (IVC) runs along the middle hepatic vein, and serves as the line of division between the right and left lobes.
  - The left lobe is divided by the falciform ligament into the medial and lateral segments.
  - Dissection along the falciform ligament should be performed carefully, so as to avoid injury to the portal venous supply to the medial segment of the left lobe.

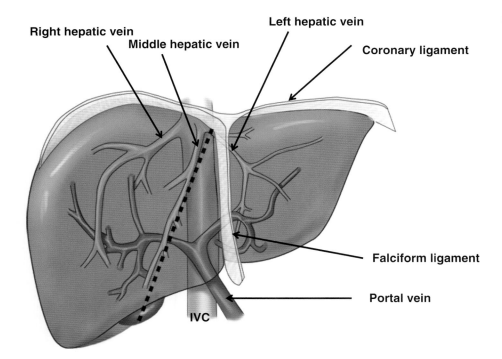

Fig. 24.1. Surgical anatomy of the liver. The plane between the gallbladder and inferior vena cava (IVC) (interrupted line) runs along the middle hepatic vein. Dissection along the falciform ligament should be done carefully, so as to avoid injury to the portal venous supply to the medial segment of the left lobe.

Atlas of Surgical Techniques in Trauma, ed. Demetrios Demetriades, Kenji Inaba, and George Velmahos. Published by Cambridge University Press. © Cambridge University Press 2015.

- The retrohepatic IVC is approximately 8–10 cm long and is partially embedded into the liver parenchyma. In approximately 7% of individuals the IVC is completely encircled by the liver.
- There are three major hepatic veins (right, middle, and left), as well as multiple accessory veins. The first 1–2 cm of the major hepatic veins are extrahepatic, with the remaining 8–10 cm intrahepatic. In approximately 70% of patients, the middle hepatic vein joins the left hepatic vein, near the IVC.
- The common hepatic artery originates from the celiac artery. It is responsible for approximately 30% of the hepatic blood flow, but supplies 50% of the hepatic oxygenation. It branches into the left and right hepatic arteries at the liver hilum in the majority of patients. In an anatomical variant, the right hepatic artery may arise from the superior mesenteric artery. Alternatively, the left hepatic artery may arise from the left gastric artery.
- The portal vein provides approximately 70% of hepatic blood flow, and the remaining 50% of the hepatic oxygenation. It is formed by the confluence of the superior mesenteric vein and the splenic vein behind the head of the pancreas. The portal vein divides into right and left extrahepatic branches at the level of the liver parenchyma.
- The porta hepatis contains the hepatic artery (left), common bile duct (right), and portal vein (posterior, between the common bile duct and the hepatic artery).
- The right hepatic duct is easier to expose after removal of the gallbladder.
- The left hepatic bile duct, the left hepatic artery, and the left portal vein enter the under-surface of the liver near the falciform ligament.

(a)

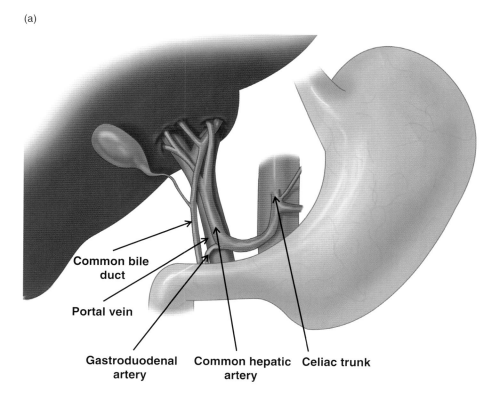

Common bile duct

Portal vein

Gastroduodenal artery   **Common hepatic artery**   **Celiac trunk**

Fig. 24.2(a). The porta hepatis contains the hepatic artery (left), common bile duct (right), and portal vein (posterior, between the common bile duct and the hepatic artery).

(b)

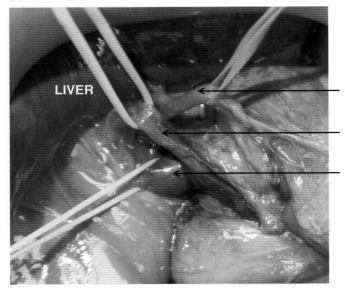

Fig. 24.2(b). Structures of the portal triad dissected out.

LIVER

Common hepatic artery

Common bile duct

Portal vein

General principles

- The liver is the most commonly injured intra-abdominal solid organ.
- Most injuries to the liver do not require operative intervention.
- Angioembolization is an effective adjunct to the non-operative management of high-grade liver injuries, especially in patients with evidence of active extravasation on contrast-enhanced CT scan. After damage control packing of complex liver injuries operatively, angioembolization may also be an effective adjunct.
- Damage control procedures have revolutionized the management of complex liver injuries and in appropriate cases they should be considered early. Packing is the mainstay of damage control for the liver and will be expanded upon below.
- A contained stable retrohepatic hematoma should not be opened. If the hematoma is expanding or leaking, and it is possible to control with packing alone, this technique should be the operative treatment of choice. The operation should then be terminated and the patient brought to the ICU for ongoing resuscitation. Angioembolization may be of use, especially if there is associated parenchymal damage that was packed. The patient can return to the operating room for pack removal after complete physiological stabilization.
- Adequate mobilization of the liver, by division of the falciform and coronary ligaments, is essential in the management of posterolateral injuries.
- If, during anterior retraction of the liver, bleeding from posterior to the liver worsens, this is suspicious for injury to the retrohepatic IVC or to the hepatic veins.
- In approximately 80%–85% of patients undergoing operation, the liver injury can be managed by relatively

simple surgical techniques, such as application of local hemostatic agents, electro-coagulation, superficial suturing, or drainage. The remaining 15%–20% of cases require more complex surgical techniques.

Special surgical instruments

- A hybrid operating room suite with angioembolization capability is highly desirable.
- A standard trauma laparotomy and thoracotomy tray, which includes vascular instruments. A sternotomy set should be available in case a median sternotomy is needed for improved exposure of the retrohepatic IVC.
- A fixed self-retaining abdominal retractor, such as an Omni-flex, Bookwalter or Gomez.
- An electrothermal bipolar vessel sealing system (LigaSure device) is desirable.
- A surgical head light.

Positioning

- Supine position, with upper extremities abducted to 90 degrees.
- Skin antiseptic preparation should include the chest, abdomen, and groin.
- Use upper and lower body warming devices.

Incisions

- The initial incision should be a midline laparotomy. This incision provides limited exposure to the posterior and lateral parts of the liver. Depending on the anatomical area, and the extent of the liver injury, additional incisions may be required.

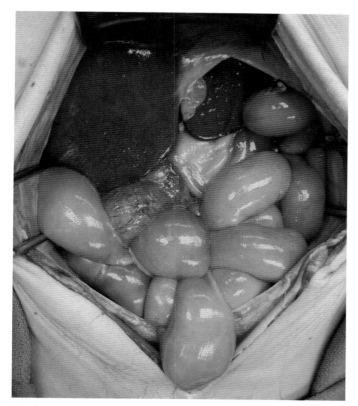

Fig. 24.3. Liver exposure thorough a midline laparotomy. This incision provides limited exposure to the posterior and lateral parts of the liver.

(a)

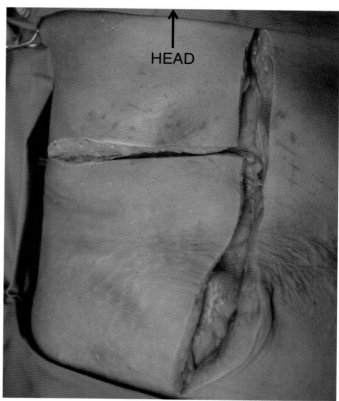

HEAD

Fig. 24.4(a). Right subcostal transverse extension of the midline laparotomy incision allows greater access to the right upper quadrant.

- To obtain better access to posterolateral liver injuries, a right subcostal incision may be required to "T-off" the initial laparotomy.
- A median sternotomy may be required to obtain access to the intrapericardial segment of the inferior vena cava for vascular occlusion of the liver, or to the heart for placement of an atrio-caval shunt.
- If the patient has undergone a right thoracotomy, access to the posterior liver and retrohepatic venous structures can best be obtained by joining the laparotomy to the thoracotomy, and dividing the diaphragm, leaving a cuff so that the diaphragm can be reconstructed.
- If the patient has a severe liver injury best handled by damage control packing, this should be recognized early, and the abdominal wall and ligaments left intact to allow for more effective packing.

(b)

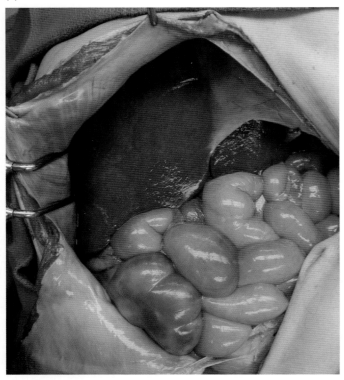

Fig. 24.4(b). Improved exposure of the posterolateral liver through combined midline and right subcostal incisions. For additional exposure, laparotomy pads can be placed between the posterior liver and the diaphragm.

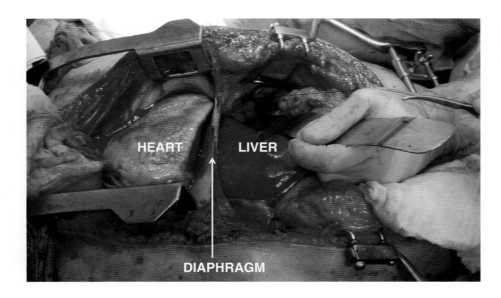

HEART   LIVER

DIAPHRAGM

Fig. 24.5. A median sternotomy may be added to the midline laparotomy in cases requiring access to the intrapericardial segment of the inferior vena cava for vascular occlusion of the liver, or to the heart for placement of an atrio-caval shunt.

Operative techniques

- The first step after entering the peritoneal cavity is to assess the extent of the liver injury, and to examine for other associated injuries.
- Temporary control of liver bleeding may be achieved by finger compression of the liver wound. If this is not effective, cross-clamping of the porta hepatis structures with a vascular clamp through the foramen of Winslow (Pringle maneuver) decreases the vascular inflow to the liver, and reduces bleeding.
  - Insert the index finger of the left hand into the foramen of Winslow and then pinch down with your thumb. This can later be replaced with a non-crushing vascular clamp or a Rummel tourniquet.
  - The duration of time for which the Pringle maneuver may be safely used is unknown, but occlusion up to 30 minutes rarely causes any problems.
  - Failure to control hemorrhage with the Pringle maneuver suggests either aberrant anatomy, or bleeding from the hepatic veins or retrohepatic vena cava.

(a)

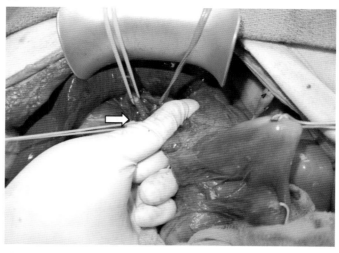

Fig. 24.7(a). Pringle maneuver. The index finger of the left hand is placed into the foramen of Winslow (arrow) and the porta hepatis structures are compressed with the thumb. This can later be replaced with a non-crushing vascular clamp or a Rummel tourniquet (portal vein: blue vessel loop; common bile duct: yellow vessel loop; hepatic artery: red vessel loop).

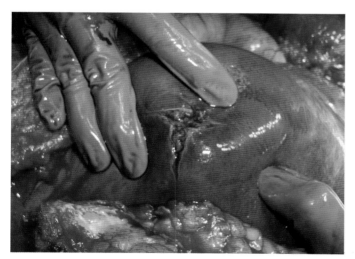

Fig. 24.6. Temporary control of liver bleeding may be achieved by finger compression of the liver wound.

(b)

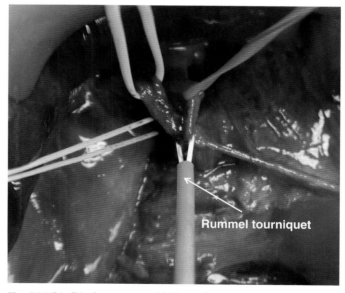

Fig. 24.7(b). Pringle maneuver with Rummel tourniquet around the porta hepatis stuctures (portal vein: blue vessel loop; common bile duct: yellow vessel loop; hepatic artery: red vessel loop).

- Adequate exposure of the liver is critical in the management of severe injuries. The first step is to place three to four laparotomy pads behind the liver, under the diaphragm, and retract the liver anteriorly and inferiorly. If this maneuver does not provide adequate exposure, the next step is mobilization of the liver by taking down the falciform and coronary ligaments. During division of the falciform ligament, care should be taken to avoid injury to the hepatic veins, as the dissection progresses posteriorly. To facilitate this in a rapid fashion, place gentle pressure down on the liver with the falciform

between two of your fingers and sharply divide the avascular ligament.
- Bleeding from deep liver lacerations can often be controlled by direct suture-ligation or clipping of any major bleeders, followed by deep, figure-of-eight, tension-free sutures, using 0-chromic on a large blunt-tip liver needle.

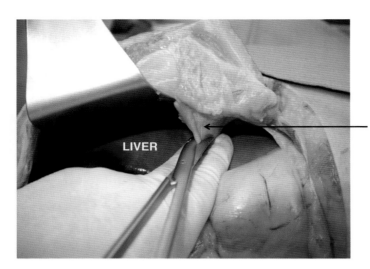

Fig. 24.8. Division of the falciform ligament: place gentle pressure down on the liver with the falciform between two of your fingers and then sharply divide this avascular ligament. Care should be taken to avoid injury to the hepatic veins, as the dissection progresses posteriorly.

———— Falciform ligament

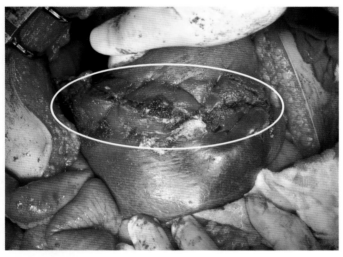

Fig. 24.9. Bleeding control from deep liver laceration with figure-of-eight, tension-free sutures and local hemostatics (circle).

o Concerns regarding intrahepatic abscess or hemobilia resulting from the placement of deep sutures have been overstated. These complications can be managed by percutaneous drainage or angiographic embolization.

o Omental packing of large liver wounds is useful for filling in defects.

• Severe bleeding from deep, bullet or knife tracts in the liver can be controlled with tractotomy and direct bleeding control or with the use of a balloon tamponade.

o Packing of the tract with hemostatic agents or gauze is usually not effective in controlling significant bleeding, but can be tried first.

o Tractotomy may be performed along the tract using sequential firings of a linear stapler, finger fracture techniques, and ligation of vessels and biliary branches, or with an electrothermal bipolar vessel sealing system

(LigaSure device). This technique is most effective for peripherally located tracts.

o For more centrally located tracts, a tractotomy will require the division of a significant volume of normal parenchyma leading to increased tissue at risk of bleeding, especially in coagulopathic patients. An alternative to the tractotomy is a damage control tamponade using a balloon catheter. A Sengstaken and Blakemore tube designed for esophageal varices, a large Foley catheter, or a custom-made balloon from a surgical glove can be used. If a Foley is used, several may be required to fully fill the tract. Once the bleeding is controlled, perihepatic damage control packing is performed. The balloon is kept in place until the patient's physiology has normalized before re-exploration and possible removal. Postoperative angiographic evaluation should be considered.

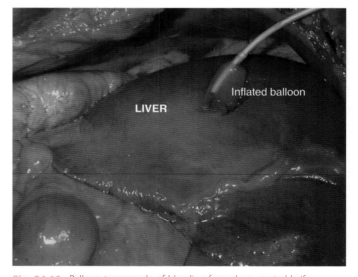

Fig. 24.10. Balloon tamponade of bleeding from deep, central knife wound tract.

- Extensive parenchymal damage, usually due to severe blunt trauma or high-velocity gunshot wounds, is often not amenable to deep suturing. Under these conditions, the bleeding can be addressed with other techniques, including perihepatic packing, liver resection, hepatic artery ligation, total vascular liver isolation, and atrio-caval shunting.

- In patients with compromised physiology and complex injuries not amenable to rapid definitive hemostasis, consider early damage control with perihepatic packing.

  o The technique of the packing is important. The presence of intact hepatic ligaments increases the effectiveness of the tamponade and they should not routinely be divided.

  o Commercially available local hemostatic products can be used if available; however, the mainstay is the use of laparotomy pads.

  o In suspected retrohepatic venous bleeding, the liver should be compressed posteriorly against the IVC, with no packs placed behind the liver.

  o In order to avoid bleeding from the raw surface of the liver during removal of the laparotomy pads at reoperation, an absorbable mesh may be laid over the raw surface of the liver, underneath the packing. The mesh is permanently left in place when the packing is removed.

(b)

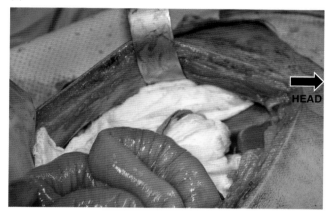

Fig. 24.11(b). Gauze packing over the perihepatic mesh.

  o If packing does not control the bleeding, it is essential to unpack and look for major surgical bleeding. The patient should never leave the operating room if packing does not control the bleeding.

  o Following perihepatic packing, the abdomen should always be left open, using a temporary abdominal wall closure, because of the high risk of development of abdominal compartment syndrome.

  o Early postoperative angiographic evaluation for possible sites of bleeding should be considered in all cases undergoing liver packing. The availability of a hybrid operating room suite facilitates the procedure.

  o The perihepatic packing should be removed as soon as the patient stabilizes physiologically, which usually occurs within 24 to 36 hours.

Non-anatomical liver resection may be needed in cases with devitalized liver parenchyma or persistent bleeding that cannot be controlled with suturing or perihepatic packing. In general, major anatomic hepatic resections are rarely indicated and should be reserved for destructive parenchymal injuries where perihepatic packing is not effective in controlling the hemorrhage.

  o Non-anatomical resections can be performed with finger dissection of the parenchyma, with suture ligation of vessels and biliary branches, or with the use of an electrothermal bipolar vessel sealing system (LigaSure device).

(a)

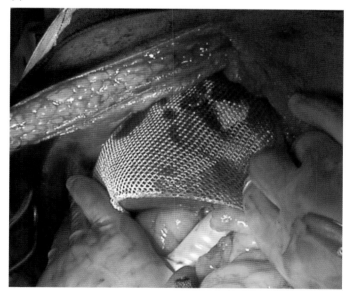

Fig. 24.11(a). Absorbable mesh may be placed over the surface of the liver, under the packing gauze. The mesh is permanently left in place when the packing is removed, after the patient stabilizes. This approach reduces the risk of recurrent bleeding during the gauze removal.

Selective hepatic artery occlusion with a hemostatic clip may be useful in rare cases. The artery should be clipped only if temporary occlusion results in reduction of the bleeding.

  o The combination of hepatic artery ligation, parenchyma injury, and hypotension, often leads to hepatic necrosis.

(a)

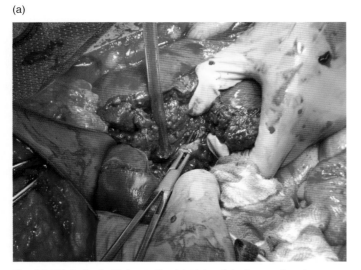

Fig. 24.12(a). Grade 4 injury to the right lobe of the liver, undergoing a non-anatomical resection. Major vessels and bile ducts are individually ligated and divided.

(b)

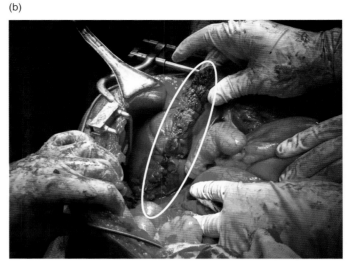

Fig. 24.12(b). Completion of non-anatomical resection of part of the right lobe (circle). The edges may be approximated with interrupted figure-of-eight sutures. Circle demonstrates the cut edge of the resected liver.

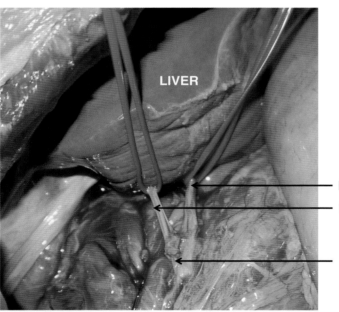

Fig. 24.13. Isolation and ligation or application of a vascular clip on one of the hepatic arteries may be useful in some cases. This approach should be considered only if temporary occlusion of the artery is effective in controlling the bleeding.

LIVER

Left hepatic artery

Right hepatic artery

Common hepatic artery

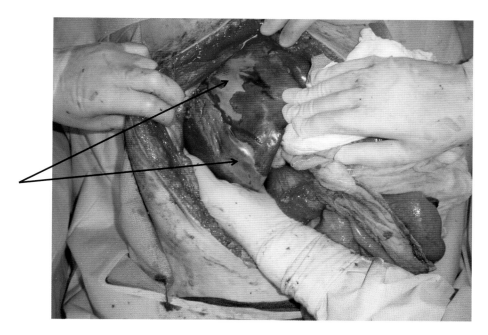

Fig. 24.14. The combination of hepatic artery ligation, parenchyma injury, and hypotension, often leads to hepatic necrosis (arrows).

○ Ligation can also be considered for the rare occasion where there is direct injury to the hepatic artery. Shunting is an alternative damage control option that may be considered, depending on the size and location of injury.

In cases of ineffective perihepatic packing when the injury is not amenable to resection, temporary control of the bleeding can be achieved by using vascular isolation of the liver. This will facilitate visualization and possible repair of the area of bleeding.

○ Vascular isolation consists of cross-clamping the aorta below the diaphragm, the suprahepatic and infraheptic IVC, and the porta hepatis.

○ Clamping the aorta is essential and should be done first in order to prevent hypovolemic cardiac arrest.

○ Suprahepatic cross-clamping of the IVC can be performed by applying a vascular clamp on the IVC, between the diaphragm and the dome of the liver. Practically, however, total hepatic vascular isolation is very rarely necessary because of the increased use of packing and is employed only for very severe injuries, often where the retrohepatic IVC or hepatic veins are injured. In these patients, attempting to place a clamp on the IVC in this location is extremely difficult due to the hematoma and bleeding, and there is a high probability of worsening the injury by clamping here. Control of the intrapericardial IVC through a limited lower sternotomy may be preferable in this situation.

The use of atriocaval shunting may be considered in selected complex retrohepatic venous injuries that cannot be managed by other less aggressive approaches.

(Details of the atriocaval shunt are shown in Chapter 30.)

○ The atriocaval shunt reduces retrohepatic venous bleeding, but does not achieve complete cessation of the bleeding.

○ The experience of the surgical team and the timing of the shunt are critical factors in determining outcome. It should be considered early, before the development of major coagulopathy and severe hypothermia.

Extrahepatic biliary tract injuries

• Most injuries to the gallbladder are best treated by cholecystectomy, although cholecystorrhaphy with absorbable sutures has been recommended for small wounds.

• Injuries to the common bile duct (CBD) are difficult to repair because of the small duct size in young, healthy individuals, and a high incidence of postoperative stenosis can be expected.

○ Complete CBD transection is best managed with a Roux-en-Y biliary enteric anastomosis.

○ Incomplete transection of the CBD may be repaired primarily. Insertion of a T-tube through a separate choledochotomy and repair of the duct injury over the T-tube can reduce the risk of stenosis.

○ In patients presenting in extremis no definitive CBD reconstruction should be attempted. In these cases the CBD can be ligated. Alternatively, a catheter can be placed into the proximal duct and brought out through the skin for external drainage. Reconstruction with a bilioenteric anastomosis is performed after patient stabilization.

Postoperative complications

- The incidence of postoperative liver-related complications in surviving patients with severe liver injuries (grades III to V) has been reported to be as high as 50%.
- These complications include early or late hemorrhage, liver necrosis, liver abscess, biloma, biliary fistula, false aneurysm, arteriovenous fistula, hemobilia, and intrahepatic biliary strictures.
- The timing of clinical presentation of liver-related complications may vary from a few days to many months. Some complications such as biloma, false aneurysm, or arteriovenous fistula may remain asymptomatic only to manifest as potentially life-threatening complications at a later stage.

Tips and pitfalls

- The anatomic division of the liver into the eight classic Couinaud segments is practical in elective liver surgery, but not in trauma.
- For approximately 80%–85% of patients undergoing operation, the liver injury can be managed by relatively simple surgical techniques, such as application of local hemostatic agents, electro-coagulation, superficial suturing, or drainage. The remaining 15%–20% of cases require more complex surgical techniques.
- Exposure of posterolateral liver injuries is difficult through the standard midline laparotomy. Addition of a right subcostal incision, division of the liver ligaments and placement of laparotomy sponges behind the liver, greatly improve the exposure.
- Perihepatic packing and angioembolization are significant surgical advances in the management of complex liver injuries. Consider these options early, before the patient is in extremis.
- For effective packing of suspected retrohepatic venous bleeding, no packs should be placed between the liver and the IVC. The liver should be compressed posteriorly, against the IVC and the hepatic veins.
- Packs placed too tightly may occlude the inferior vena cava and impair venous return leading to hemodynamic instability and kidney dysfunction.
- Stable retrohepatic hematomas should not be explored. In cases with bleeding, if packing is effective, do not pursue further exploration.
- Use closed-suction drains in all complex injuries.

Chapter

25

Splenic injuries

Demetrios Demetriades and Matthew D. Tadlock

Surgical anatomy

- The spleen lies under the ninth to eleventh ribs, under the diaphragm. It is lateral to the stomach and anterosuperior to the left kidney. The tail of the pancreas is in close anatomical proximity to the splenic hilum and amenable to injury during splenectomy or hilar clamping.
- The spleen is held in place by four ligaments, which include the splenophrenic and splenorenal ligaments posterolaterally, the splenogastric ligament medially, and the splenocolic ligament inferiorly. The splenorenal ligament begins at the anterior surface of Gerota's fascia

of the left kidney and extends to the splenic hilum, as a two-layered fold that invests the tail of the pancreas and splenic vessels. The splenophrenic ligament connects the posteromedial part of the spleen to the diaphragm, and the splenocolic ligament connects the inferior pole of the spleen to the splenic flexure of the colon. The splenogastric ligament is the only vascular ligament and contains five to seven short gastric vessels, which originate from the distal splenic artery and enter the greater curvature of the stomach. Excessive retraction of the splenic flexure or the gastrosplenic ligaments can easily tear the splenic capsule and cause troublesome bleeding.

(a)

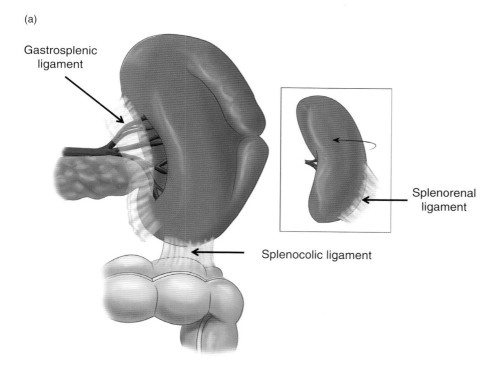

Gastrosplenic ligament

Splenorenal ligament

Splenocolic ligament

Fig. 25.1(a). The spleen is held in place by four ligaments: the splenophrenic and splenorenal ligaments posterolaterally, the splenogastric medially, and the splenocolic inferiorly. Medial rotation of the spleen (inset) exposes the splenophrenic and splenorenal ligaments.

Atlas of Surgical Techniques in Trauma, ed. Demetrios Demetriades, Kenji Inaba, and George Velmahos. Published by Cambridge University Press. © Cambridge University Press 2015.

(b)

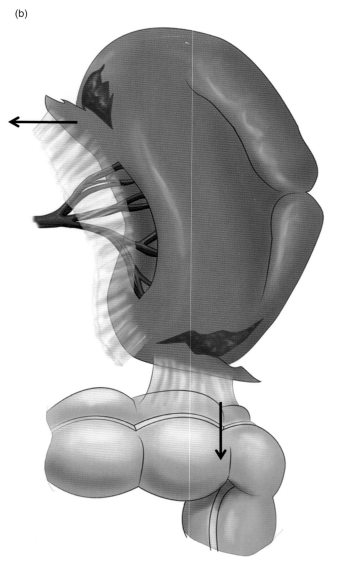

(a)

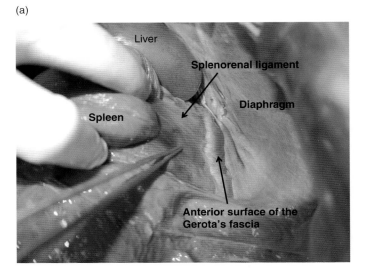

(b)

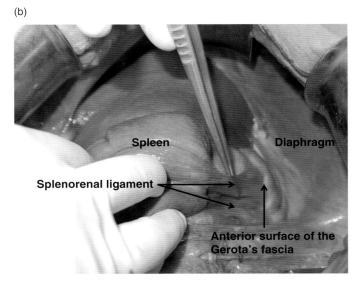

Fig. 25.1(b). Undue traction on the spleen, the stomach, or the colon may cause capsular avulsion and bleeding.

Fig. 25.2(a),(b). Medial rotation of the spleen exposes the splenorenal ligament, which begins at the anterior surface of the Gerota's fascia of the left kidney and extends to the splenic hilum.

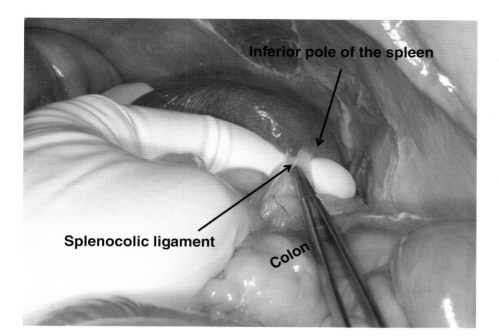

Fig. 25.3. The splenocolic ligament connects the inferior pole of the spleen to the splenic flexure of the colon and is avascular. Excessive traction may cause capsular avulsion and bleeding.

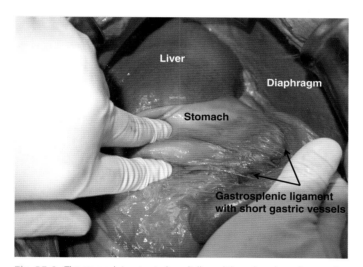

Fig. 25.4. The stomach is retracted medially and the spleen laterally, revealing the gastrosplenic ligament and the short gastric vessels.

- The mobility of the spleen depends on the architecture of these ligaments. In patients with short and well-developed ligaments mobilization is more difficult and requires careful dissection in order to avoid further splenic damage.
- The splenic hilum contains the splenic artery and vein and is often intimately associated with the tail of the pancreas. The extent of the space between the tail of the pancreas and the splenic hilum varies from person to person.
- The splenic artery is a branch of the celiac axis that courses superior to the pancreas towards the splenic hilum where it divides into an upper and lower pole artery. There is significant variability in where this branching occurs.

Most people, approximately 70%, have a distributed or medusa-like branching that occurs 5–10 cm from the spleen. Simple branching occurs in approximately 30%, 1–2 cm from the spleen.

- The splenic vein courses posterior and inferior to the splenic artery, receives the inferior mesenteric vein, and joins the superior mesenteric vein to form the portal vein.

General principles

- The spleen is the second most commonly injured abdominal solid organ after blunt trauma and the second most commonly injured after penetrating trauma.
- Nearly 80% of patients with splenic injury after blunt trauma can be managed non-operatively, but only if they are hemodynamically stable with a stable hemoglobin and without peritonitis. Non-operative management of splenic injuries is ill-advised in patients with a significant injury burden, coagulopathy, or a severe traumatic brain injury.
- Angioembolization is an adjunct to the non-operative management of high-grade splenic injuries, especially in patients with evidence of active extravasation on contrast-enhanced CT scan.
- All patients who undergo emergent splenectomy should receive vaccinations for encapsulated organisms prior to hospital discharge.

Special surgical instruments

- A standard trauma laparotomy tray, which includes vascular instruments.

- A fixed self-retaining retractor such as a Bookwalter retractor is very helpful.
- An electrothermal bipolar vessel sealing system device (LigaSure device) is desirable.
- An absorbable mesh or pre-formed mesh splenic pouch should be available in cases where splenic preservation is to be attempted.

Positioning and incision

- The patient should be placed in the supine position with arms out and prepped from nipples to knees. For trauma, entry into the abdomen should be through a midline incision, starting high, at the xiphoid process.

Exposure

- Upon entry into the peritoneal cavity, the surgeon often encounters a significant amount of blood. The blood should be removed quickly and the left upper quadrant packed with laparotomy pads, to temporarily control the bleeding.
- The next step is full exposure and inspection of the spleen in order to plan the definitive management of the injury. The surgeon should slide his hand gently over the posterolateral surface of the spleen and exert slight medial and downward traction. Three or four laparotomy pads are then placed under the left diaphragm and behind the spleen, providing excellent exposure.
- The surgeon should be gentle during exposure of the spleen because undue traction on the stomach or the splenic

(a)

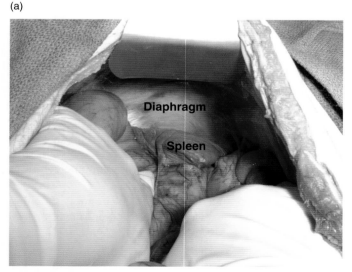

Fig. 25.5(a)–(c). View of the spleen, deep in the left hypochondrium from the right side of the operating room table. Note the deep and posterior position of the spleen, which makes exposure difficult.

(b)

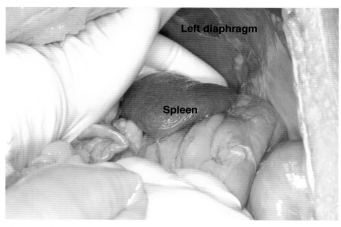

Fig. 25.5(b). With the surgeon's left hand, the spleen is gently rotated medially and downward to facilitate the placement of laparotomy pads.

(c)

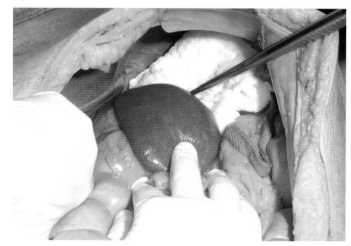

Fig. 25.5(c). Laparotomy pads are placed above and behind the spleen, to keep the spleen in a downward and medial position. Note the significantly improved exposure.

flexure of the colon or excessive medial rotation of the spleen may cause avulsion of the delicate splenic capsule, aggravating the bleeding and decreasing the possibility of splenic preservation.

- Profuse bleeding can temporarily be controlled with digital compression of the hilum between the second and third fingers of the surgeon's left hand or by direct digital compression of the splenic parenchyma. A vascular clamp can also be placed across the hilum, taking care not to injure the tail of the pancreas.
- Mobilization of the spleen is not necessary for simple repairs and in some cases it may worsen the splenic injury.

- In order to facilitate splenectomy or complex splenic preservation operations using splenic mesh or partial splenectomy, the spleen should be adequately mobilized. The first step is division of the splenophrenic and splenorenal ligaments posterolaterally. These ligaments are avascular and can be divided sharply. The next step is the en-bloc medial mobilization of the spleen and the tail of the pancreas. Mobilization of the tail of the pancreas may not be necessary in patients with a short pancreas and a long distance between the tail and the hilum. The next step is division of the vascular gastrosplenic ligament, as far away from the stomach as possible, in order to avoid injury or ischemic necrosis of the gastric wall. The final step is division of the splenocolic ligament. Although this stepped approach for the mobilization of the spleen is applicable to most patients, the surgeon should have in mind that the order of taking down the splenic ligaments should be flexible and determined by the local anatomy, and may vary from patient to patient. For the patient with a partially avulsed spleen that is actively hemorrhaging, rapid hilar vascular control takes precedence over meticulous ligament identification and division.

system such as the LigaSure device may be used as a safe and faster alternative to vessel ligation and division.

- The spleen now is attached only by the splenic vessels, along with the tail of the pancreas, at the hilum.

(a)

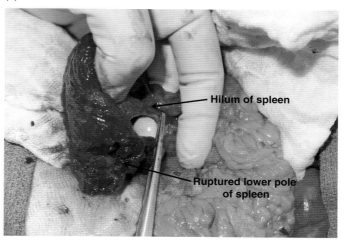

(b)

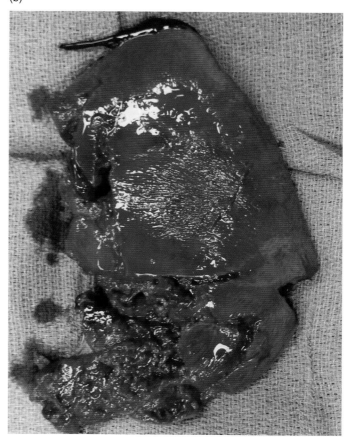

Fig. 25.6. The spleen is mobilized, reflected medially, and the splenic vessels dissected.

- Once adequate exposure is obtained, the salvageability of the spleen is assessed.

Splenectomy

- The first step is adequate mobilization of the spleen and delivery of the spleen towards the midline. Temporary bleeding control and division of the ligaments are performed as described. The short gastric vessels in the gastrosplenic ligament should be ligated away from the stomach, in order to avoid damage or ischemic necrosis of the gastric wall. An electrothermal bipolar vessel sealing

Fig. 25.7(a),(b). After division of the splenic ligaments and medial rotation, the spleen remains attached only by the splenic vessels. Bleeding control is achieved by compressing the hilar structures between the fingers. The vessels are individually ligated and divided (b). Splenectomy specimen (b).

- The splenic artery and vein should be individually ligated as close to the hilum as possible to avoid injuring the pancreas. Use of an electrothermal bipolar vessel sealing system is an alternative to ligation and division of the vessels.
- Occasionally, the splenic hilum and tail of the pancreas are so intimately related that a small portion

of the distal pancreas may need to be resected to safely perform the splenectomy. This can be done with a TA stapling device or an electrothermal bipolar vessel sealing system. In these cases care should be taken to ensure hemostasis of the superior pancreatic artery that runs along the superior portion of the pancreas.

(a)

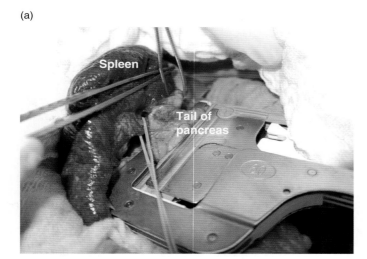

(b)

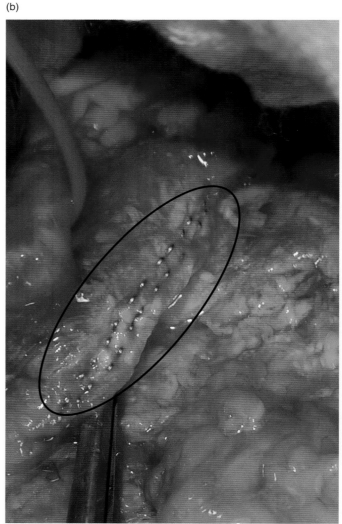

Fig. 25.8(a),(b). Stapled splenectomy technique. Sometimes the tail of the pancreas is so intimately related to the splenic hilum, that it may be necessary to remove a small part of the pancreas with the spleen. A stapled en-masse resection is an effective resection technique. (The splenic artery is shown encircled with a red vessel loop and the splenic vein with a blue vessel loop.) The photo shows medial mobilization of the spleen and pancreas and application of the TA stapler on the tail of the pancreas. Circle shows staple line of the distal pancreas after distal pancreatectomy.

- Mass ligation of the artery and vein together may be considered in unstable patients, although there is concern about the rare complication of arteriovenous fistula.
- After the removal of the spleen, meticulous hemostasis should be performed. The most common sites of incomplete hemostasis are the areas near the tail of the pancreas and the greater curvature of the stomach, at the insertion of the short gastric vessels. The stomach should be inspected for any ischemic damage. Likewise, the tail of the pancreas should also be examined for any iatrogenic injury.
- In a damage control setting, there is no role for spleen preserving operations. The splenic bed is at risk of bleeding and should be packed with several laparotomy pads.
- Although the routine placement of closed suction drains in the splenic bed is a controversial issue, it is advisable to place a closed drain in cases where there is concern about incomplete hemostasis or possible injury to the tail of the pancreas.

(a)

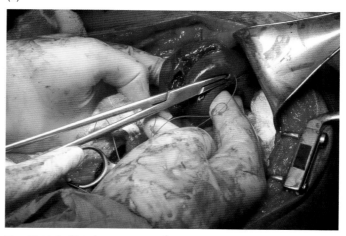

Fig. 25.9(a). Digital compression of the injured spleen by the assistant provides temporary bleeding control, while the surgeon places the sutures.

(b)

Splenorrhaphy

- The size, site, and shape of the splenic injury and the hemodynamic condition of the patient will determine the feasibility of a spleen-preserving operation.
- For capsular avulsions or superficial parenchymal lacerations, there is no need for full splenic mobilization with division of the splenic ligaments. Placement of two to three laparotomy pads behind the spleen usually provides adequate exposure.
- For complex repairs, full mobilization of the spleen, as described above, may be necessary.
- In cases with avulsion of the splenic capsule or minor lacerations, hemostasis can be achieved with local hemostatic agents.
- Superficial lacerations may be repaired with figure-of-eight or horizontal mattress absorbable sutures, on a blunt liver needle. The presence of an intact splenic capsule makes the placement of the sutures technically easier, because it prevents tearing of the parenchyma. If the parenchyma is fragile and does not hold sutures, pledgets may be used.

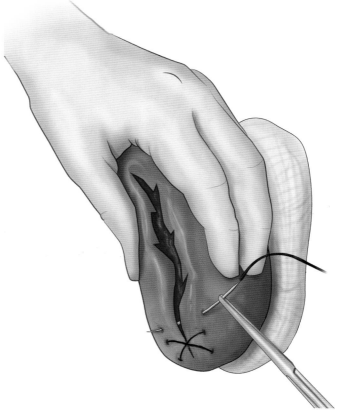

Fig. 25.9(b). Alternatively, the surgeon compresses the spleen with the non-dominant hand and places the sutures with the dominant hand.

o In deep lacerations with active bleeding, temporary control may be achieved by finger compression of the injured site or the hilum. Any major bleeders are suture ligated individually and the laceration is then repaired with interrupted figure-of-eight sutures, as described above. Failure to individually ligate any major bleeders before suturing a deep laceration may result in intrasplenic hematoma or false aneurysm. An omental patch may be sutured into areas with tissue loss.

Partial splenectomy

- A partial splenectomy is possible because of the segmental blood supply of the spleen, with the vessels traveling in a parallel fashion. It should be considered in injuries localized to either the upper or lower pole of the spleen.
- Full splenic mobilization, as described above, is essential before attempting partial splenic resection.
- If the individual vessels to the injured pole can be identified, they should be ligated at the hilum before entering the spleen, for better hemostasis.

(a)

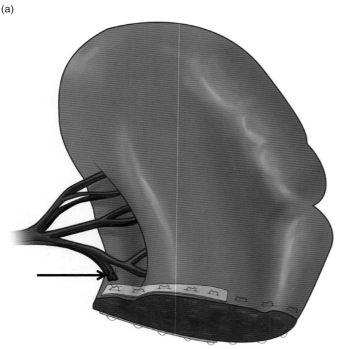

Fig. 25.10(a). Partial splenectomy is a viable option in splenic injuries involving the poles. The procedure may be performed with finger dissection and ligation of individual intrasplenic vessels or electrothermal bipolar vessel sealing system (LigaSure device) or a TA stapling device. Ligation of segmental vessels in the hilum (arrow) reduce bleeding. If there is persistent oozing from the cut edges, vertical mattress sutures may be applied, with or without pledgets.

(b)

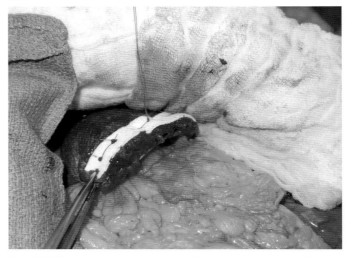

Fig. 25.10(b). Vertical mattress sutures with pledgets may be used for persistent oozing from the cut edge.

- A capsular incision is made with electrocautery, parallel to the lobar arteries. Using blunt finger dissection or fine-tipped suction, the underlying parenchyma of the avascular tissues is divided and individual intrasplenic vessels are identified and ligated with a 3–0 or 4–0 silk. Alternatively an electrothermal bipolar vessel sealing system (LigaSure device) or a TA stapling device may be used.

(a)

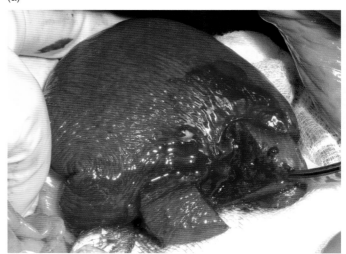

Fig. 25.11(a)–(c). Partial splenectomy of the lower pole with a TA-90 stapler; injury to the inferior pole of the spleen, not amenable to repair (a). Application of TA-90 stapler proximal to the injury's inferior pole (b). Completion of partial splenectomy with complete hemostasis (c).

(b)

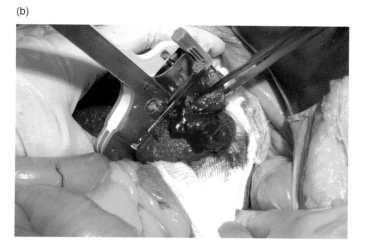

(c)

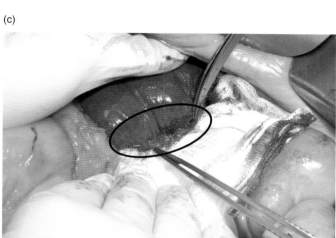

Fig. 25.11(a)–(c). *(cont.)*

- If there is persistent oozing from the cut edges, hemostatic vertical mattress sutures may be applied, with or without pledgets.

Splenic mesh

- An absorbable mesh can also be utilized for splenic salvage, in cases with multiple stellate parenchymal injuries or with extensive avulsion of the splenic capsule.
- Bean-shaped mesh pouches are commercially available, or a mesh wrap can be constructed by the surgeon. Local hemostatic agents may be used as adjuncts to the mesh.

(a)

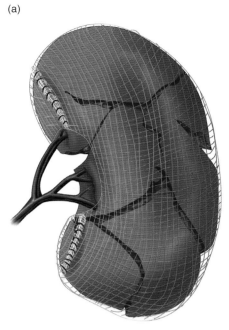

(b)

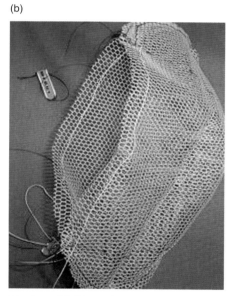

Fig. 25.12(a),(b). Application of a splenic mesh may be a good adjunct in splenic preservation operations, in multiple stellate parenchymal lacerations, or in extensive capsular avulsion (a). Commercially available splenic mesh (b).

Tips and pitfalls

- Non-operative management of severe blunt splenic injuries in patients with traumatic head injury or coagulopathy is generally not recommended.
- Splenic salvage is a reasonable option in stable patients, if the injury is amenable to simple repair, splenic mesh, or partial splenectomy. In unstable or coagulopathic patients, splenectomy is the procedure of choice.
- Full mobilization of the spleen is mandatory before attempting splenorrhaphy of deep or complex lacerations, placement of a splenic mesh, or a partial splenectomy. Mobilization of the spleen improves the exposure, but it has the potential of making the injury worse, if done incorrectly.
- During splenectomy, ligation of the short gastric vessels should be performed close to the spleen to avoid damage to the greater curvature of the stomach. These vessels can be very short and there is little or no space between the stomach and the spleen. In these cases leave a thin rim of splenic tissue distally. If there is concern about damage to the stomach, it is advisable to oversew the area with Lembert sutures.
- During splenectomy, the splenic vessels should be ligated very close to the spleen to avoid injury to the tail of the pancreas. If a rim of pancreatic tissue has to be removed with the spleen, suture-ligate or use an electrothermal bipolar vessel sealing system to prevent pancreatic leaks or bleeding from the superior pancreatic artery.
- The most common sites of persistent postoperative bleeding are the areas near the tail of the pancreas from the superior pancreatic artery and at the insertion of the short gastric vessels into the stomach.
- All severe splenic injuries managed with splenic preservation should undergo a postoperative CT scan with intravenous contrast to rule out false aneurysms or arteriovenous fistulas.
- Remember to vaccinate splenectomy patients for encapsulated organisms prior to discharge.

Chapter

26

Pancreas

Demetrios Demetriades, Emilie Joos, and George Velmahos

Surgical anatomy

- The pancreas lies transversely in the retroperitoneum, at the L_1–L_2 vertebral level, between the duodenum and the hilum of the spleen.
- The head of the pancreas lies over the inferior vena cava (IVC), right renal hilum, and the left renal vein at its junction with the IVC.
- The uncinate process extends to the left and wraps from around the superior mesenteric vessels. It is in close proximity to the inferior pancreaticoduodenal artery.
- The neck of the pancreas lies over the superior mesenteric vessels and the proximal portal vein. The space between the neck and the superior mesenteric vessels is avascular and allows blunt dissection without bleeding. The area to either side of the midline is vascular and should be avoided.
- The body of the pancreas lies over the suprarenal aorta and the left renal vessels. It is intimately related to the splenic artery and vein.
- The major pancreatic duct (Wirsung duct) traverses the entire length of the pancreas and drains into the ampulla of Vater, approximately 8 cm below the pylorus. The lesser duct of Santorini branches off the superior aspect of the major duct, at the level of the neck of the pancreas, and drains separately into the duodenum, approximately 2–3 cm proximal to the ampulla of Vater.
- The pancreas receives its blood supply from both the celiac artery and the superior mesenteric artery.
  - The head of the pancreas and the proximal part of the duodenum receive their blood supply from the anterior and posterior pancreaticoduodenal arcades. These arcades lie on the surface of the pancreas, close to the duodenal loop. Any attempts to separate the two organs result in ischemia of the duodenum.
  - The body and tail of the pancreas receive their blood supply mainly from the splenic artery. The splenic artery originates from the celiac artery and courses to the left, along the superior border of the pancreas. It follows a tortuous route, with parts of it looping above and below the superior border of the pancreas. It gives numerous small and short branches to the body and tail of the pancreas.
  - The splenic vein courses from left to right, superiorly and posteriorly to the upper border of the pancreas, inferiorly to the splenic artery. It is not tortuous like the artery. It joins the superior mesenteric vein, at a right angle, behind the neck of the pancreas, to form the portal vein. The inferior mesenteric vein crosses behind the body of the pancreas and drains into the splenic vein.
- The portal vein is formed by the junction of the superior mesenteric and splenic veins, in front of the inferior vena cava and behind the neck of the pancreas.
- The common bile duct (CBD) courses posterior to the first part of the duodenum, in front of the portal vein, continues behind the head of the pancreas, often partially covered by pancreatic tissue, and drains into the ampulla of Vater, in the second part of the duodenum.

Atlas of Surgical Techniques in Trauma, ed. Demetrios Demetriades, Kenji Inaba, and George Velmahos. Published by Cambridge University Press. © Cambridge University Press 2015.

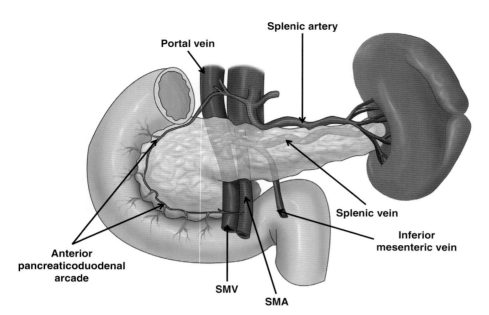

Portal vein

Splenic artery

Anterior pancreaticoduodenal arcade

SMV

SMA

Splenic vein

Inferior mesenteric vein

Fig. 26.1. Surgical anatomy of the pancreas. The head of the pancreas and the proximal part of the duodenum share blood supply from the anterior and posterior pancreaticoduodenal arcades. (SMA = superior mesenteric artery, SMV = SMA = superior mesenteric vein.)

General principles

- The management of pancreatic trauma is determined by the presence or absence of pancreatic duct injury. Patients with pancreatic contusions or lacerations without duct involvement may be managed non-operatively. If these injuries are discovered during the operation, drainage with closed suction drain is usually sufficient. Conversely, almost all patients with pancreatic duct transection require operative management and pancreatic resection.

- The pancreas is surgically divided into a distal and proximal part. The distal pancreas consists of all pancreatic tissue (body and tail) to the left of the superior mesenteric vessels. The proximal pancreas is composed of all pancreatic tissue (head and neck) to the right of the superior mesenteric vessels.

  o In distal pancreatic injuries involving the pancreatic duct, a distal pancreatectomy is the procedure of choice. A spleen-preserving distal pancreatectomy can be considered in stable patients. However, in the presence of severe associated injuries or hemodynamic instability a distal pancreatectomy with splenectomy should be performed because it is a much faster and easier procedure.

  o Distal pancreatectomy rarely results in permanent diabetes or in pancreatic exocrine insufficiency. Hyperglycemia may be observed in the early postoperative period, but it usually resolves spontaneously.

  o For injuries involving the head of the pancreas, if the integrity of the duct cannot be confirmed, pancreatic drainage alone should be considered. Radical resections should be avoided because of the associated high morbidity and mortality.

  o Freeing of the lateral aspect of the head of the pancreas from the duodenum results in ischemia of the duodenum and it should never be considered.

  o Pancreaticoduodenectomy should rarely be considered because of its complexity and the associated high morbidity and mortality. It should be considered primarily in cases with severe combined pancreaticoduodenal trauma.

  o In cases with pancreatic injury selected for non-operative management, evaluation by means of endoscopic retrograde cholangiopancreatography (ERCP) or magnetic resonance cholangiopancreatography (MRCP) is important in order to assess the integrity of the pancreatic duct. In addition, for selected cases, ERCP can be used for therapeutic stent placement.

- Missed pancreatic injuries with ductal involvement may result in complications such as pancreatitis, pancreatic ascites, pancreatic pseudocyst, abscess, or erosion of the adjacent vessels with life-threatening bleeding.

- Pancreatic injuries without ductal involvement rarely cause significant problems and do not require operation.

Special surgical instruments

- Standard exploratory laparotomy tray can be used for this approach.
- Self-retaining Bookwalter or Omni-flex retractor can greatly facilitate surgical exposure.
- Head light.

Positioning

- The patient should be in supine position, with arms abducted at 90 degrees. Preparation and draping should be done in the usual fashion.

Incision

- A standard midline trauma laparotomy incision.

Exposure

- A pancreatic injury should be suspected by the presence of fluid collection or hematoma in the lesser sac, and by fat necrosis of the surrounding tissues.
- Most of the pancreas can be exposed through the lesser sac. The stomach is retracted upward and toward the patient's head and the transverse colon is retracted towards the pelvis. The gastrocolic ligament is divided, starting from the left side where the ligament is usually thin and transparent. An electrothermal bipolar vessel sealing system (LigaSure device) may be used as a safe and rapid alternative to vessel ligation and division. The lesser sac is then entered and any attachments between the pancreas and the posterior wall of the stomach are divided. This approach exposes the anterior, superior, and inferior surfaces of the body and tail of the pancreas.
- The posterior pancreas can be inspected by incising the peritoneum over the inferior border of the pancreas and by gentle upward retraction. In cases where a detailed examination of the posterior distal pancreas is required, the spleen and tail of the pancreas are mobilized and retracted medially en-bloc (see Chapter 25).
- The head and uncinate process of the pancreas can be exposed with an extended Kocher maneuver. The hepatic flexure of the colon is mobilized and retracted medially and inferiorly. The second and third portion of the duodenum comes into view, and the peritoneum over the lateral wall of the duodenum is incised. Using blunt dissection, the second and third part of the duodenum, and the head of the pancreas, are mobilized en-bloc from their retroperitoneal position and rotated to the left. This exposure allows inspection and palpation of the anterior and posterior surfaces of the head and uncinate process.
- In penetrating injuries, associated vascular injuries to the superior mesenteric vessels or the portal vein are common and hemostasis is difficult. In these cases, division of the neck of the pancreas with a stapling device may achieve adequate exposure of the vessels with a stapling device. This can be done by dissecting the avascular plane between the posterior surface of the neck of the pancreas and the portal vein and the superior mesenteric vessels, creating a tunnel to pass the stapler. Care should be taken to stay in the avascular midline to avoid bleeding.
- All peripancreatic hematomas should be explored to evaluate the integrity of the pancreatic duct. However, some surgeons recommend that isolated hematomas in the head of the pancreas with no associated injuries may be left undisturbed, because the duct in this area is deep in the parenchyma and the surgical management if undertaken, would include major resections, such as pancreaticoduodenectomy. These patients should be evaluated postoperatively using MRCP or ERCP. In cases with ductal injury, an ERCP-placed stent should be considered.
- Normal size pancreatic ducts may be difficult to visualize. The use of magnifying glasses and administration of secretin may facilitate visualization of smaller ductal injuries.
- Radiological and endoscopic methods of intraoperative pancreatography are rarely used in trauma.

(a)

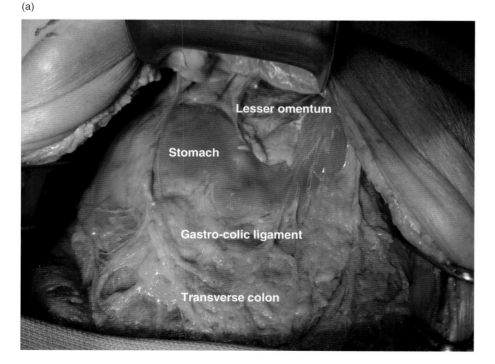

Fig. 26.2(a). Most of the pancreas can be exposed through the lesser sac, by dividing the gastrocolic ligament.

(b)

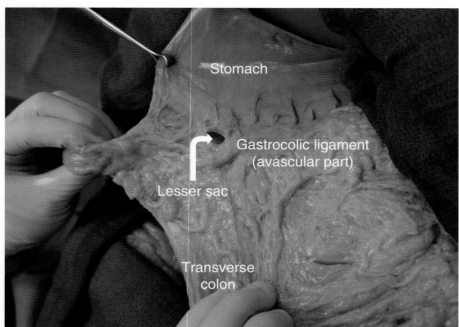

Fig. 26.2(b). Opening of the lesser sac: the stomach is retracted upward and toward the patient's head and the transverse colon is retracted toward the pelvis. The gastrocolic ligament is divided, starting from the left side where the ligament is usually thin and transparent.

(a)

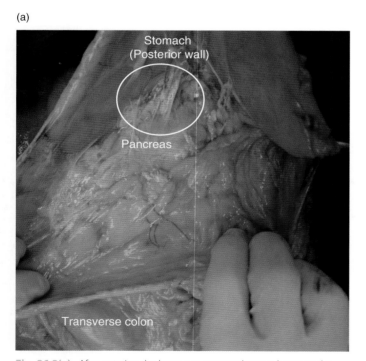

Fig. 26.3(a). After entering the lesser sac, any attachments between the pancreas and the posterior wall of the stomach (circle) are divided.

(b)

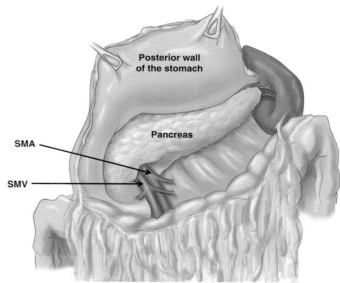

Fig. 26.3(b). Complete exposure of the body and tail of the pancreas, after opening the lesser sac and dividing any attachments between the posterior wall of the stomach and the pancreas (SMA = superior mesenteric artery, SMV = superior mesenteric vein.)

(a)

(b)

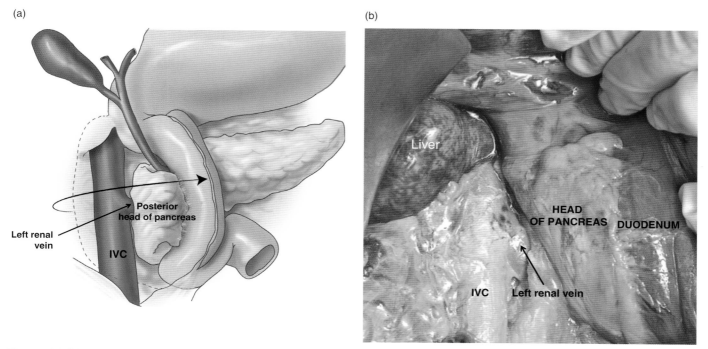

Fig. 26.4(a),(b). Kocher maneuver: the posterior aspect of the head of the pancreas is exposed after medial rotation of the second portion of the duodenum. The IVC and left renal vein are directly under the head of the pancreas.

(a)

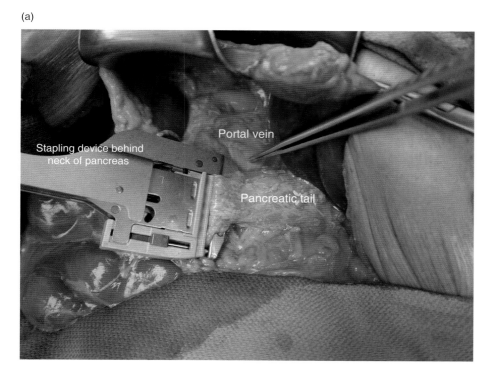

Fig. 26.5(a). Exposure of the superior mesenteric vessels and the portal vein: division of the neck of the pancreas with a stapling device. The stapling device should be placed in the avascular plane between the posterior surface of the neck of the pancreas and the portal vein and the superior mesenteric vessels.

(b)

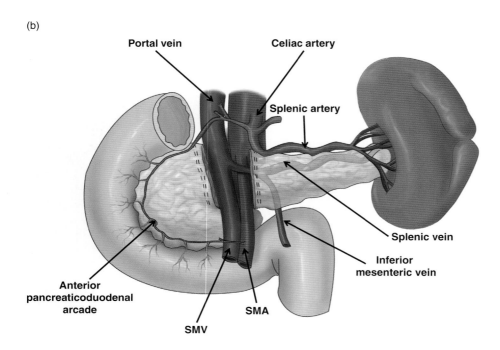

Portal vein

Celiac artery

Splenic artery

Splenic vein

Inferior mesenteric vein

Anterior pancreaticoduodenal arcade

SMA

SMV

Fig. 26.5(b). Exposure of the superior mesenteric vessels and the portal vein after division of the neck of the pancreas with a stapling device.

Management of pancreatic injuries

- Low-grade injuries without ductal injury are best managed with conservative debridement of non-viable tissue, hemostasis, and external drainage with closed suction drains. Repair of the pancreatic capsule is possible, although it is controversial because of concerns about increased risk of pseudocyst formation. Diffuse bleeding may be managed with application of topical hemostatics and tissue glue.
- High-grade injuries with ductal involvement or associated severe duodenal injuries require more complex procedures. The choice of procedure depends on the hemodynamic condition of the patient, the site of the pancreatic injury (head and neck versus tail of the pancreas), and the experience of the surgeon.

- Pancreatic injuries to the left of the superior mesenteric vessels are best treated by distal pancreatectomy, often en-bloc with the spleen. The first step is to mobilize the body or tail of the pancreas, starting at the point of the injury. The peritoneum at the inferior border of the pancreas is incised and the plane behind the pancreas is developed using blunt dissection, taking care to avoid injury to the splenic vessels, which are near the superior border and behind the pancreas. A vessel loop is then placed around the pancreas. The resection of the pancreas is performed just proximal to the injury, through healthy tissues, using a GIA or TA stapling device (see Fig. 26.5 a,b). If the proximal end of the pancreatic duct is visible, it should be suture ligated with figure-of-eight non-absorbable sutures. The splenic artery and vein are then individually suture ligated with figure-of-eight sutures. The pancreatectomy is

(a)

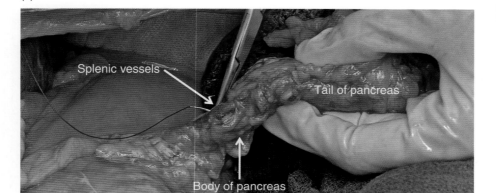

Splenic vessels

Tail of pancreas

Body of pancreas

Fig. 26.6(a). Technique of distal pancreatectomy: after mobilization of the tail, the splenic artery and vein are individually suture-ligated.

(b)

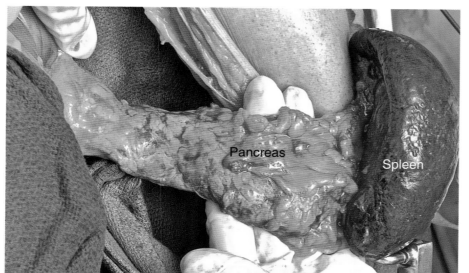

Fig. 26.6(b). Mobilization of the pancreatic tail and the spleen.

(a)

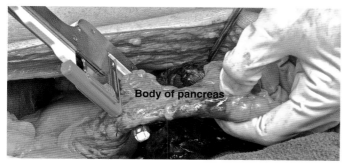

(b)

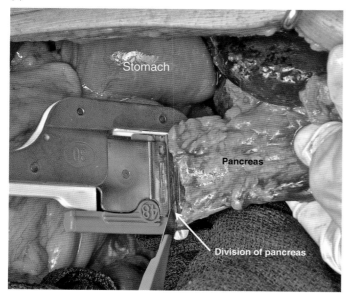

(c)

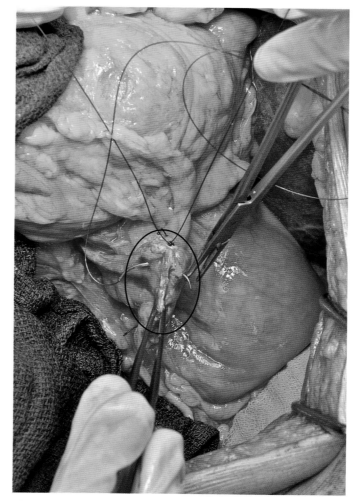

Fig. 26.7(a),(b). Placement of TA stapling device and division of the body of the pancreas.

Fig. 26.7(c). The pancreatic stump is oversewn (circle) with non-absorbable sutures.

(d)

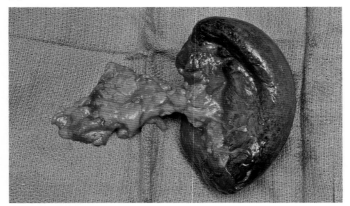

Fig. 26.7(d). En-bloc distal pancreatectomy and splenectomy.

completed by mobilizing the pancreas distally towards the spleen. After the dissection reaches the hilum of the spleen, the spleen is mobilized by dividing the vascular gastrosplenic ligament first, followed by division of the splenocolic, splenorenal, and splenodiaphragmatic ligaments (see Chapter 25). An alternative aproach for distal pancreatectomy is to start with mobilization of the spleen, en-bloc medial rotation of the spleen with the tail of the pancreas and a stapled resection proximal to the site of injury.

- Distal pancreatectomy with splenic preservation may be considered in selected hemodynamically stable patients, especially in children. The peritoneum is incised at the inferior border of the pancreas, near the area of the injury, and the surgeon dissects the plane behind the pancreas with the index finger or a right-angle forceps. A vessel loop is applied around the pancreas and the splenic artery and vein are dissected free, taking care to clip or ligate and divide the numerous small branches to the pancreatic parenchyma. When the dissection reaches the splenic hilum, the pancreas is removed.

- Pancreatic resection extending to the right of the neck may lead to diabetes and exocrine insufficiency. Preservation of at least 1 cm of pancreatic tissue from the duodenal wall is important in order to maintain the blood supply to the duodenum and avoid ischemic necrosis. In these cases, after debridement of any damaged tissue, the distal pancreas may be preserved and anastomosed to a Roux-en-Y jejunal loop, using an end-to-end pancreaticojejunostomy. Closed suction drains should always be placed.

- Injuries to the head of the pancreas may require complex operations associated with high mortality and morbidity. In the presence of hemodynamic instability or major associated injuries, or if the surgeon has no experience with these injuries, the safest option is hemostasis and liberal external drainage. Damage control with packing and temporary abdominal closure may be necessary in cases with difficult, persistent bleeding.

(a)

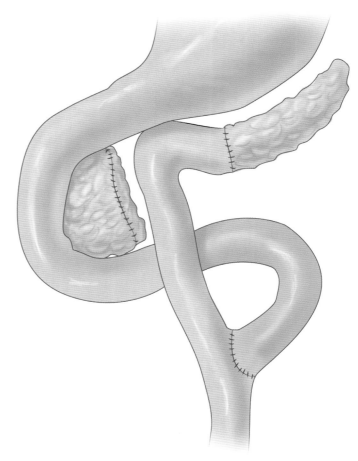

Fig. 26.8(a). Oversewn proximal pancreatic stump and distal Roux-en-Y end-to-end pancreaticojejunostomy.

(b)

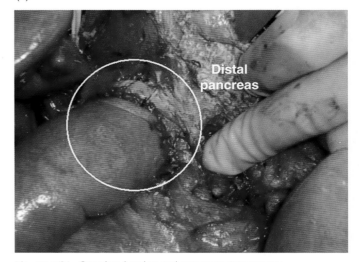

Fig. 26.8(b). Completed end-to-end pancreaticojejunostomy.

- In destructive injuries to the head of the pancreas or the duodenum, a pancreaticoduodenectomy may be necessary. It should only be performed as a primary procedure in hemodynamically stable patients by an experienced surgeon. In coagulopathic or physiologically compromised patients the surgeon should opt for damage control and a two-stage procedure. At the initial operation, damage control surgery should be performed to control the hemorrhage and any intestinal spillage. The definitive Whipple's pancreaticoduodenectomy should be deferred for 24 to 48 hours after restoration of hemodynamic stability, and after correction of any coagulopathy and hypothermia. The reconstruction, including pancreaticojejunostomy, choledochojejunostomy, and gastroenterostomy, is similar to that in elective cases and will not be discussed in the current Atlas.
- Insertion of a jejunal feeding tube beyond the ligament of Treitz is recommended in cases undergoing pancreaticoduodenectomy or complex duodenal repairs, in order to allow enteral nutrition in cases with postoperative anastomotic leaks.

Tips and pitfalls

- Pancreatic injuries without ductal involvement rarely cause significant problems and do not require an operation.
- Distal pancreatectomy (to the left of the neck of the pancreas) rarely results in permanent diabetes or pancreatic exocrine insufficiency.
- Mobilization and separation of the head of the pancreas from the medial aspect of the duodenal loop results in duodenal ischemia and necrosis. A minimum of 1 cm of pancreatic tissue should be left behind in order to preserve the pancreaticoduodenal vascular arcades.
- In isolated injuries involving the head of the pancreas, if the integrity of the duct cannot be confirmed, pancreatic drainage alone should be considered. Radical resections should be avoided because of the high mortality and morbidity. The pancreatic duct should be evaluated postoperatively by means of MRCP or ERCP. In cases with ductal injury, ERCP-placed stenting may be considered.
- During tunneling between the neck of the pancreas and the superior mesenteric vessels and portal vein, stay in the midline, directly under the neck. This area is avascular.

Urological trauma

Charles Best and Stephen Varga

Surgical anatomy

Kidney

- Both kidneys have similar muscular surroundings. Posteriorly, the diaphragm covers the upper third of each kidney. Medially, the lower two-thirds of the kidney lie against the psoas muscle, and laterally, the quadratus lumborum.
- The right kidney borders the duodenum medially. Its lower pole lies behind the hepatic flexure of the colon.
- The left kidney is bordered superiorly by the tail of the pancreas, the spleen superolaterally, and the splenic flexure of the colon inferiorly.
- Gerota's fascia encloses the kidney and is an effective barrier for containing blood or a urine leak.
- The renal artery and vein travel from the aorta and IVC just below the SMA at the level of the second lumbar vertebra. The vein lies anterior to the artery. The renal pelvis and ureter are located posterior to the vessels.
- The right renal artery takes off from the aorta with a downward slope under the IVC into the right kidney. The left renal artery courses directly off the aorta into the left kidney. Each renal artery branches into five segmental arteries as it approaches the kidney.
- The right renal vein is typically 2–4 cm in length, does not receive any branches and enters into the lateral edge of the IVC. Ligation of the vein causes hemorrhagic infarction of the kidney because of the lack of collaterals.
- The left renal vein is typically 6–10 cm in length, passes posterior to the SMA and anterior to the aorta. The left renal vein receives branches from the left adrenal vein superiorly, lumbar veins posteriorly, and the left gonadal vein inferiorly. This allows for ligation of the left renal vein proximal to the kidney close to the IVC.

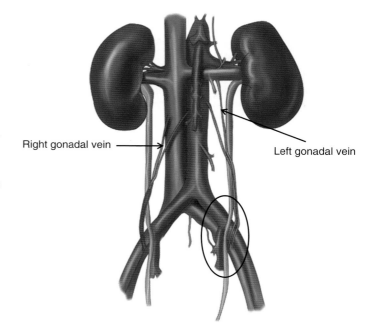

Right gonadal vein

Left gonadal vein

Fig. 27.1. Anatomy of the kidneys and ureters and their relationship with the major vessels. Note the right renal artery coursing under the inferior vena cava. The ureters cross over the bifurcation of the common iliac arteries (circle).

Ureter

- The ureter courses posterior to the renal artery and travels along the anterior edge of the psoas muscle.
- The gonadal vessels cross anterior to the ureter.
- The ureter crosses over the bifurcation of the common iliac artery.

Atlas of Surgical Techniques in Trauma, ed. Demetrios Demetriades, Kenji Inaba, and George Velmahos. Published by Cambridge University Press. © Cambridge University Press 2015.

Bladder

- The superior surface of the bladder is covered by peritoneum. Posteriorly, the peritoneum passes to the level of the seminal vesicles (in males) and meets the peritoneum on the anterior rectum.
- The bladder neck rests approximately 3–4 cm behind the midpoint of the symphysis pubis.

Kidney injuries

General principles

- In hemodynamically stable patients the vast majority of blunt and a significant proportion of penetrating renal injuries can be managed non-operatively. Gerota's fascia effectively contains bleeding and urine leaks. CT scan evaluation is important in assessing the severity and location of the injury. The addition of a delayed CT scan allows for the evaluation of the collecting system and proximal ureter.
- If no pre-operative imaging is available and the patient is undergoing exploratory laparotomy, it is important to assess by palpation the presence and size of the contralateral kidney.
- Intraoperatively, in a hemodynamically stable patient, in the absence of active bleeding or expanding hematoma or injury to the hilar vessels, Gerota's fascia should not be opened as it increases the probability of nephrectomy.
- Nephrectomy should be reserved for life-threatening hemorrhage or renal injuries that are beyond repair: approximately 10% of renal injuries. Uncontrolled hemorrhage is the most common reason for unplanned nephrectomy in a trauma setting.
- If time allows, proximal vascular pedicle control should be considered before kidney exploration, in order to reduce the need for nephrectomy.

Patient positioning

- The patient is placed in the standard trauma laparotomy position supine with both arms abducted at 90 degrees to allow access to the extremities.

Incision

- Standard midline trauma laparotomy incision. A Bookwalter or other fixed abdominal retractor facilitates the exposure.

Kidney exposure

- Proximal vascular control, before opening the Gerota's fascia, may be considered in stable patients if a kidney-preserving operation is planned. This approach increases the chances of kidney salvage.

- In unstable patients or in those undergoing a planned nephrectomy, a direct approach through Gerota's fascia without prior vascular control is faster and preferable.

Proximal renal vascular control

- Proximal control of both the left and right renal vessels can be obtained directly through a single incision of the retroperitoneum over the abdominal aorta.

  o The transverse colon is retracted anteriorly and superiorly, towards the patient's chest. The small intestine is wrapped in a moist towel and retracted superiorly and to the right to expose the ligament of Treitz, the root of the mesentery, and the underlying great vessels.

  o An incision is made in the posterior peritoneum, over the aorta, just above the inferior mesenteric vein. The dissection continues superiorly along the aorta until the left renal vein is identified, crossing over anteriorly. A vessel loop is placed around the vein for retraction. Once the left renal vein is mobilized and retracted, dissect out the left renal artery, which is located posterior to the renal vein.

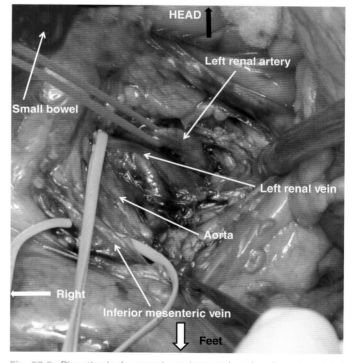

Fig. 27.2. Dissection in the posterior peritoneum lateral to the aorta and just above the inferior mesenteric vein, and continuing superiorly along the aorta, will identify the left renal vein crossing the aorta anteriorly. The left renal artery is located posterior to the vein.

- After vascular control has been achieved, a medial visceral rotation is performed by mobilizing the left colon along the white line of Toldt and reflecting the colon medially. The kidney is then exposed by making an anterior vertical incision in Gerota's fascia.

(a)

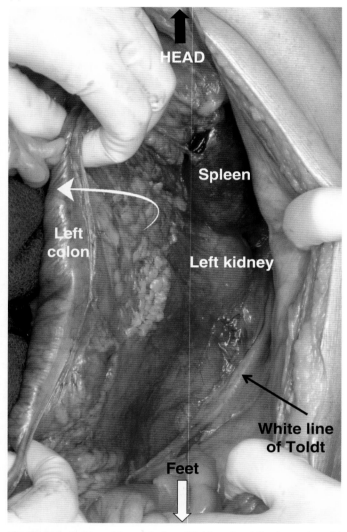

Fig. 27.3(a). Incision of the white line of Toldt, and mobilization and medial rotation of the left colon, exposes the left kidney.

(b)

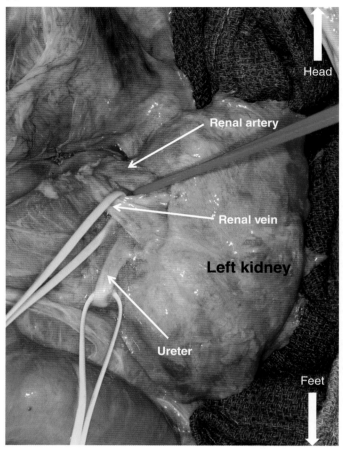

Fig. 27.3(b). Exposure of the left kidney and the hilum after medial rotation of the left colon (artery in red, vein in blue and ureter in yellow loop).

(c)

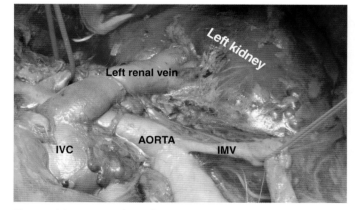

Fig. 27.3(c). Exposure of the left kidney and the hilum after medial rotation of the left colon. Note the left renal vein crossing over the aorta. (IVC: inferior vena cava, IMV: inferior mesenteric vein.)

- The right renal vessels can be exposed through the same posterior peritoneal incision, described above. The right renal artery originates from the right side of the aorta and courses under the inferior vena cava and behind the renal vein.

- As described above, the left renal vein is mobilized and retracted as it crosses over the aorta. The right renal artery, which is located posterior to the vein and to the right of the aorta, is identified.
- Finally, identify the right renal vein traveling to the inferior vena cava and control with a vessel loop.
- After vascular control has been achieved, perform a right medial visceral rotation, mobilizing the right colon by incising the white line of Toldt and reflecting it medially.
- Explore the right kidney by making an anterior vertical incision in Gerota's fascia. Completely expose the kidney, mobilizing it and lifting it anteriorly into the wound.

(a)

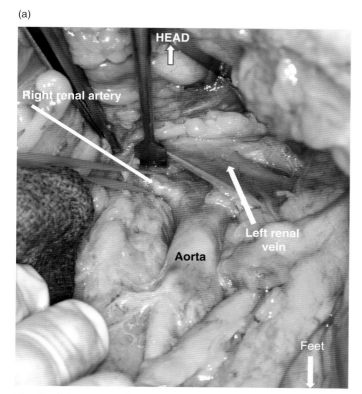

Fig. 27.4(a). Exposure of the right renal vessels through a midline retroperitoneal dissection. The left renal vein is identified as it crosses over the aorta and is retracted to expose the underlying right renal artery (red loop).

Direct kidney exposure without prior vascular control

- This is a common approach to the kidney and the preferred approach in patients with hemodynamic instability or unsalvageable renal injuries.
- A medial visceral rotation is performed by mobilizing the left or right colon, after incising the white line of Toldt.
- Gerota's fascia is opened with an anterior vertical incision and the kidney is exposed and delivered anteriorly.
- The blood supply and ureter can then be controlled.

(b)

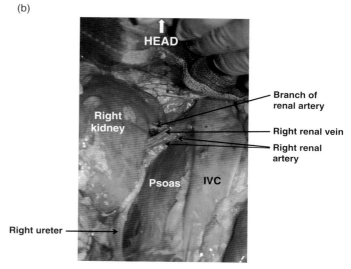

Fig. 27.4(b). Exposure of the right kidney and the hilum after medial rotation of the right colon. Note the renal vein anteriorly, the artery posteriorly and the ureter inferiorly.

Renal injury repair

- After opening Gerota's fascia and exposing the kidney, the extent of the injury is assessed. In cases with significant bleeding from the parenchyma, the renal vessels are clamped for bleeding control. Manual compression of the bleeding parenchyma is often adequate for temporary control of the hemorrhage. Any significant bleeders are controlled by suture ligation or by electrocautery.
- Once hemorrhage is controlled, any devitalized tissue is sharply excised. The collecting system is carefully examined and any injury is repaired watertight with a 4–0 absorbable suture.

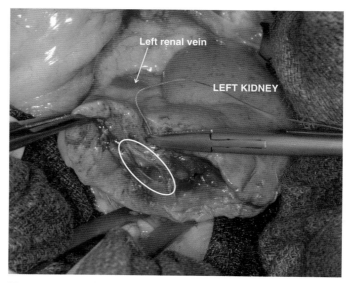

Fig. 27.5. Repair of injury to the collecting system (circle), of the lower pole of the left kidney, with 4–0 absorbable suture.

- If unsure of the presence of a collecting system injury or to check if the collecting system repair is watertight, methylene blue can be used to look for a leak. Place a bulldog clamp on the proximal ureter and, using a 22-gauge or smaller butterfly needle, directly inject 2 to 3 mL methylene blue into the renal pelvis to look for further leaks or injury. If identified, close the leaks or repair the injury with figure-of-eight, 4–0 absorbable sutures.

(a)

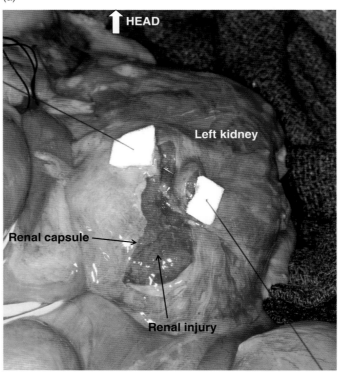

Fig. 27.7(a). Suturing of pledgets on intact renal capsule edges, for primary repair of injury.

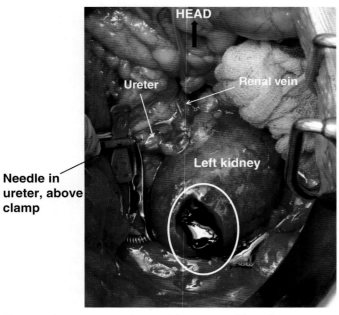

Fig. 27.6. Intraoperative evaluation of the integrity of the collecting system: insertion of a 22-gauge needle into the proximal ureter, with bulldog clamp applied distally, and injection of 2–3 mL of methylene blue into the renal pelvis. Extravasation of the methylene blue (circle) confirms injury to the collective system.

- If possible, the renal capsule should be primarily closed, without tension, using pledgets.
- If the defect in the capsule is large, an omental pedicle flap, fibrin sealant, or thrombin-soaked GelFoam bolsters can be used to fill the defect. The capsule should then be closed over the bolster or flap with pledgeted 4–0 polypropylene sutures.
- If other intra-abdominal injuries are present, an omental interposition flap should be placed over the renal injury to separate the kidney from the other injuries.
- A retroperitoneal drain should be placed at the end of the operation.

Partial nephrectomy

- Extensive damage to the upper or lower poles of the kidney requires partial nephrectomy rather than primary repair.

First, attempt to dissect the capsule off the damaged parenchyma for assistance with closure later.

- Perform a guillotine transection of the renal parenchyma back to healthy bleeding tissue. Control small bleeding vessels with figure-of-eight 4–0 absorbable sutures, and close the collecting system in a watertight fashion with a 4–0 absorbable suture. Topical hemostatics may be placed on the renal parenchyma to aid in hemostasis.
- If the renal capsule has been preserved, close the capsule over the raw surface of the kidney with a 3–0 polypropylene or vicryl suture with or without pledgets. If the capsule could not be preserved or if the injury is too extensive to cover completely, the defect can be covered by an omental flap or absorbable material such as GelFoam, which can be sutured to the remaining renal capsule with 3–0 polypropylene or vicryl sutures.
- A retroperitoneal drain should be placed at the end of the operation.

Nephrectomy

- If the injury to the kidney is too extensive for repair, a nephrectomy is warranted. If the patient is unstable, and the kidney is the source of hemorrhage, likewise nephrectomy is warranted. No preliminary vascular isolation is needed. After medial visceral rotation, Gerota's

(b)

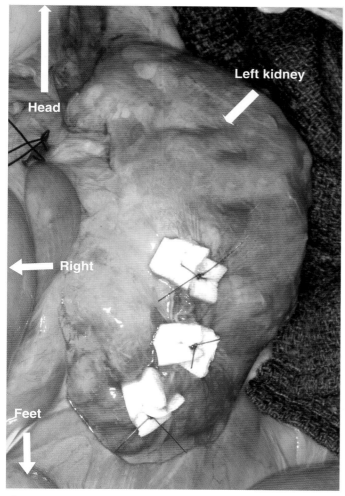

Fig. 27.7(b). Definitive, tension-free, repair of left kidney injury using pledgets.

fascia is opened and the kidney is delivered anteriorly. Digital compression of the hilum is applied to control the bleeding. Ligate the artery and the vein, near the kidney hilum, with 0 silk ties. The ureter should be identified and ligated with a 2–0 silk tie.

Tips and pitfalls

- Failure to identify a collecting system injury or failure to perform a watertight closure of the collecting system may result in a urinoma postoperatively.
- Parenchymal tissue typically will not hold a suture, so capsular tissue approximation should be used.
- During debridement or partial nephrectomy, preserve as much renal capsule as possible for repair or cover of the raw surface.
- Attempting to close the capsule primarily over a large defect will cause tearing of the capsule and further bleeding

(a)

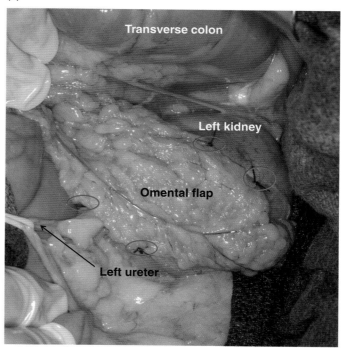

Fig. 27.8(a). Omental pedicle flap may be used to fill in large parenchymal defects, not amenable to primary repair. The flap is anchored to the capsule with sutures (red circles).

(b)

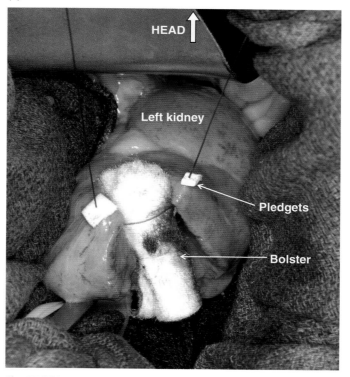

Fig. 27.8(b). Hemostatic bolster used to repair a large defect that cannot be closed primarily without tension with closure of the capsule over the bolster.

(a)

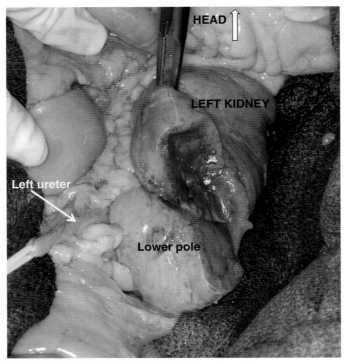

Fig. 27.9(a). Extensive damage to the lower poles of the kidney is best managed with partial nephrectomy.

(b)

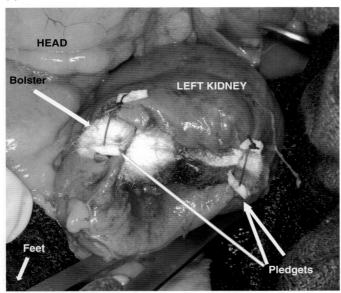

Fig. 27.9(b). Partial lower pole nephrectomy with the raw surface covered with absorbable materials such as GelFoam, which can be sutured to the remaining renal capsule.

(c)

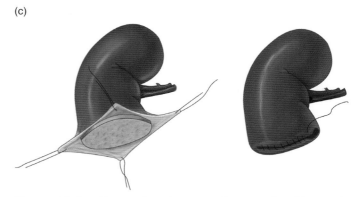

Fig. 27.9(c). Partial lower pole nephrectomy with preservation of the capsule: the capsule can close over the raw surface of the kidney.

or injury. Omentum or GelFoam can be utilized to cover the bare area.

- Postoperative urine leak increases the risk of breakdown of any adjacent hollow viscus or vascular anastomosis or repair. Separate the renal repair from other organ injuries with omentum or other available tissue. Routine closed suction drains should be placed.

Postoperative care

- Patients who have undergone kidney repair should be followed with periodic urinalysis, blood pressure monitoring, and CT scan with intravenous contrast, in order to rule out early or late complications such as a urinoma, kidney infarct, false aneurysm, arteriovenous fistula, or secondary hypertension.
- Urinomas are the most common complication, and they can be managed by endoscopic stenting with or without percutaneous drainage.
- False aneurysms, or arteriovenous fistulas can be managed by angioembolization.
- Hypertension can be managed medically, but if medical management fails, a delayed nephrectomy may be indicated.

Ureter injury

General principles

- Early recognition and treatment of ureteral injuries is important because failure to recognize these injuries can result in loss of renal function, sepsis, or death.
- In patients undergoing laparotomy for penetrating trauma, all retroperitoneal hematomas should be explored and the ureter examined for any injury. The ureter can be inspected with or without the use of intravenous or intraureteral dye.

- The ureter can be divided into three separate anatomical areas when considering repair, including the proximal, mid and distal ureter. The proximal ureter is the segment above the iliac bifurcation. The mid ureter is the segment between the iliac bifurcation and the deep pelvis. The distal ureter is defined as the segment of ureter below the internal iliac artery. Each of these anatomic areas requires a different type of repair.
- The type of ureteral repair depends on the level of the injury, the amount of ureteral loss, and the condition of the patient. The general principles for all ureteral repairs are debridement to healthy tissue with a tension-free watertight repair over a stent.
- In severe trauma the patient may not be stable enough to undergo extensive ureteral repair during the initial operation. In these cases a damage control procedure should be considered. If a ureteral transection is identified, the proximal and distal ends of the ureter can be ligated and tagged and left in place to be repaired semi-electively after the patient has stabilized. Alternatively, an external stent can be placed in the proximal ureter and brought out through the abdominal wall through a separate stab incision in the abdomen to allow for monitoring of urine output during resuscitation. Immediate diversion is not necessary, as the affected kidney can tolerate complete obstruction for several days until a definitive repair can be performed. If repair will be significantly delayed for clinical reasons, a percutaneous nephrostomy tube should be considered.

Repair of the proximal and mid ureter

- Explore the retroperitoneum by performing a medial visceral rotation, mobilizing the ipsilateral colon by incising the white line of Toldt and reflecting it medially.
- Identify the ureter and trace it proximally and distally to examine the extent of injury.

- The injured part of the ureter should be debrided to viable tissue.
- Take care not to injure or devitalize the ureter.
- The ureter is mobilized to allow the proximal and distal ends to come together without tension.
- Spatulate the ends of the ureter to prevent stenosis at the suture line.
- Place an indwelling double-J-type stent into the proximal and distal ends of the ureter.
- Perform a tension-free, mucosa-to-mucosa anastomosis using an interrupted 4–0 or 5–0 absorbable suture.
- Place a retroperitoneal drain near the repair site. In the case of bowel or pancreatic injuries in addition to ureteral injuries, every attempt should be made to isolate the ureteral repair from the other injuries by covering it with an omental flap or local tissue.

Repair of the distal ureter

- Distal ureter injuries usually occur in the setting of a pelvic hematoma, making the dissection difficult. If an injury is identified, direct re-implantation of the distal ureter into the bladder is preferable if it can be performed tension-free. This should be done in an anti-refluxing fashion if possible over a stent.
- Although anti-refluxing is not crucial in the adult patient, an attempt should be made to perform an anti-refluxing tunnel with an extravesical reimplant if a psoas hitch is not required. Once the ureter has been adequately mobilized, a tunnel is created in the posterolateral dome, by dissecting off the detrusor muscle, leaving small muscle flaps on either side. A hole can be made in the bladder mucosa at the apex of this trough, and the spatulated ureteral end can be anastomosed over a stent with interrupted 4–0 vicryl suture. The muscle flaps are then laid over the ureter in this trough, and secured with 3–0 vicryl absorbable suture.

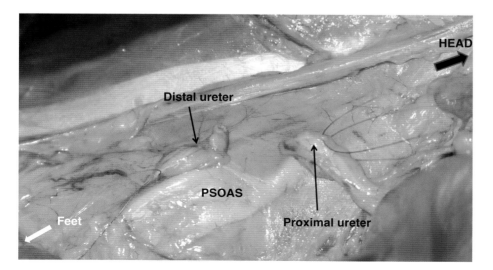

Fig. 27.10. Ureter transection sharply debrided to healthy tissue prior to anastomosis.

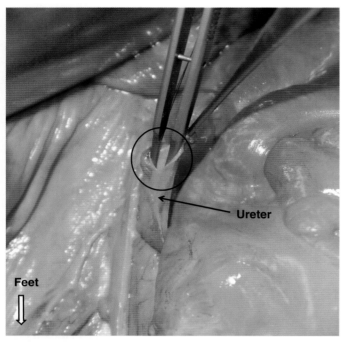

Fig. 27.11. Spatulated end (circle) of the transected ureter.

- If the distal anastomosis cannot be performed tension-free, the bladder may be mobilized to the transected ureter to perform a "psoas hitch." The bladder is opened vertically

and obliquely toward the side of the injury. The lateral peritoneal attachments are then divided as needed for mobilization. The bladder body can then be displaced towards the side of the injury and sutured to the psoas muscle with a 2–0 non-absorbable suture. The distal ureter can then be re-implanted into the bladder using a tunneled anti-reflux anastomosis with a stent. The bladder is then closed in two layers with a 2–0 or a 3–0 absorbable suture.

- If there are adjacent vascular or visceral repairs, every attempt should be made to isolate the ureteral repair by placing an omental pedicle flap over the repair to prevent fistula formation.

- Tissue sealant may be applied to the area of anastomosis.

- Place drains after the repair.

Tips and pitfalls

- Avoid extensive dissection of the surrounding tissues during mobilization of the ureter. The ureter receives its blood supply from the surrounding tissues medially, and extensive dissection may cause ischemia of the repair site and either stricture or breakdown of the anastomosis.

- Failure to use a double-J stent or to spatulate the ends of the ureter when doing the primary repair increases the risk of anastomotic stricture.

- When performing re-implantation, ensure there is no acute angulation of the ureter as it enters the bladder, as acute angulation will prevent adequate drainage of the ureter.

Fig. 27.12. Placement of an indwelling double-J-type stent into the proximal and distal ends of the ureter.

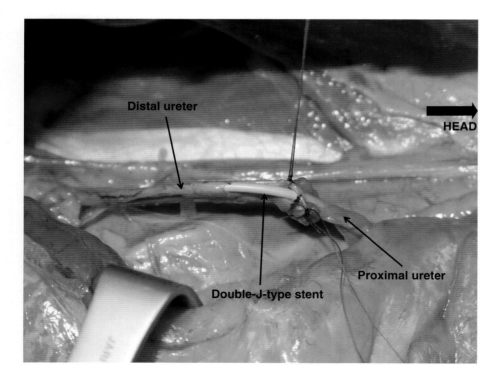

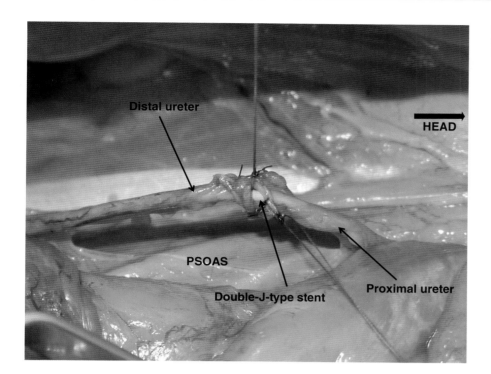

Fig. 27.13. Tension-free, mucosa-to-mucosa anastomosis using interrupted 4–0 absorbable sutures over double-J-type stent.

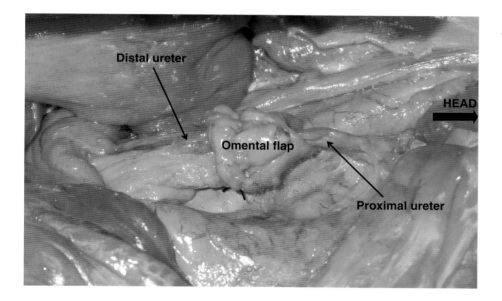

Fig. 27.14. Omental flap covering ureteral anastomosis.

Postoperative care

- Drains should be left in the retroperitoneum until the output is minimal. Internal stents should be removed endoscopically through the bladder 4–6 weeks postinjury, followed by excretory urography or retrograde pyelography to demonstrate a patent anastomosis without any evidence of urine leak. Ureteral patency should be reassessed again after 3 months with excretory urography, or renal ultrasound to assess for hydronephrosis.

(a)

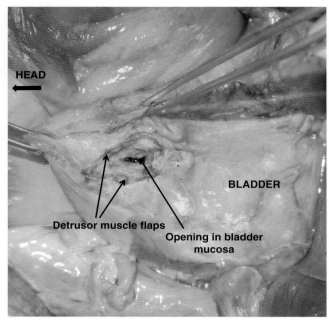

Fig. 27.15(a). Preparation of the bladder for distal ureter anastomosis. A tunnel is made in the ipsilateral, posterolateral dome by dissecting off the detrusor muscle, leaving small muscle flaps on either side to cover anastomosis later. A hole is made in the bladder mucosa at the apex of this trough.

(b)

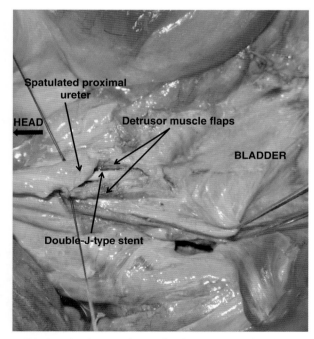

Fig. 27.15(b). Spatulated proximal ureteral end is anastomosed to the bladder mucosa over a stent with interrupted 4–0 absorbable sutures.

(c)

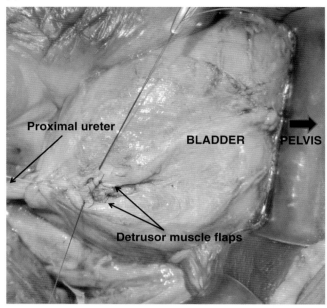

Fig. 27.15(c). Closure of detrusor muscle flaps over the ureteral anastomosis with 3–0 absorbable sutures.

Bladder injury
General principles

- Injuries to the bladder are classified according to the location of rupture. Intraperitoneal bladder rupture always requires operative repair. Extraperitoneal ruptures can be managed with urethral catheter drainage alone. Some bladder injuries can be a combination of both intraperitoneal and extraperitoneal ruptures and should be fixed surgically.

Repair of bladder injury

- Intraperitoneal bladder ruptures almost always involve the dome of the bladder. Inspect and palpate the bladder through the laceration to verify that there are no other injuries and that there is clear efflux from both ureteral orifices. If necessary, the laceration can be extended, to adequately visualize the inner surface of the bladder.
- Debride any devitalized tissue.
- If extraperitoneal lacerations are seen on examination, close them from inside the bladder with a single layer of interrupted 3–0 or 4–0 absorbable sutures.
- Once inspection and repair of extraperitoneal lacerations is complete, close the laceration in two layers using 2–0 or 3–0 absorbable sutures.
- Place a drain near the repair.

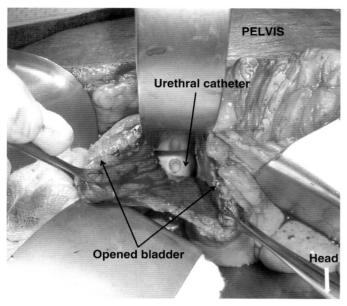

Fig. 27.16. Intraperitoneal bladder rupture with laceration extended into an anterior midline cystotomy to fully visualize the inside of the bladder.

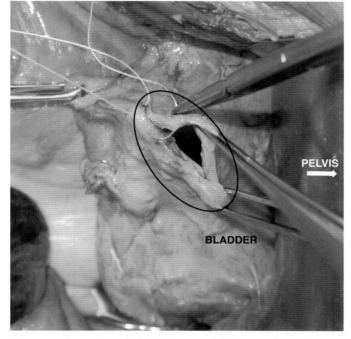

Fig. 27.17. Intraperitoneal bladder laceration (circle) repaired in two layers using 3–0 absorbable sutures.

Tips and pitfalls

- In penetrating injuries with no accountable second bladder wound, always examine the bladder from the inside, in order to avoid missed injuries.
- Test the closure by instilling the bladder with sterile irrigation through the existing urethral catheter. Any significant leaks may be oversewn with 3–0 absorbable sutures in a figure-of-eight fashion. Tiny leaks will most likely seal on their own. Tissue sealant may be applied.

Postoperative care

- Intraperitoneal drains should be left in place until output is minimal. The urethral catheter should be left in place for 7 to 10 days. If there is any concern about bladder healing, a cystogram can be performed to evaluate for urine leakage from the repair. This should be considered for all complex repairs, and for those involving the trigone of the bladder.

Chapter

28

Abdominal aorta and visceral branches

Pedro G. Teixeira and Vincent L. Rowe

Surgical anatomy

- For vascular trauma purposes, the abdomen is conventionally divided into four retroperitoneal anatomical areas.

  o *Zone I.* The midline retroperitoneum from the aortic hiatus to the sacral promontory is broken into the supramesocolic and inframesocolic areas. The supramesocolic area contains the suprarenal aorta and its major branches (celiac artery, superior mesenteric artery, and renal arteries), the supramesocolic segment of the inferior vena cava with its major branches, and the superior mesenteric vein. The inframesocolic area contains the infrarenal aorta and the inferior vena cava.

  o *Zone II (left and right).* This is the paired right and left region lateral to Zone 1 and contains the kidneys with the renal vessels.

  o *Zone III.* The pelvic retroperitoneum, which contains the iliac vessels.

  o *Zone IV.* This is the retrohepatic area containing the retrohepatic inferior vena cava and the hepatic veins.

- The abdominal aorta originates between the two crura of the diaphragm at the T12 to L1 level and bifurcates into the common iliac arteries at the L4 to L5 level. The external landmark for the bifurcation is the umbilicus. The first branches are the phrenic arteries, which originate from its anterolateral surface. Immediately below this is the origin of the celiac trunk, and 1 to 2 cm below this is the superior mesenteric artery. The renal arteries originate 1 to 1.5 cm below the origin of the superior mesenteric artery at the level of L2. Finally, the inferior mesenteric artery originates 2 to 5 cm above the aortic bifurcation.

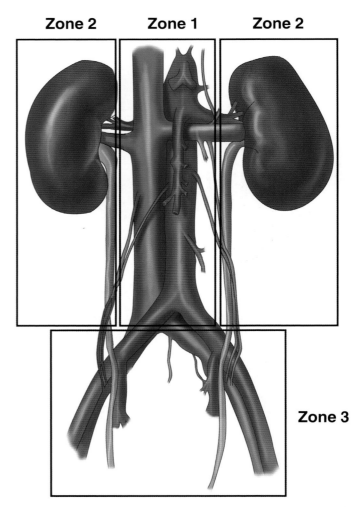

Zone 2   **Zone 1**   **Zone 2**

Zone 3

Fig. 28.1. Retroperitoneal vascular zones: Zone I includes the midline vessels from the aortic hiatus to the sacral promontory; Zone II the paracolic gutter and the kidneys; Zone III the pelvic retroperitoneum.

Atlas of Surgical Techniques in Trauma, ed. Demetrios Demetriades, Kenji Inaba, and George Velmahos. Published by Cambridge University Press. © Cambridge University Press 2015.

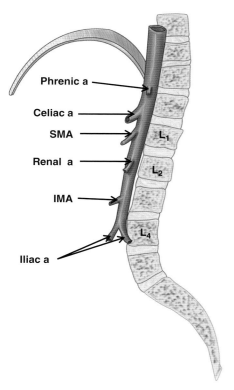

Fig. 28.2. Lateral view of the major visceral branches of the abdominal aorta. Note the tight concentration of the supramesocolic vessels: celiac artery, superior mesenteric artery (SMA), and renal vessels.

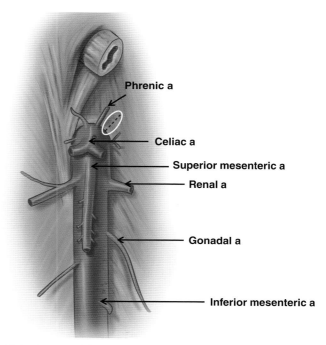

Fig. 28.3. Anatomy of the major branches of the abdominal aorta. Note the site of division (dashed line) of the left crux of the diaphragm, at the avascular 2 o'clock, for exposure of the lower thoracic aorta.

- *Celiac artery.* The main trunk is 1 to 1.5 cm long and at the upper border of the pancreas it separates into three branches (the tripod of Haller), which includes the common hepatic, left gastric, and splenic arteries. Due to the extensive fibrous, ganglionic, and lymphatic tissues which surround the trunk, surgical dissection in this area is difficult.
- *Superior mesenteric artery (SMA).* The SMA originates from the anterior surface of the aorta, 1 cm to 2 cm below the celiac artery, behind the pancreas, at the level of L1. It then courses over the uncinate process of the pancreas and the third part of the duodenum and enters into the root of the mesentery. Branches include the inferior pancreaticoduodenal artery, the middle colic artery, an arterial arcade with 12–18 intestinal branches, the right colic artery, and the ileocolic artery.
- *Renal arteries.* The right renal artery emerges at a slightly higher level and is longer than the left and courses under the inferior vena cava. Approximately 30% of the population have more than one renal artery, usually an accessory artery supplying the lower pole of the kidney. The renal vein lies in front of the renal artery. The left renal vein is significantly longer than the right and courses in front of the aorta and drains the left gonadal vein inferiorly, the left adrenal vein superiorly, and a lumbar vein posteriorly.
- *Inferior mesenteric artery (IMA).* The IMA provides blood supply to the left colon, sigmoid, and upper part of the rectum. It communicates with the SMA through the marginal artery of Drummond.

General principles

- Hemorrhage resulting from abdominal vascular injuries is not amenable to temporary control by application of external pressure. Immediate operative intervention is the cornerstone of survival.
- Penetrating abdominal vascular injuries are usually associated with hollow viscus injuries, which increase the complexity of the operation and expose the vascular repairs to contamination from enteric contents.
- In physiologically compromised patients, if the injured vessel cannot be ligated, temporary stenting with delayed definitive reconstruction should be utilized.
- Abdominal arterial and venous injuries occur with the same incidence. The most commonly injured abdominal vessel is the inferior vena cava, followed by the aorta.
- In suspected abdominal vascular injuries, where the IVC or iliac veins may be injured, the femoral veins should not be used for venous access.
- During induction of anesthesia in patients with severe intra-abdominal bleeding, there is a high risk of rapid hemodynamic decompensation or even of cardiac arrest. The patient should be prepared and draped and the surgical team ready to enter prior to the induction of anesthesia.
- The value of systemic heparin is limited because of the trauma-induced coagulopathy. Local heparinized saline (5000 units in 100 mL saline) however, should be used liberally.
- About 15% of patients with intra-abdominal vascular injuries are in cardiac arrest on arrival. These patients may benefit from a left anterolateral resuscitative thoracotomy and cross-clamping of the aorta above the diaphragm (see Chapter 4).

Special surgical instruments

- In addition to a standard trauma laparotomy instrument tray, vascular clamps with multiple lengths and angulations must be available.
- A self-retaining retractor, such as Omni-Tract® or Bookwalter® can aid in providing exposure.
- A U-shaped aortic compression device should be available for temporary aortic control below the diaphragm. If this is not available, a sponge stick or manual pressure can be used.
- Surgical head light and magnifying loupes should be available.
- A thoracotomy instrument tray with a Finochietto retractor should be available, should a left anterolateral thoracotomy be necessary for aortic cross-clamping.

Positioning

- Supine, with upper extremities abducted to 90 degrees. Skin antiseptic preparation should include the chest, abdomen, and groin, in anticipation of a possible thoracotomy or venous conduit harvesting.

Incision

- Extended midline trauma laparotomy, from xiphoid to pubic symphysis.
- For proximal aortic control in cases with high supramesocolic bleeding or hematoma, a left anterolateral thoracotomy through the fifth intercostal space may be needed. The technical aspects are described in Chapter 4.

Exposure

- In penetrating trauma, upon entering the peritoneal cavity, the usual findings include free intraperitoneal bleeding or a retroperitoneal hematoma or a combination of the two. In blunt trauma the most likely finding is a retroperitoneal hematoma, which may or may not be expanding or pulsatile.
- The management of retroperitoneal hematomas depends on the mechanism of injury.
  - As a general rule, almost all hematomas due to penetrating trauma should be explored, irrespective of size. Often, underneath a small hematoma there is a vascular or hollow viscus perforation. The only exception to this recommendation is a stable and non-expanding retrohepatic Zone IV hematoma. Surgical exploration of the retrohepatic vena cava or the hepatic veins is challenging and may cause harm.
  - Retroperitoneal hematomas due to blunt trauma rarely require exploration because of the very low incidence of underlying vascular or hollow viscus injuries requiring surgical repair. The only indications for exploration of hematomas due to blunt trauma include a paraduodenal hematoma, large expanding or leaking hematoma, and a hematoma in the region of the superior mesenteric artery associated with ischemic bowel.

Exploration of Zone I

Supraceliac aortic control

- Proximal control and direct compression or cross-clamping of the distal thoracic and proximal abdominal aorta can be achieved below the diaphragm, through a midline laparotomy, in most cases.
- At the aortic hiatus of the diaphragm, the aorta is surrounded by dense connective, nervous, and lymphatic tissue, which makes the exposure difficult. However, more proximally, at the distal thoracic aorta level, the vessel is free from this dense periaortic tissue and can be more easily exposed. This segment is accessible through the esophageal hiatus.

○ The first step for this approach is to mobilize the left lobe of the liver. The round ligament of the liver is divided between clamps and ligated, and the falciform ligament is divided with electrocautery. The left triangular ligament of the liver is then divided. This maneuver is facilitated by positioning the surgeon's right hand behind the left lobe of the liver, using the right thumb to retract the liver caudad. The left triangular ligament is then divided with electrocautery over the surgeon's right index finger and the left lateral segment of the liver is folded medially, exposing the esophageal hiatus.

○ While the left lobe of the liver is folded medially, the stomach is retracted to the patient's left and downward to expose the gastrohepatic ligament. The ligament is then opened and the crux of the diaphragm is exposed.

○ The esophagus is circumferentially dissected at the gastroesophageal junction and encircled with a Penrose drain for traction.

○ The left diaphragmatic crux is then divided at the avascular 2 o'clock position.

○ Using blunt digital dissection, the distal thoracic aorta is isolated and a DeBakey or Cooley aortic aneurysm clamp is applied. After adequately positioning, the clamp should be stabilized using an umbilical tape or a vessel loop secured to the surgical drapes. Blind application of a clamp in this area is ineffective and may cause iatrogenic injury.

● An alternative strategy for rapid temporary supraceliac aortic control is the utilization of a U-shaped aortic compression device. This handheld device is positioned over the supraceliac aorta through the lesser sac. Applying constant anteroposterior pressure, the device compresses the aorta against the spine until definitive control of the bleeding is achieved. The advantage of this technique is the minimal dissection needed for application of the device, but a second assistant is required to hold pressure while definitive bleeding control is pursued.

● In cases with a high supramesocolic hematoma where infradiaphragmatic exposure of the aorta is difficult or not possible, a left thoracotomy may be necessary for aortic control.

(a)

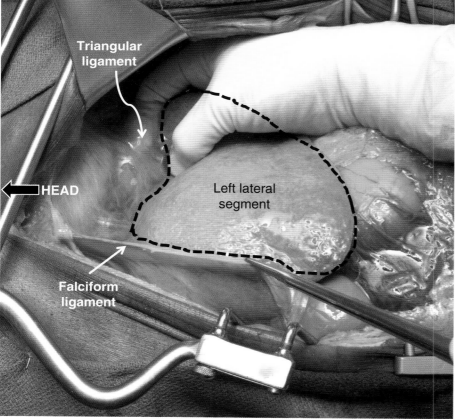

Fig. 28.4(a). Mobilization of the left lateral segment of the liver to expose the area of the esophageal hiatus. The falciform ligament has been divided and the surgeon's right index finger is positioned posteriorly to the left triangular ligament of the liver.

(b)

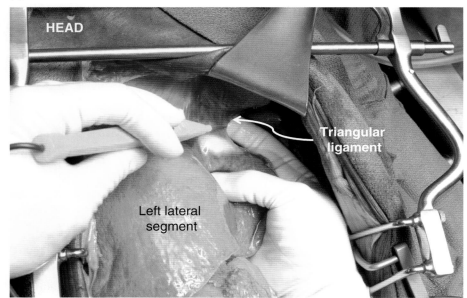

Fig. 28.4(b). Division of the left triangular ligament of the liver with electrocautery. This maneuver allows the left lateral segment to be retracted medially to expose the area of the gastroesophageal junction.

(c)

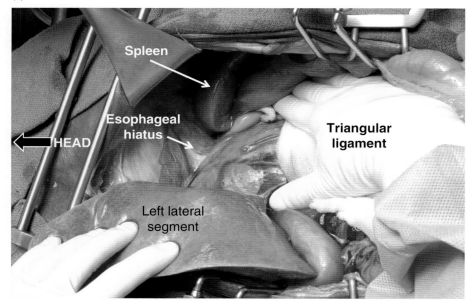

Fig. 28.4(c). The left lateral segment of the liver has been retracted medially, exposing the esophageal hiatus.

(a)

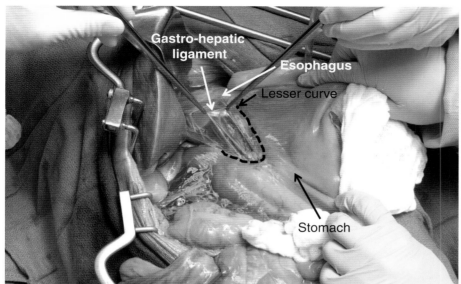

Fig. 28.5(a). The stomach is retracted caudad and the gastrohepatic ligament is divided.

(b)

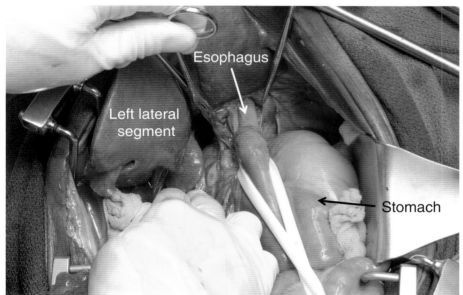

Fig. 28.5(b). After the esophagus is circumferentially dissected at the gastroesophageal junction, a Penrose drain is positioned around it for traction. Note the use of Allis clamps to retract the diaphragmatic crus fibers.

(a)

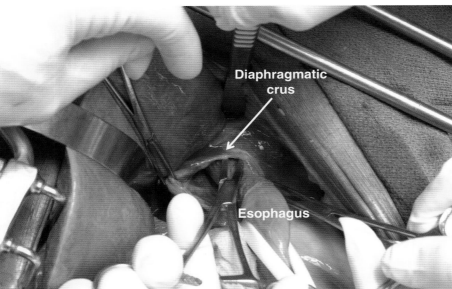

Diaphragmatic crus

Esophagus

Fig. 28.6(a). With the esophagus retracted downwards, a Peon clamp is advanced into the esophageal hiatus of the diaphragm to facilitate the division of the muscle fibers.

(b)

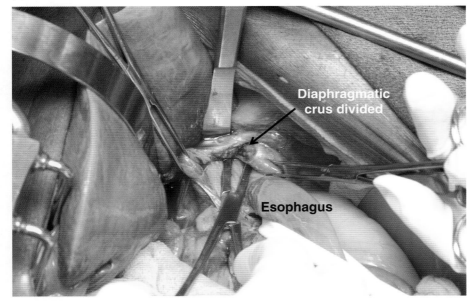

Diaphragmatic crus divided

Esophagus

Fig. 28.6(b). The right diaphragmatic crus is divided at the 2 o'clock position.

(a)

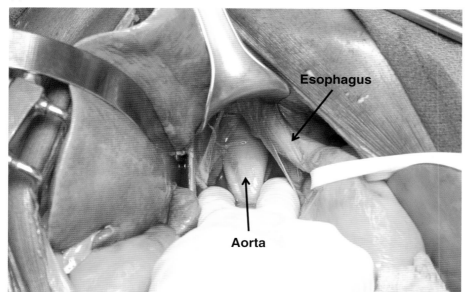

Fig. 28.7(a). The distal thoracic aorta has been identified and isolated. Note how, at this level, the aorta is free from surrounding connective, nervous, and lymphatic tissue.

(b)

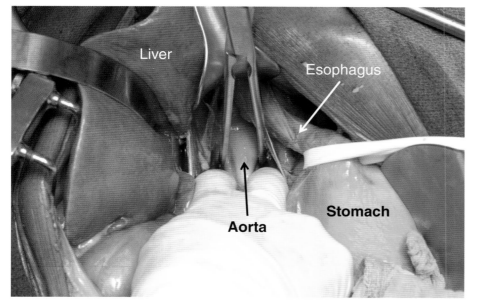

Fig. 28.7(b). A vascular clamp is applied to the aorta. Note the esophagus retracted laterally and protected from inadvertent injury with the application of the clamp.

(c)

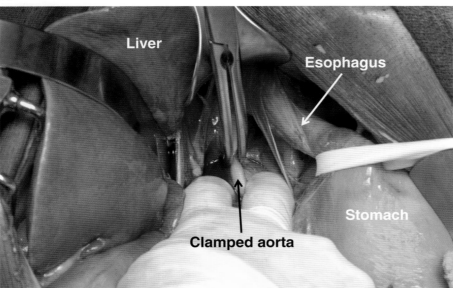

Liver

Esophagus

Stomach

Clamped aorta

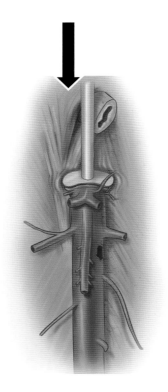

Fig. 28.8. Aortic compression device applied on the supraceliac aorta through the lesser sac. The aorta is compressed against the spine.

Exposure of the supramesocolic aorta and visceral branches

- Zone I supramesocolic bleeding or hematomas are the most difficult to approach because of the dense concentration of major vessels (aorta, celiac artery, superior mesenteric artery, renal vessels, inferior vena cava), the difficult exposure of many of these vessels, and the difficult proximal control of the infradiaphragmatic aorta.

- The supramesocolic aorta with the origins of its major visceral branches is best exposed by mobilization and medial rotation of the viscera, with or without mobilization of the left kidney.

  o The first step of this approach is the division of the peritoneal reflection lateral to the left colon (white line of Toldt) and dissection of the left colon from the lateral abdominal wall. This retroperitoneal plane is developed anteriorly to the Gerota's fascia if the intention is to leave the left kidney in place.

  o The retroperitoneal dissection is continued cephalad and the spleen is completely mobilized after division of the splenophrenic ligament. Avoid excessive traction to the splenic flexure of the colon or the spleen in order to prevent inadvertent avulsion of the splenic capsule and bleeding. The spleen, fundus of the stomach, pancreas, colon, and small bowel are then rotated en-bloc medially, exposing the aortic hiatus and origins of the celiac axis, superior mesenteric artery, and left renal artery.

  o Exposure of the aorta directly under the left renal vein may be difficult. In this case, there are three possible options: (1) include the left kidney in the visceral rotation, (2) mobilize the left renal vein, often after ligation and division of its three tributaries (left gonadal vein, left adrenal vein, and ascending lumbar vein), (3) division of the left renal vein. In this case the tributaries must be preserved and the left renal vein ligated and divided as close to the inferior vena

(a)

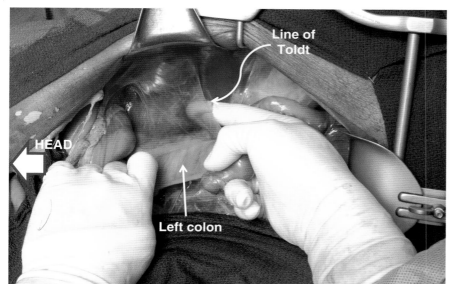

Fig. 28.9(a). Left visceral rotation: traction of the descending colon exposes the left peritoneal reflection and the white line of Toldt is identified.

(b)

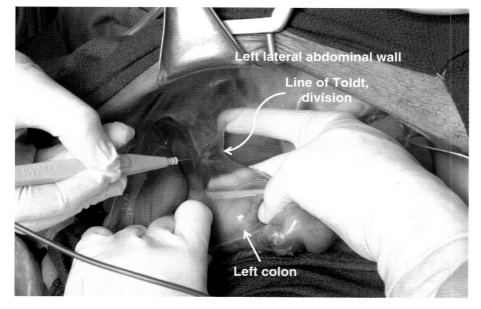

Fig. 28.9(b). The white line of Toldt being divided with cautery and the left colon is mobilized away from the lateral abdominal wall.

cava as possible in order to maintain venous outflow from the left kidney.

o The left visceral rotation provides good exposure to the supramesocolic aorta and its major branches. However, it is associated with a significant risk of

iatrogenic injury to the spleen and the tail of the pancreas.

o Following medial visceral rotation, the exposure of the abdominal aorta is carried out by division of the tissues overlying its anterolateral surface.

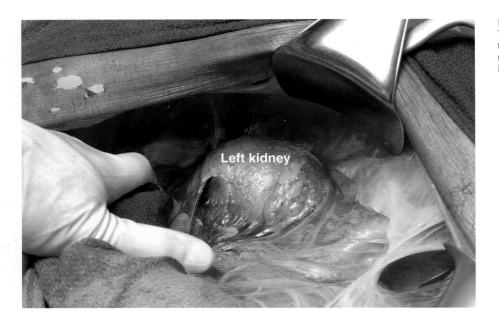

Fig. 28.10. After division of the white line of Toldt, the plane between the left mesocolon and the left kidney in entered and the left colon mobilized medially. Note that the kidney was left at its original position.

(a)

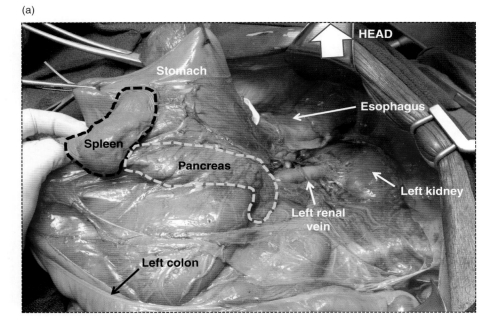

Fig. 28.11(a). Medial visceral rotation has been performed after division of the splenorenal and splenophrenic ligaments. The pancreas and the spleen have been rotated medially en bloc. The posterior surface of the pancreas and its anatomical relationship with the spleen is depicted. The left kidney remains at its original position in the retroperitoneal area. Note the left renal vein crossing anteriorly over the aorta.

(b)

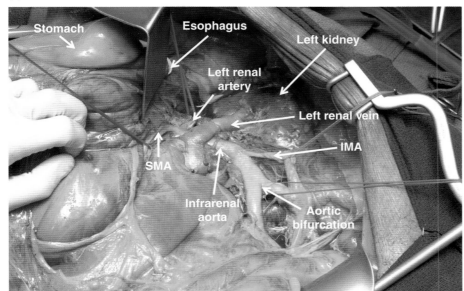

Fig. 28.11(b). Anatomy and visceral branches of the abdominal aorta.

Exposure of the inframesocolic aorta

- The inframesocolic abdominal aorta can be exposed directly by retracting the transverse colon cephalad and displacing the small bowel to the right. The peritoneum over the aorta is then incised and the aorta is exposed. An alternative approach is medial rotation of the left colon.

Exploration of Zone II

- Zone II is explored by mobilization and medial rotation of the right colon, the duodenum, and the head of the pancreas on the right side or the left colon on the left side. The source of bleeding in Zone II is usually the kidney and the renal vessels.

Exploration of Zone III

- The source of Zone III bleeding is usually the iliac vessels in penetrating injury and the pelvic soft tissue and venous plexus in blunt injury. This area is explored by incising the paracolic peritoneum and medial rotation of the right or left colon. An alternative approach is by direct dissection of the peritoneum over the vessels (see Chapter 29).

Celiac artery

- The celiac artery and its three proximal branches can be approached directly through the lesser sac. Alternatively, exposure may be achieved through the previously described left medial visceral rotation. The rotation need not include the left kidney.

- It is rare that the celiac artery needs complex reconstruction. Ligation should be performed in all cases requiring anything more than simple arteriorrhaphy. Ligation is unlikely to result in ischemic sequelae to the stomach, liver, or spleen, because of the rich collateral circulation. The left gastric and splenic arteries may also be ligated. The common hepatic artery is the largest of the celiac artery branches and can be repaired with lateral arteriorrhaphy, end-to-end anastomosis or venous graft interposition. However, ligation of the artery proximal to the origin of the gastroduodenal artery, is often well tolerated because of collateral blood supply. Transient elevation of liver enzymes lasting for a few days is common, but rarely has any clinical significance. However, in some cases, especially in the presence of prolonged hypotension or associated liver injuries, segmental necrosis may be seen.

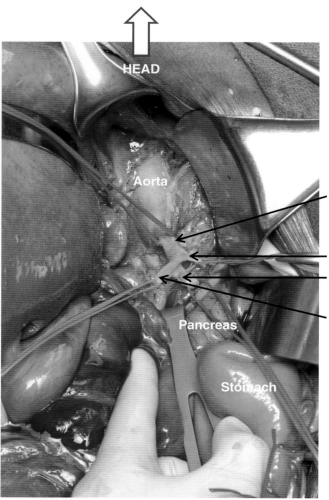

Superior mesenteric artery

- Anatomically, the SMA is divided into four zones: Zone I, from the aortic origin to the inferior pancreaticoduodenal branch; Zone II, from the inferior pancreaticoduodenal artery to the middle colic artery; Zone III, distal to middle colic artery; and Zone IV, the segmental intestinal branches.

- An alternative anatomical classification system uses only two zones, the short retropancreatic segment and the segment below the body of the pancreas, where it courses over the uncinate process of the pancreas and the third part of the duodenum.

- Exposure of the SMA differs according to the site of the injury.

  o Exposure of the retropancreatic SMA can be achieved by medial visceral rotation, as described above. The kidney does not need to be included in the rotation, unless there is a suspicion of injury to the posterior wall of the aorta.

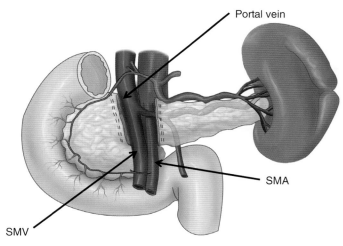

Fig. 28.13. In cases with severe bleeding where immediate exposure of the retropancreatic SMA is critical, stapled division (GIA stapler) of the neck of the pancreas provides fast and direct exposure of the SMA and the portal vein.

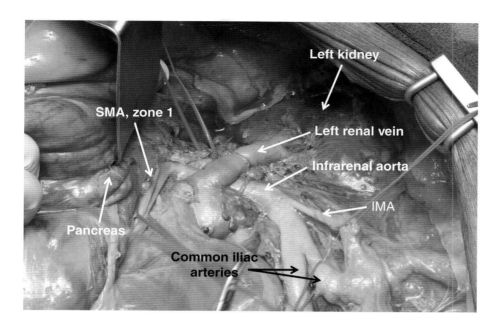

○ In cases with severe bleeding where immediate exposure of the retropancreatic SMA is critical, stapled division of the neck of the pancreas provides fast and direct exposure of the SMA and the portal vein.

○ Exposure of the infrapancreatic SMA can be achieved by cephalad retraction of the inferior border of the pancreas and direct dissection of the vessel. For more distal injuries, exposure can be achieved with dissection through the root of the small bowel mesentery, to the right of the ligament of Treitz.

• In contrast to the celiac artery, ligation of the SMA results in variable degrees of ischemia according to the zone involved. Ligation at Zones I and II leads to extensive ischemia to the entire small bowel and right colon. Ligation at Zones III and IV results in segmental small bowel ischemia. Unless irreversible bowel ischemia is present at laparotomy, ligation of the SMA, especially in Zones I and II, should generally be avoided, if possible.

• Primary repair of the SMA may be possible in selected cases of sharp transection of the vessel, usually inflicted by knife wounds. The repair can be performed with 6–0 vascular sutures.

• In the presence of even limited tissue loss, an end-to-end anastomosis is rarely possible, because mobilization of the SMA is restricted due to the surrounding dense neuroganglionic tissue and its multiple branches.

• The management of complex SMA injuries not amenable to simple arteriorrhaphy should be determined by the condition of the patient, the site of the injury, and the experience of the surgeon. The surgical options for these patients include reconstruction with an interposition graft, ligation, or damage control with temporary shunting.

○ Reconstruction of the very proximal SMA is usually performed with an autologous venous or synthetic graft, between the distal stump of the SMA and the anterior surface of the aorta. For more distal injuries, an interposition venous graft between the transected ends of the vessel is usually required.

○ For patients in critical condition with severe hypothermia, acidosis, and coagulopathy, a damage control procedure with temporary endoluminal shunting should be considered. This is preferable to ligation. Definitive reconstruction is performed at a later stage after resuscitation and correction of the physiologic parameters of the patient. The technique of temporary endoluminal shunt placement is described in other chapters.

○ Ligation of the SMA below the middle colic artery is usually associated with a moderate risk of ischemia of the bowel. However, ligation of the proximal SMA results in ischemic necrosis involving the small bowel and the right colon. The first 10 to 20 cm of the jejunum may survive via collaterals from the superior pancreaticoduodenal artery. Ligation of the SMA proximal to the origin of the inferior pancreaticoduodenal artery may preserve critical collateral circulation to the proximal jejunum and is preferable to a more distal ligation. Ligation of the proximal SMA should be performed only in the presence of necrotic bowel. Ligation should be avoided in all other circumstances because of the catastrophic consequences of short bowel syndrome.

○ In the presence of an associated pancreatic injury the vascular anastomosis should be performed away from the pancreas, if possible. The anastomosis should be protected with the use of omentum and surrounding soft tissues.

- Postoperatively, the patient should be monitored closely for any signs of bowel ischemia (lactic acid, leukocytosis, physiological deterioration). In the presence of any of these signs, a second look laparotomy should be performed to rule out bowel ischemia. If in doubt, the abdomen should be left open during the original operation.

Renal artery

- The left renal artery is more likely to sustain blunt trauma than the right renal artery. The right renal artery is better protected from deceleration injuries because of its course underneath the IVC.
- The management of renovascular injuries depends on the mechanism of injury, the ischemia time, the general condition of the patient, and the presence of a contralateral normal kidney.

  o Penetrating trauma always requires emergency operative intervention because of severe bleeding.

  o Blunt trauma to the renal artery often results in thrombosis without bleeding. These cases may be managed non-operatively or with endovascular stenting. In cases with avulsion of the artery there is severe bleeding and an emergency operation is required.

  o In emergency operations for bleeding, a nephrectomy is usually the procedure of choice.

  o Ligation of the right renal vein results in hemorrhagic infarction of the kidney and should always be followed by nephrectomy. However, ligation of the left renal vein near the IVC without nephrectomy may be possible because of collateral venous drainage through the left gonadal, adrenal, and lumbar veins.

- Exposure of the renal vessels.

  o The left kidney and renal vessels may be exposed quickly by mobilization and by medial rotation of the left colon. On the right side, mobilization of the right colon combined with a Kocher maneuver provides excellent visualization of the renal system. Bleeding control is then achieved by digital compression or application of a vascular clamp on the renal hilum. This is the most commonly used approach in trauma surgery.

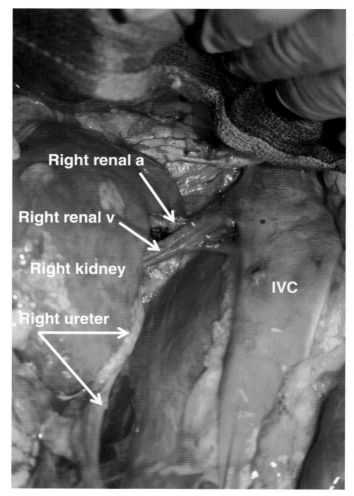

Fig. 28.15. After right medial rotation, the right renal hilum is identified. The IVC is exposed. Note the position of the right renal artery, posterior to the right renal vein and to the IVC. The right ureter is demonstrated posterior to the hilar vessels.

  o An alternative approach to the exposure and proximal control of the renal arteries is through a midline retroperitoneal exploration. The transverse colon is retracted anteriorly and cephalad, placing the transverse mesocolon under tension. The ligament of Treitz is divided and the duodenum is retracted caudad and to the right. The left renal vein is identified and mobilized as needed to expose the origins of bilateral renal arteries.

(a)

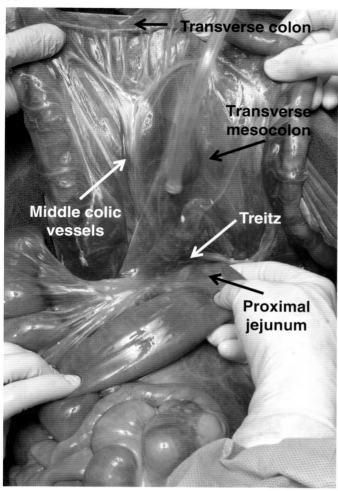

Fig. 28.16(a). Transverse colon is retracted anteriorly and cephalad, placing the transverse mesocolon under tension, exposing the fourth portion of the duodenum and the ligament of Treitz.

(b)

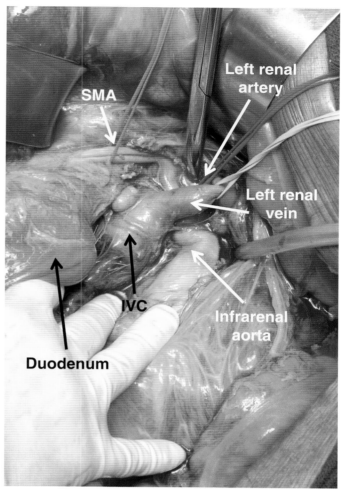

Fig. 28.16(b). Midline retroperitoneal exploration after the ligament of Treitz had been divided and the duodenum retracted caudad and to the right. Note the left renal vein crossing over anteriorly to the aorta. Mobilization of the left renal vein provides access to the origin of bilateral renal arteries.

(c)

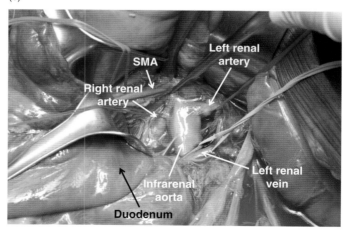

Fig. 28.16(c). Through a midline retroperitoneal exploration, the left renal vein has been retracted caudad and the origin of both renal arteries is noted. Note the close proximity between the origins of the SMA and the renal arteries.

Inferior mesenteric artery

- Injury to the inferior mesenteric artery is managed by ligation.

Tips and pitfalls

- In patients with suspected abdominal vascular injuries where the IVC or iliac veins may be injured, the femoral veins should not be used for venous access.
- In a young trauma patient, a small and constricted aorta may be difficult to identify within a large retroperitoneal hematoma. Likewise, the choice of conduit size for reconstruction acutely should take this vasoconstriction into account.
- During control of the aorta at the hiatus, the esophagus should be carefully retracted laterally to avoid inadvertent injury during application of the vascular clamp.
- Division of the left crux of the diaphragm for exposure of the distal thoracic aorta should be performed at 2 o'clock, which is an avascular plane.
- During left medial visceral rotation, complete division of the splenic attachments to the diaphragm and careful mobilization of the spleen decreases the chance of capsular avulsion and bleeding.
- The descending lumbar vein is at risk of injury during mobilization of the left kidney to expose the lateral wall of the aorta. It should be identified, ligated, and divided to avoid laceration and unnecessary additional blood loss.
- In order to obtain increased exposure to the peri-renal aorta and renal arteries, the inferior mesenteric vein may need to be ligated.

Iliac injuries

Demetrios Demetriades and Kelly Vogt

Anatomy of the iliac vessels

- The abdominal aorta bifurcates into the two common iliac arteries at the level of the fourth to the fifth lumbar vertebrae (surface landmark is the umbilicus). The common iliac arteries are about 5–7 cm in length.
- At the level of the sacroiliac joint, the common iliac arteries bifurcate to the external and the internal iliac arteries.
- The external iliac artery runs along the medial border of the psoas muscle and goes underneath the inguinal ligament to become the common femoral artery. It gives two major branches: the inferior epigastric artery, just above the inguinal ligament; and the deep iliac circumflex artery which arises from the lateral aspect of the external iliac artery, opposite the inferior epigastric artery.
- The internal iliac artery is a short and thick vessel, about 3–4 cm in length. It divides into the anterior and posterior branches at the sciatic foramen. These branches provide blood supply to the pelvic viscera, perineum, pelvic wall, and the buttocks.
- The ureter crosses over the bifurcation of the common iliac artery.
- The common iliac veins lie mostly medial and posterior to the common iliac arteries. They join to form the inferior vena cava at the level of the fifth lumbar vertebrae, posterior to the right common iliac artery.
- The left external iliac vein runs medial to the artery along its entire length. The right external iliac vein above the inguinal ligament is medial to the artery and, as it courses proximally, it moves to the right, posterior to the artery.

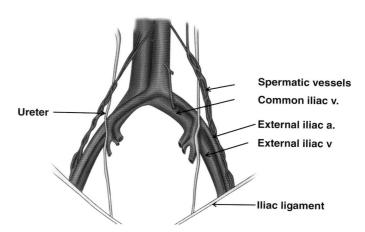

Fig. 29.1. Schematic anatomy of the iliac arteries, veins, and ureter crossing over the common iliac bifurcation. The left external iliac vein runs medial to the artery along its entire length. The right external iliac vein, above the inguinal ligament is medial to the artery and, as it courses proximally, it moves to the right, posterior to the artery.

General principles

- For effective iliac vascular control, the internal iliac artery should always be included, because bleeding may persist despite proximal and distal clamping of the vessels.
- Control of any enteric injuries and removal of enteric spillage should be done before definitive vascular reconstruction.
- The presence of enteric contamination is not a contraindication for the use of synthetic grafts and there is no need for routine extraanatomical bypass procedures.

Atlas of Surgical Techniques in Trauma, ed. Demetrios Demetriades, Kenji Inaba, and George Velmahos. Published by Cambridge University Press. © Cambridge University Press 2015.

Copious irrigation and washout of the peritoneal cavity before arterial reconstruction and tissue coverage with adjacent peritoneum or omentum reduces the risk of graft infection.

- Extra-anatomical bypass procedures are rarely indicated at the acute stage, because of the critical condition of the patient. They should be considered only in patients with graft infection.
- Ligation of the common or external iliac arteries should never be done because of the high incidence of limb loss and systemic complications. In patients in extremis a damage control procedure with a temporary shunt should be considered.
- The internal iliac artery can be ligated with impunity.
- Ligation of the common or external iliac veins is usually tolerated well. In most patients there is transient leg edema, which resolves with elevation and elastic stockings. In rare cases there is development of extremity compartment syndrome requiring fasciotomy.
- Following arterial or venous injuries, the patient should always be monitored for extremity compartment syndrome. The combination of arterial and venous injuries is associated with a high risk of compartment syndrome, and liberal fasciotomy should be considered.
- Venous repairs producing more than 50% narrowing are associated with a high incidence of pulmonary embolism. In these cases consider ligation or a caval filter.

Special surgical instruments

- The surgeon should have available a complete vascular tray, along with a laparotomy tray.
- If possible, operations should be performed in a suite with angiographic capabilities.

Positioning

- The patient should be supine on the operating table, prepped to include access to the lower extremities.

Incisions

- The majority of injuries can be adequately managed using an extended midline laparotomy incision.
- If the exposure of the distal iliac vessels is difficult, usually due to a narrow pelvis, extension of the midline incision by adding a transverse lower abdominal incision or longitudinal incision over the groin and division of the inguinal ligament may be necessary.

Operative technique

- The usual operative finding in iliac vascular injuries is severe intraperitoneal bleeding or a large retroperitoneal hematoma, or a combination of the two.
- Although proximal and distal control is desirable, in the presence of severe bleeding direct entry into the hematoma with exposure and compression control is often faster and more effective. Although exposure of the vessels may be achieved through a peritoneal incision over the distal aorta and the iliac vessels, a medial rotation of the cecum and ascending colon on the right or the sigmoid and descending colon on the left, provide a better exposure of the vessels and the ureters. The small bowel is rotated cephalad and to the opposite side of the vascular injury and held in place with warm, wet sponges. The paracolic peritoneal reflexion is incised and the cecum or sigmoid is mobilized medially. The bleeding is controlled by direct pressure, and proximal and distal control is achieved with vascular clamps or vessel loops.

(a)

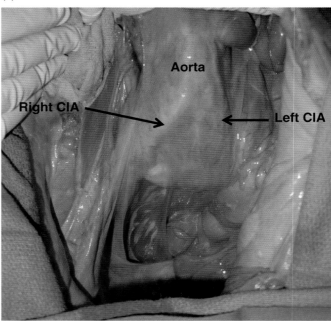

Fig. 29.2(a). Exposure of the retroperitoneum with underlying distal aorta and iliac vessels after retraction of the bowel cephalad and toward the opposite side.

(b)

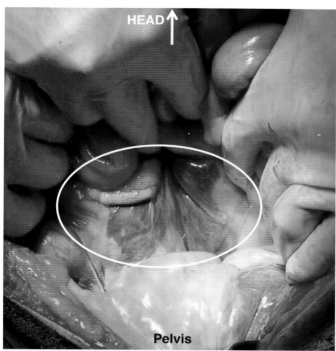

HEAD↑

Pelvis

Fig. 29.2(b). Retraction of the bowel cephalad and exposure of the retroperitoneum with underlying hematoma, secondary to iliac vascular injury. The vessels can be exposed with an incision on the peritoneum, directly over the vessels, or by medial rotation of the left or right colon.

- The ureter crosses over the bifurcation of the common iliac artery and should be gently retracted with a vessel loop and protected from accidental injury.

(a)

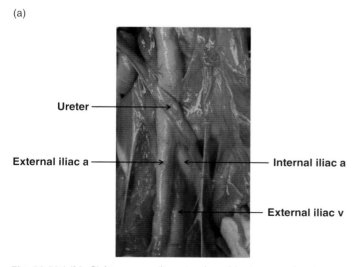

Ureter

External iliac a — Internal iliac a

— External iliac v

Fig. 29.3(a),(b). Right common iliac artery branching to external and internal iliac arteries. The external iliac vein is identified medial to the artery. The common iliac vein courses under the artery. The ureter crosses over the bifurcation of the common iliac artery to the internal and external iliac arteries.

(b)

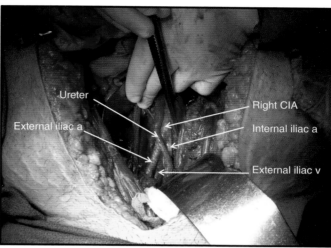

Ureter — Right CIA

External iliac a — Internal iliac a

— External iliac v

Fig. 29.3(a),(b). (cont.)

(a)

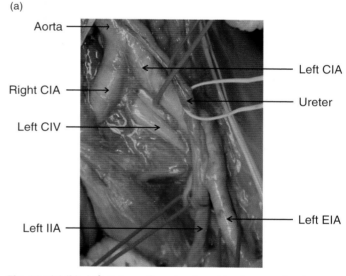

Aorta — — Left CIA

Right CIA — — Ureter

Left CIV —

Left IIA — — Left EIA

Fig. 29.4(a),(b). Left common iliac artery branching to external and internal iliac arteries. The iliac veins are identified medial and posterior to the arteries. The ureter crosses over the bifurcation of the common iliac artery to the internal and external iliac arteries.

- Exposure of the iliac veins is technically more challenging than the iliac arteries, because of their position underneath the arteries, especially on the right side. Some authors even recommend transection of the artery in order to gain adequate access to the underlying vein. This approach is not recommended, especially in a critically injured and coagulopathic patient! Adequate venous exposure can be achieved with mobilization of the artery and gentle traction with vessel loops. Ligation and division of the internal iliac artery provides additional mobilization and better venous exposure.

(b)

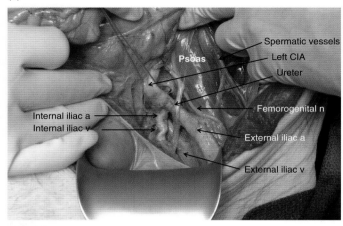

Fig. 29.4(a),(b). (*cont.*)

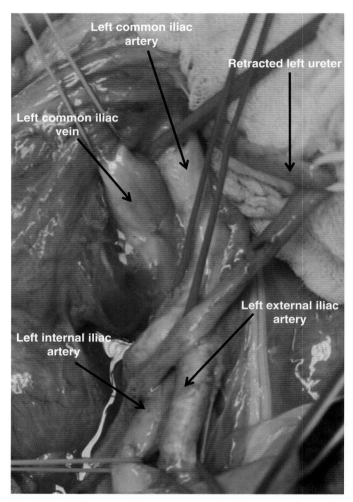

Fig. 29.5. Mobilization and lateral retraction of the left common iliac artery allows good exposure of the common iliac vein. Additional mobilization of the common iliac artery can be obtained by ligating and dividing the internal iliac artery.

- Small arterial injuries without significant tissue loss may be repaired with adequate mobilization of the vessel and primary suturing. However, in most cases a more complex reconstruction with a size 6–8 synthetic graft is necessary. Due to size mismatch, it is rarely possible to use a saphenous vein autologous graft.

- Iliac artery transposition may be a reconstruction option in selected stable patients. The procedure involves ligation of the proximal common iliac artery, near the aortic bifurcation. The distal external and internal iliac arteries are mobilized to allow for adequate length. The contralateral common and external iliac arteries are exposed. The injured artery is then anastomosed end-to-side to the contralateral common or external iliac artery (depending on anatomy), using a running, 4–0 monofilament non-absorbable suture.

- In patients in extremis consider early damage control with temporary shunting. Semi-elective definitive reconstruction is performed after patient stabilization.

- Venous repair with lateral venorrhaphy should be considered in small injuries that can be repaired without producing significant stenosis (<50% of the lumen). In most cases the vein can safely be ligated. These patients should be monitored closely for extremity compartment syndrome. In rare cases with post-ligation massive edema of the leg, reconstruction with ring graft may be necessary.

- The management of iliac venous injuries in the presence of associated iliac artery injuries is controversial. Some authors recommend venous reconstruction with patch venoplasty or PTFE grafts, although there is no evidence of improved outcome with this approach. Most surgeons do not recommend complex venous reconstructions, because these patients are often in extremis and any procedures that prolong the operation may be counterproductive.

- The best damage control option is temporary shunting. Ligation of the common or external iliac artery should be avoided whenever possible to prevent irreversible limb ischemia.

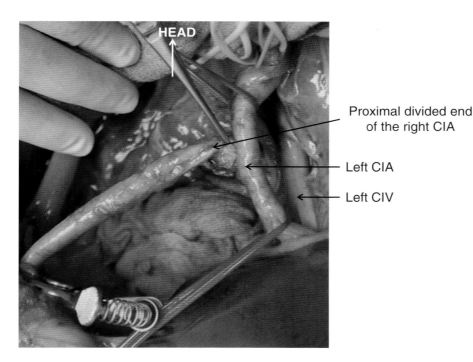

Fig. 29.6. The right common iliac artery after transection and set-up for transposition to the left common iliac artery.

HEAD

Proximal divided end of the right CIA

Left CIA

Left CIV

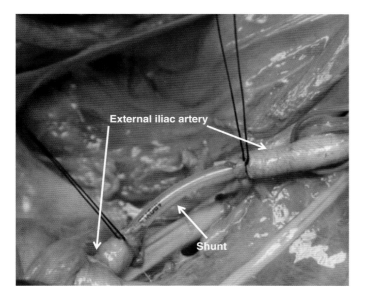

External iliac artery

Shunt

Fig. 29.7. External iliac artery injury with a damage control shunt in place.

Tips and pitfalls

- When clamping or mobilizing the iliac artery, proceed cautiously to avoid iatrogenic injury to the underlying vein.
- The ureter crosses over the bifurcation of the common iliac artery and is at risk of iatrogenic injury. Retract it out of the way with a vessel loop.

- Exposure of the iliac veins is more difficult than exposure of the arteries, because of their anatomic position. Good mobilization of the artery and retraction with vessel loops allows venous exposure. Ligation and division of the internal iliac artery improves the exposure. Avoid the recommendation by some authors to divide the common or external iliac artery in order to improve the exposure of the underlying vein.
- Extra-anatomical bypass (axillofemoral or femorofemoral) is rarely indicated at the acute stage. Its main indication is in patients with postoperative graft infection.
- If repair of the iliac vein produces significant stenosis, consider anticoagulation and inferior vena cava filter placement to prevent pulmonary embolism.
- Some patients with iliac vascular injuries (especially in combined arterial and venous injuries or prolonged ischemia) develop extremity compartment syndrome. In these cases a therapeutic fasciotomy should be performed without delay, often before arterial reconstruction.
- The role of prophylactic fasciotomy is controversial and has been challenged by many authors. If it is elected not to perform a fasciotomy, the patient should be monitored closely with frequent clinical examinations, serial CPK levels, and in the appropriate cases with compartment pressure measurements. Fasciotomy should be performed at the first signs of compartment syndrome.

30

Inferior vena cava

Lydia Lam and Matthew D. Tadlock

Surgical anatomy

- The inferior vena cava (IVC) is formed by the confluence of the common iliac veins, just anterior to the L5 vertebral body, and posterior to the right common iliac artery. As it courses superiorly towards the diaphragm, it lies to the right of the lumbar and thoracic vertebral bodies. It enters the thorax at T8, where the right crus of the diaphragm separates the IVC and aorta. In most individuals, there is a small segment of suprahepatic IVC, about 1 cm in length, between the liver and diaphragm, which is amenable to cross clamping.

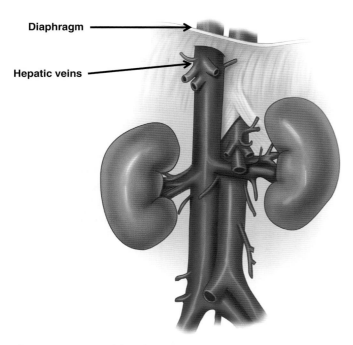

Diaphragm

Hepatic veins

Fig. 30.1. Anatomy of the inferior vena cava (IVC). Note the right renal artery coursing behind the IVC.

- The IVC receives four or five pairs of lumbar veins, the right gonadal vein, the renal veins, the right adrenal vein, the hepatic veins and the phrenic veins. It is of practical importance to remember that all lumbar veins are below the renal veins and that between the renal veins and the hepatic veins, besides the right adrenal vein there are no other venous branches. The left lumbar veins pass behind the abdominal aorta.
- The confluence of the renal veins with the IVC lies posterior to the duodenum and the head of the pancreas.
- The retrohepatic IVC is about 8–10 cm in length and is adhered to the posterior liver, helping to anchor the liver in place. In this liver "tunnel" several accessory veins from the caudate lobe and right lobe drain directly into the IVC.
- There are three major hepatic veins that drain the liver into the IVC. The extrahepatic portion of these veins is short, measuring about 0.5 to 1.5 cm in length. The right hepatic vein is the largest. In about 70% of individuals, the middle vein drains into the left hepatic vein to enter the IVC as a single vein.
- The thoracic IVC is almost entirely in the pericardium.

General principles

- The IVC is the most frequently injured abdominal vessel following penetrating trauma.
- Blunt trauma to the IVC usually involves the retrohepatic part of the vein.
- Patients with intra-abdominal IVC injury, who present to the hospital alive, typically have a contained retroperitoneal hematoma and therefore may initially appear to be hemodynamically stable.
- Avoid femoral vein catheters in patients with penetrating abdominal trauma, because of the possibility of proximal iliac or IVC injury.
- In abdominal gunshot wounds obtain a plain abdominal radiograph prior to going to the operating room if time

Atlas of Surgical Techniques in Trauma, ed. Demetrios Demetriades, Kenji Inaba, and George Velmahos. Published by Cambridge University Press. © Cambridge University Press 2015.

permits, as it helps determine missile trajectory and other structures at risk.

- During induction of anesthesia in patients with severe intra-abdominal bleeding, there is a high risk of rapid hemodynamic decompensation or even of cardiac arrest. The surgical team should be ready and the skin preparation should be performed before induction of anesthesia.
- During exploration of a caval injury, there is high risk for air embolism. Prevent this complication by early direct compression, followed by proximal and distal control.
- Because of the extensive collateral circulation below the renal veins, the infrarenal cava can be safely ligated with acceptable morbidity of lower extremity swelling that is usually temporary.
- Following IVC ligation, the lower extremities and feet should be wrapped with elastic bandages to reduce edema. Monitor closely for extremity compartment syndrome.
- Following packing or repair of IVC injuries, the patient should not be over-resuscitated.

Special surgical instruments

- In addition to a standard trauma laparotomy instrument tray, vascular clamps with multiple lengths and angulations must be available.
- A self-retaining retractor, such as Omni-Tract® or Bookwalter®.
- A sternotomy set should be available in case a median sternotomy is needed for improved exposure of the retrohepatic IVC.
- A surgical head light is important.

Patient positioning

- Supine, with upper extremities abducted to 90 degrees. Skin antiseptic preparation should include the chest, abdomen, and groin.
- Use upper and lower body warming devices.

Incisions

- Extended midline trauma laparotomy, from xiphoid to pubic symphysis.
- The laparotomy may be extended through a subcostal incision to provide exposure to the retrohepatic IVC (see Chapter 20).

(a)

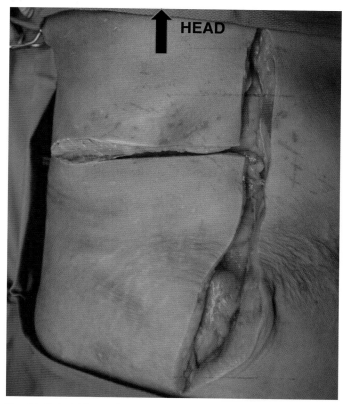

Fig. 30.2(a). Addition of a right subcostal incision to the standard midline laparotomy, for improved exposure of the liver. The subcostal incision is made one to two finger breadths below the costal margin. Avoid an acute angle between the two incisions to prevent ischemic necrosis of the skin.

(b)

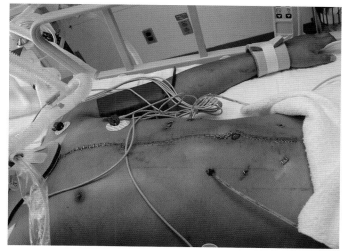

Fig. 30.2(b). A median sternotomy may be added to the midline laparotomy in cases requiring access to the intrapericardial segment of the inferior vena cava for vascular occlusion of the liver, or to the heart for placement of an atrio-caval shunt.

Exposure

- In penetrating trauma, upon entering the peritoneal cavity, the usual findings include a large retroperitoneal hematoma with or without free intraperitoneal bleeding. In blunt trauma the most likely finding is a retroperitoneal hematoma, usually retrohepatic.
- Almost all retroperitoneal hematomas due to penetrating trauma should be explored, irrespective of size, to rule out an underlying vascular or hollow viscus injury. The only exception is a stable and non-expanding retrohepatic hematoma. Surgical exploration of the retrohepatic vena cava or the hepatic veins is difficult and potentially dangerous.

- Retroperitoneal hematomas due to blunt trauma rarely require exploration. However, large expanding or leaking hematomas should be explored.
- The infrarenal and juxtarenal IVC is best exposed by mobilization and medial rotation of the right colon, the hepatic flexion of the colon, and the duodenum.
- The small bowel is eviscerated to the left of the patient and kept in place with warm and moist towels. The avascular white line of Toldt, lateral to the colon, is divided, using sharp dissection or electrocautery. The cecum, right colon, and hepatic flexure are mobilized and retracted medially.
- Following the medial visceral rotation, the second portion of the duodenum, the Gerota's fascia of the right kidney, and the iliopsoas muscle are exposed.
- The duodenum is then mobilized medially with the Kocher maneuver, by incising the lateral peritoneal attachments of the first, second, and proximal third portions of the duodenum. The C-loop of the duodenum and the pancreatic head are retracted medially to expose the inferior vena cava posteriorly.

(a)

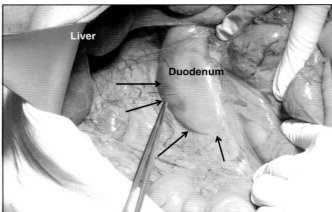

Fig. 30.4(a). Kocher maneuver: the lateral attachments of the duodenum (arrows) are sharply divided, exposing the lateral and posterior surfaces of the second portion of the duodenum.

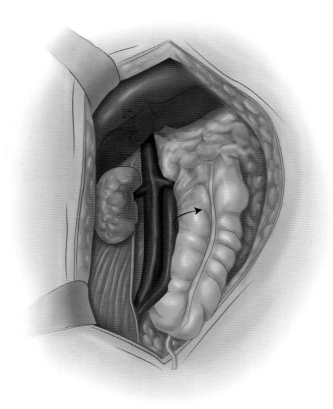

Fig. 30.3. Medial rotation of the right colon combined with Kocher mobilization of the duodenum provides good exposure of the inferior vena cava, the right renal vessels, and the right iliac vessels.

(b)

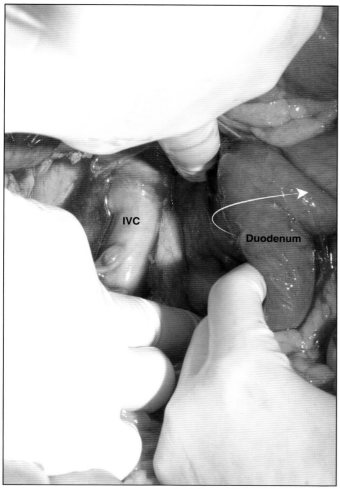

Fig. 30.4(b). The duodenum is mobilized medially and the IVC is exposed.

- The IVC is then visualized with the aorta to the left of the IVC. The paired renal veins and the right gonadal vein are visualized draining into the IVC.

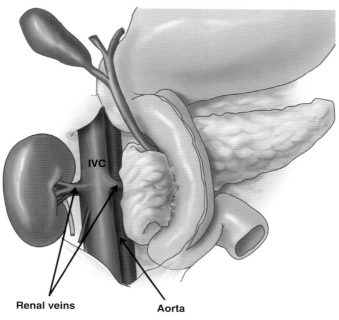

Fig. 30.5. Kocher maneuver with medial mobilization of the duodenum exposes the inferior vena cava (IVC) and the renal veins.

Fig. 30.6. Exposure of the juxtarenal IVC, after Kocher maneuver and medial visceral rotation.

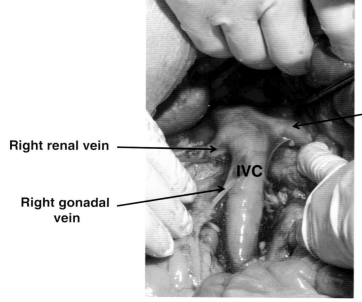

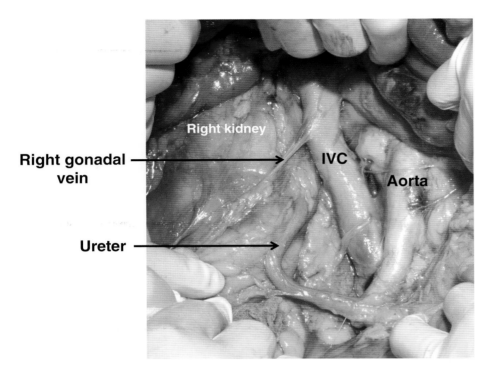

Fig. 30.7. Exposure of the IVC after medial visceral rotation and Kocher mobilization of the duodenum.

- Circumferential infrarenal IVC control may be necessary in cases where larger injuries or concern for posterior injury is suspected. The IVC should be carefully encircled with a right angle, taking care to avoid injury to the lumbar veins.

- The initial hemorrhage control can be achieved by direct digital compression and subsequent application of a side vascular clamp, if possible. Alternatively, two sponge sticks are placed above and below the IVC injury compressing the vein against the vertebral bodies. Ligation or clipping of some of the lumbar veins may be necessary for complete vascular control.

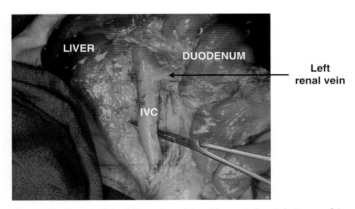

Fig. 30.8. Control of the IVC can be achieved by encircling it, being careful not to avulse any of the lumbar veins. Taking a medial to lateral approach will ensure no injury to the aorta.

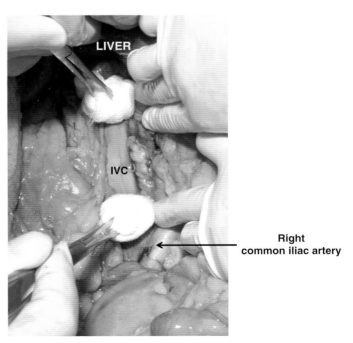

Fig. 30.9. Temporary bleeding control and prevention of air embolus with compression with two sponge sticks, above and below the IVC injury, compressing the vein against the spine.

Hemorrhage control and caval repair
Suprarenal, juxtarenal, and infrarenal IVC

- In the unstable patient in extremis aortic inflow control by either resuscitative thoracotomy (Chapter 4) or through the abdomen at the diaphragm (Chapter 19) may be necessary prior to IVC exposure.

- Many IVC lacerations can be repaired primarily with a 4–0 or 5–0 non-absorbable monofilament suture.

(a)

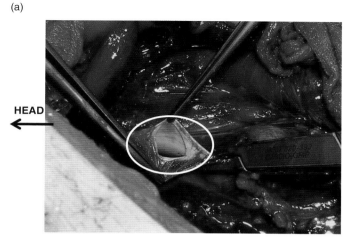

Fig. 30.10(a). Primary repair of the IVC with nonabsorbable 4–0 or 5–0 monofilament is usually possible in most knife wounds and in some low-velocity gunshot wounds.

(b)

Fig. 30.10(b). Primary repair of the IVC with no significant stenosis.

(c)

Fig. 30.10(c). Primary repair of the IVC with significant stenosis. If the stenosis is >50% of the lumen, there is an increased risk of thrombosis and pulmonary embolism.

- While some stenosis of the IVC after repair is of little consequence, more than 50% stenosis is associated with a significant risk of thromboembolism. In these cases, other options should be considered:

  (a) Repair of the IVC with an autologous venous or biologic or synthetic patch, sutured in place with a 4–0 or 5–0 non-absorbable monofilament suture.

(a)

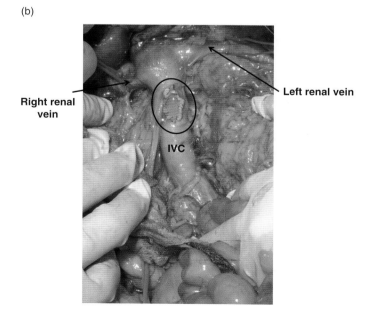

(b)

Fig. 30.11(a),(b). Synthetic or venous patches can be used to avoid >50% stenosis for repair of the IVC. The patch is sutured in using a 5–0 or 6–0 non-absorbable monofilament suture.

(b) Place a caval filter above the area of stenosis. This can be done intraoperatively with the application of a caval clip or postoperatively with the insertion of a caval filter.

(c) Ligation of the infrarenal IVC should be considered in cases with extensive tissue loss or if the patient is in extremis.

- The graft or patch should be covered with any surrounding tissues or omentum, to protect from infection or pancreatic leaks.

- Exposure of posterior IVC injuries can be achieved through circumferential mobilization of the IVC or within the lumen through an anterior venotomy.

  o Mobilize the IVC, rotate it medially, and repair the injury being cautious of avulsing the lumbar veins.

  o An anterior caval venotomy is another option to access a posterior injury. Once the posterior cava is repaired, the anterior injury can be repaired primarily or with a vascular patch, depending on the degree of stenosis that results after primary repair.

- Complete reconstruction of the IVC with a prosthetic interposition graft inserted to re-establish IVC continuity, in selected cases involving the suprarenal IVC, which are not amenable to simpler repairs. The injured portion is resected and an end-to-end anastomosis to the IVC is performed with a Dacron or PTFE graft. The graft must be 6 mm or larger.

(a)

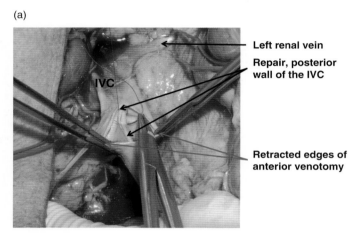

Fig. 30.12(a). Posterior IVC injury can be repaired through an anterior venotomy. The anterior venotomy is usually present in penetrating injuries and can easily be extended.

(b)

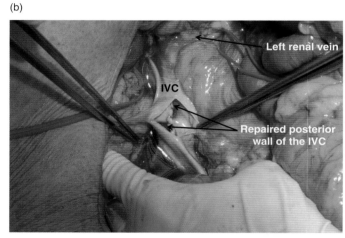

Fig. 30.12(b). Completed repaired wound of the posterior wall of the IVC.

Fig. 30.13. Methods of reconstruction in complex IVC injuries: interposition synthetic graft (A), synthetic patch (B), repair of posterior wall through anterior venotomy (C).

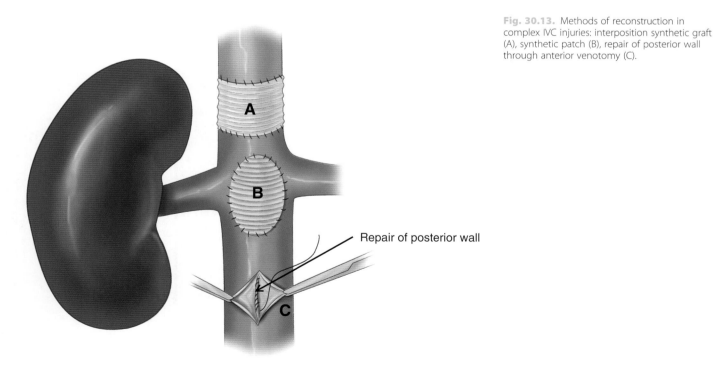

○ For juxtarenal injuries, ligation of the right renal vein necessitates a right nephrectomy. The left renal vein can be ligated close to the IVC, preserving the left gonadal vein, which provides adequate venous drainage.

• The suprarenal cava is a very short segment of IVC just below the liver and above the renal veins that is difficult to expose.

○ Repair should be attempted, if technically possible. The exposure of the laceration can be improved by applying Allis or Babcock traumatic clamps, to control the bleeding and pull down suprarenal injuries, facilitating venorrhaphy.

(a)

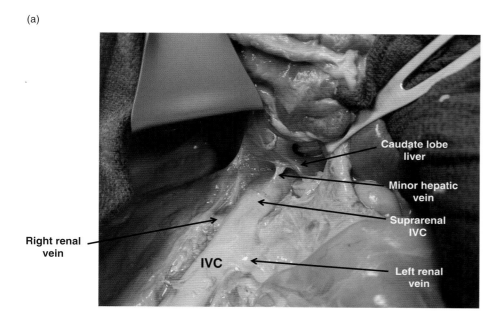

Right renal vein

Caudate lobe liver

Minor hepatic vein

Suprarenal IVC

IVC

Left renal vein

Fig. 30.14(a). The suprarenal IVC has no lumbar veins and thus poor collaterals. Ligation of the IVC in this location leads to renal failure, and increased morbidity and mortality to the patient.

(b)

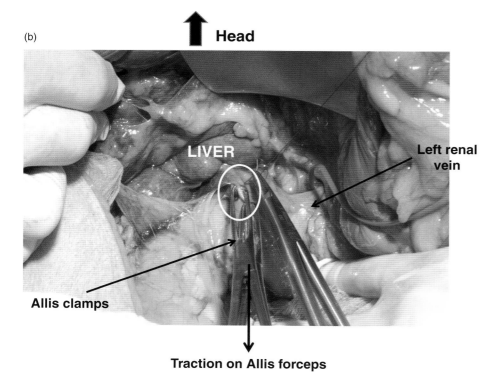

Head

LIVER

Left renal vein

Allis clamps

Traction on Allis forceps

Fig. 30.14(b). Repair of high suprarenal IVC injury (circle): using Allis or Babcocks to approximate the edges of the wound and pull it down, facilitating exposure and repair.

o In cases with significant tissue loss a vascular patch can be placed. For complex injuries not amenable to simple venorrhaphy or a vascular patch, a synthetic interposition or native vein graft can be utilized.

o Ligation of the suprarenal cava should be avoided because it results in renal failure in all cases. However, in patients in extremis it might be the only option.

• Damage control procedures should be considered in patients in extremis with severe coagulopathy, hemodynamic instability, or acidosis. They include the following.

(a) Ligation of the infrarenal IVC.

(b) Placement of a temporary shunt and semi-elective reconstruction at a later stage. A chest tube can be used, being mindful to include vents near the renal veins if the shunt traverses them. The shunt is secured with either vessel loops that are double looped and secured with clips, or with a braided suture anchoring the shunt in place.

Retrohepatic IVC

• A retrohepatic hematoma or bleeding are suggestive of an injury to the retrohepatic IVC or hepatic veins. Characteristically, the bleeding becomes worse when the liver is retracted anteriorly, and the Pringle maneuver is not effective in controlling bleeding.

• Exposure of the retrohepatic IVC is technically very difficult and should be avoided, if possible. If the hematoma is not bleeding actively or expanding rapidly, it should be left undisturbed. The liver ligaments should not be divided.

• If the retrohepatic bleeding can be controlled with gauze packing, this technique should be the operative treatment of choice and the operation should be terminated. The patient should be returned to the operating room for removal of the packing after complete physiological stabilization of the patient, usually after 24–36 hours after the initial procedure. If after removal of the packs there is still bleeding, repacking should be done.

• The effective packing of the retrohepatic bleeding requires posterior compression of the liver. The packs should be placed between the liver and the anterior abdominal wall and also under the inferior surface of the liver. This packing compresses the liver posteriorly, against the IVC, and produces a more effective tamponade. No packs should be placed between the liver and IVC.

• If the perihepatic packing is not effective in controlling bleeding, exposure and repair of the venous bleeding remain the only option. The standard midline laparotomy alone does not provide appropriate exposure. Additional exposure through a subcostal incision, or a median

sternotomy, or a right thoracotomy, is needed for good visualization of the retrohepatic vessels.

o A subcostal incision (see Fig. 30.2a) is the most common option and provides good exposure to the posterior right lobe of the liver and to the retrohepatic vessels. Division of the falciform and coronary ligaments should be performed to allow inferior-medial rotation of the liver.

o A right thoracotomy incision, through the 6–7 intercostal space to join up with the midline laparotomy incision, and division of the diaphragm straight down to the IVC diaphragmatic foramen, allows exposure of the entire length of the retrohepatic and suprahepatic IVC.

o Extension of the laparotomy incision into a median sternotomy (see Fig. 30.2b) should be done only if an atriocaval shunt is planned.

• Complete vascular control of the retrohepatic IVC requires many steps: infradiaphragmatic clamping of the aorta, followed by clamping of the infrahepatic IVC, the suprahepatic IVC, and the portal triad (Pringle maneuver, for hepatic artery and portal vein control).

o Aortic control should always be done first, in order to reduce the risk of hypovolemic cardiac arrest. The technique is described in Chapter 28.

o Suprahepatic IVC control can be achieved at two different locations:

– Between the liver and the diaphragm. In most individuals there is typically a 0.5–1.0 cm portion of the IVC where a vascular clamp can be placed. Follow the falciform ligament posteriorly until the hepatic veins and IVC is encountered and apply a vascular clamp.

– In the pericardium: this approach requires the addition of a right thoracotomy or a median sternotomy, as decribed above.

o Infrahepatic IVC control is achieved by placing a suprararenal vascular clamp.

o The portal triad control, or the Pringle maneuver, is performed through the foramen of Winslow. The portal triad can be clamped or encircled with a vessel loop (see Chapter 24).

• In extreme situations, the retrohepatic IVC injury can be bypassed with the insertion of an atrio-caval shunt.

o The laparotomy incision is extended into a median sternotomy and the pericardium is opened.

o A tape tourniquet is then applied around the intrapericardial IVC. The right atrial appendage is occluded with a vascular clamp and a 2-0 silk purse-string suture is placed in the appendage. A size 8 endotracheal tube with a side hole cut at about 8 to 10 cm from the clamped proximal end of the tube is then inserted through the purse-string. The tube is guided by the surgeon into the IVC, the balloon is inflated just above the renal veins, and the tape tourniquet around the intra-pericardial IVC is tightened.

o Alternatively, a size 36 chest tube, with cut fenestrations in its proximal part, to allow blood from the IVC to drain into the right atrium, might be used as a shunt. A second tape tourniquet placed around the suprarenal IVC is applied.

(a)

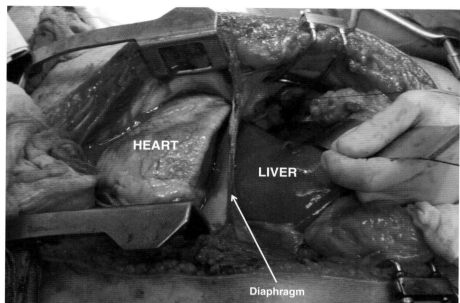

Fig. 30.15(a). Exposure for placement of atriocaval shunt requires extension of the midline laparotomy into a median sternotomy.

(b)

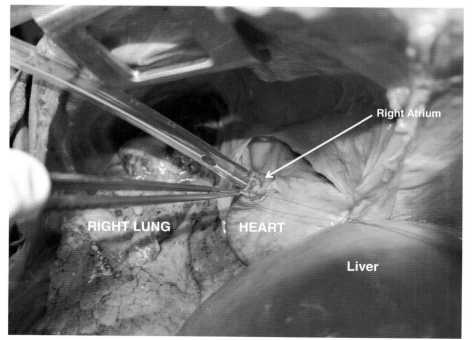

Fig. 30.15(b). Atriocaval shunt: a purse-string suture is placed in the right atrium and the shunt is inserted carefully caudad until the shunt is beyond the renal veins.

(c)

Fig. 30.15(c). Atriocaval shunt in place.

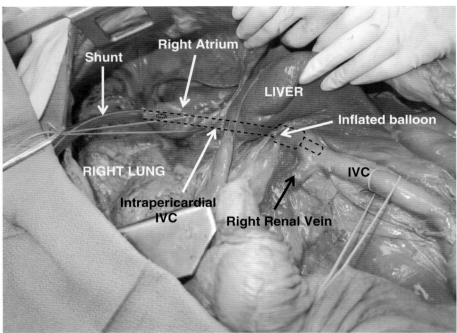

(d)

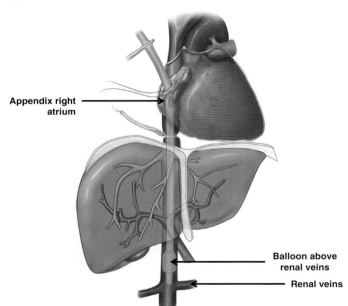

Fig. 30.15(d). Illustration of atriocaval shunt in place.

- After control of the inflow to the retrohepatic IVC is achieved, the retroperitoneal vessels are accessed by inferomedial retraction of the liver, and the venous injury is repaired with an interrupted or running 3–0 or 4–0 non-absorbable monofilament suture.

Tips and pitfalls

- In suspected abdominal vascular injuries, the femoral veins should not be used for line placement, in case the victim has an injury to the inferior vena cava or the iliac veins.
- Resist the temptation to expose a contained retrohepatic IVC injury! A disaster is likely to occur!
- In damage control, do not place packs behind the liver! The liver should be compressed posteriorly against the IVC.
- During mobilization of the infrarenal IVC, proceed carefully to avoid injury to the lumbar veins. The avulsed vein retracts and it is difficult to find it.
- During exploration of a caval injury, there is high risk for air embolism. Prevent this complication by early direct compression, followed by proximal and distal control.
- Following IVC ligation, the lower extremities and feet should be wrapped with elastic bandages to reduce edema. Monitor closely for extremity compartment syndrome.
- Following damage control packing or repair of IVC injuries, the patient should not be over-resuscitated.
- In the appropriate cases, consider placement of the atriocaval shunt early, before the patient is in extremis. During placement of the atriocaval shunt, manually guide the tube into the IVC. It often curls into the heart!

31

Surgical control of pelvic fracture hemorrhage

Peep Talving and Matthew D. Tadlock

Surgical anatomy

- Severe bleeding in complex pelvic fractures usually originates from branches of the internal iliac artery, the presacral venous plexus, the fractured bones, and the soft tissues. On rare occasions, it could be due to tear of the major iliac arteries and veins.

- The abdominal aorta bifurcates into the two common iliac arteries at the L_4–L_5 level. The iliac veins are located posterior and to the right of the common iliac arteries. The ureter crosses over the bifurcation of the common iliac artery into the external and internal iliac arteries.

- The internal iliac artery is about 4 cm long. At the level of the greater sciatic foramen, it divides into the anterior and posterior trunks. It gives numerous splanchnic and muscular branches and terminates as an internal pudendal artery, which is a potential source of hemorrhage in

anterior ring disruptions. Hemorrhage following pelvic fracture can occur from any branch.

- The most commonly injured internal iliac artery branches (in decreasing order of frequency) are the superior gluteal, internal pudendal, and obturator arteries.

  - The superior gluteal artery is the largest branch of the internal iliac artery. It exits the pelvis through the greater sciatic foramen, above the piriformis muscle. It provides blood supply to the gluteus medius and minimus muscles.

  - The internal pudendal artery passes through the greater sciatic foramen, courses around the sciatic spine, and enters the perineum through the lesser sciatic foramen.

  - The obturator artery courses along the lateral pelvic wall and exits the pelvis through the obturator canal. In about 30% of cases the obturator artery is perfused from both internal and external iliac arteries, making angioembolization more complicated.

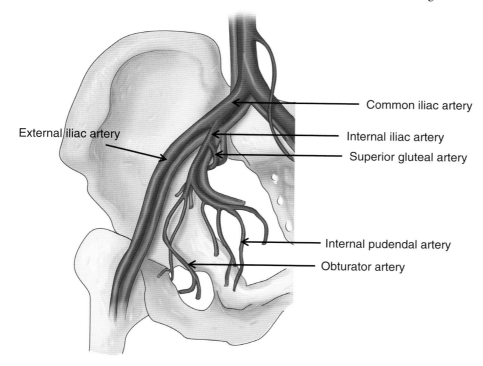

Fig. 31.1. Anatomy of the internal iliac artery. The most commonly injured internal iliac artery branches (in decreasing order of frequency) are the superior gluteal, internal pudendal, and obturator arteries.

External iliac artery

Common iliac artery

Internal iliac artery

Superior gluteal artery

Internal pudendal artery

Obturator artery

Atlas of Surgical Techniques in Trauma, ed. Demetrios Demetriades, Kenji Inaba, and George Velmahos. Published by Cambridge University Press. © Cambridge University Press 2015.

General principles

- The pelvic retroperitoneal space can accommodate 3–4 liters of blood before venous tamponade occurs. Any significant (>3 cm) pubic symphysis diastasis increases significantly the pelvic volume and reduces the effectiveness of tamponade.
- Complex pelvic fractures are associated with a high incidence of intra-abdominal injuries and significant blood loss. Nearly 30% of these fractures are associated with intra-abdominal injuries and about 80% have multisystem trauma.
- The most common associated intra-abdominal injuries are bladder and urethral injuries, followed by injuries to the liver, small bowel, spleen, and diaphragm.
- Patients with severe pelvic fractures should be admitted under Trauma Surgery, for close monitoring for major bleeding or possible intra-abdominal injuries, for at least 24 hours before transferring to the orthopedic service.
- Hemorrhage in pelvic fractures originates from the cancellous bone surfaces, pelvic vein plexuses, internal iliac artery branches (15%–20%), and soft tissue injuries. Pelvic vascular injuries involving the major iliac veins and arteries occur in about 4%–10% of severe fractures.
- Independent predictors of severe hemorrhage from the pelvic fracture include persistent hypotension, contrast extravasation on CT-imaging, large pelvic sidewall hematoma, sacroiliac joint disruption, symphysis diastasis ≥ 2.5 cm, bilateral and concomitant superior and inferior pubic rami fractures ("Butterfly fracture"), age ≥ 55 years, and female sex.
- While the open anteroposterior compression, i.e., open book pelvic fractures, are frequently associated with pelvic vascular injury and hemodynamic compromise, whereas closed book fractures are often associated with injuries to urogenital and gastrointestinal structures.
- A pelvic radiograph is useful in determining the need or contraindication for application of a pelvic binder. Pubic symphysis diastasis is an excellent indication for pelvic binder application, while a fracture of the iliac wing is an absolute contraindication. However, it often underestimates the severity of the fracture and may miss posterior fractures.

Management of pelvic fracture bleeding

- The majority of patients with bleeding from pelvic fractures can safely be managed with supportive measures, such as pelvic immobilization, blood transfusions, and angioembolization. A massive transfusion protocol should be followed in the appropriate cases.
- Pelvic binder is the first treatment to reduce the pelvic ring volume in an open book type pelvic fracture. Pelvic binders should be applied over the greater trochanters to appropriately reduce pelvic volume and allow laparotomy

and femoral artery access for catheter-based angiographic embolization. Pelvic binders are contraindicated in major iliac wing fractures and has no role in closed book fractures.

(a)

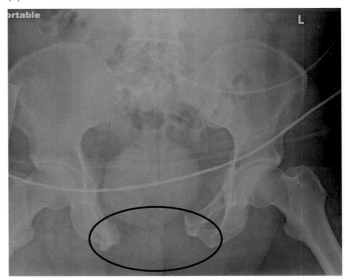

Fig. 31.2(a). Open book fracture with severe pubic symphysis diastasis is the ideal indication for pelvic binder application.

(b)

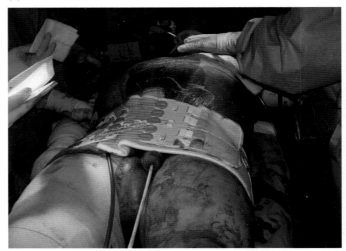

Fig. 31.2(b). A pelvic binder is applied to open book pelvic fractures, reducing pelvic ring volume and hemorrhage.

- External pelvic fixation in the emergency room is rarely indicated or performed, and there is no evidence that it is of any benefit.
- In a small number of patients with severe bleeding not responding to conventional therapeutic interventions, damage control with pelvic packing may be life-saving. The indications for operative management include severe hemodynamic instability, need for laparotomy for associated intra-abdominal injuries, and failed or non-availability of angioembolization.

Damage control operations

There are two methods of damage control in severe pelvic fracture bleeding: the extra-peritoneal approach and the intra-peritoneal approach.

Special instruments

- The optimal operating room is the hybrid operating room with surgical and interventional radiology capabilities simultaneously available.
- Operating-table mounted laparotomy retractor systems facilitate surgical exposure.
- Major trauma laparotomy tray and vascular tray must be available.
- Large and medium clips and applier.
- Vessel loops.
- Local hemostatic sealants based on fibrin, thrombin, collagen sponge, cellulose, microfibrillar collagen, and bone wax facilitate local hemostasis and effective packing.
- Angiography equipment with embolization coils and Gelfoam particles.

Patient positioning

- The patient is positioned in the supine position for trauma laparotomy and resuscitative thoracotomy when warranted. Skin preparation should include the chest, abdomen, and lower extremities to the knees.
- Access to the femoral artery below the inguinal ligament should be available for interventional radiology.

Incision

Extra-peritoneal pelvic packing

- An 8–10 cm skin incision is made midline below the umbilicus.

(a)

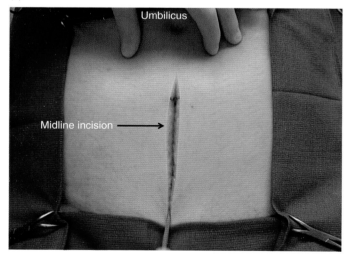

Fig. 31.3(a),(b). Extra-peritoneal pelvic packing: a 8–10 cm skin incision is made at the midline below the umbilicus to gain access to the preperitoneal space.

(b)

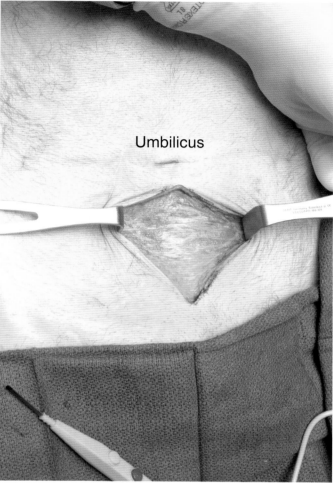

Umbilicus

Fig. 31.3(a),(b). (cont.)

- The midline fascia is exposed and incised down to the peritoneum. The peritoneum is not entered. The prevesical space of Retzius is now exposed.
- While the clots are removed from the prevesical space, the bladder and peritoneum are swept posteriorly to allow effective packing.

(a)

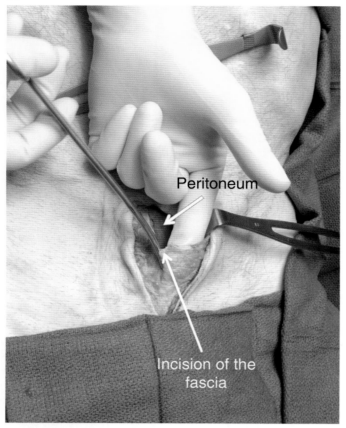

Peritoneum

Incision of the fascia

Fig. 31.4(a). The midline fascia is exposed and incised down to the peritoneum. The peritoneum is not entered.

(b)

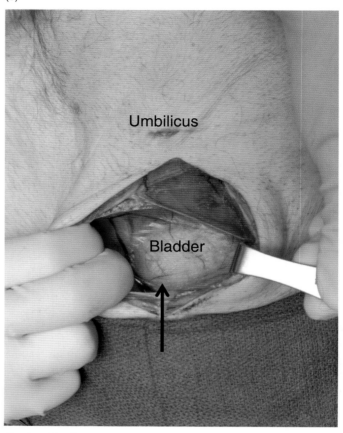

Umbilicus

Bladder

Fig. 31.4(b). The prevesical space of Retzius (arrow).

(c)

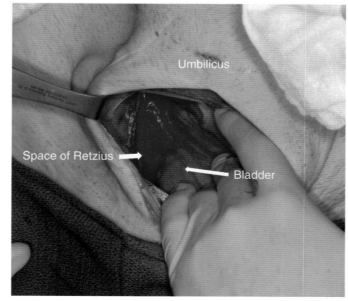

Umbilicus

Space of Retzius

Bladder

Fig. 31.4(c). Blood is seen in the preperitoneal space (space of Retzius). Peritoneal contents and the bladder are reflected posteriorly to facilitate extraperitoneal pelvic packing.

- Three laparotomy packs are inserted extraperitoneally along the pelvic sidewall on both sides of the bladder, towards the sacroiliac joint and internal iliac vessels to control bleeding originating from internal iliac arteries and vein plexuses.

(a)

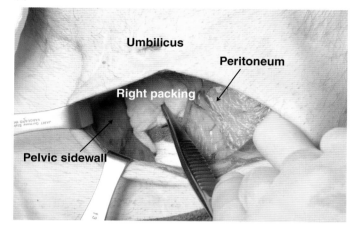

(b)

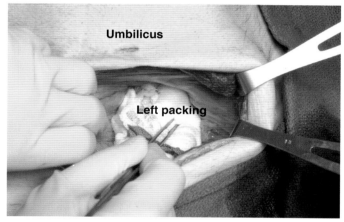

Fig. 31.5(a),(b). Packs are placed posteriorly towards the sacroiliac joint and internal iliac vessels. Three packs are placed on each pelvic sidewall.

- Following the packing, the rectus sheath is closed with a running suture to facilitate effective tamponade.
- Early angiography should be considered after the extraperitoneal packing.

(a)

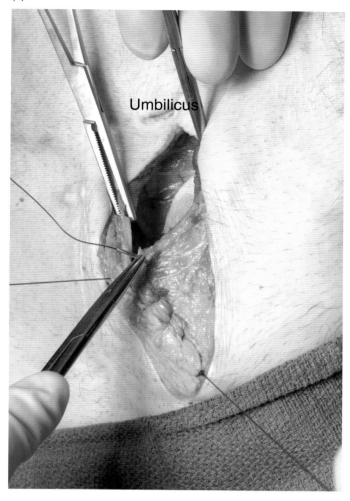

Fig. 31.6(a),(b). The fascia is closed over the extraperitoneal pelvic packing.

(b)

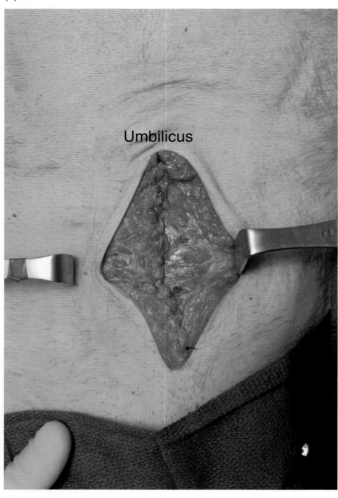

Umbilicus

Fig. 31.6(a),(b). (cont.)

Intraperitoneal damage control

- Rationale for intraperitoneal damage control: exploration and management of associated abdominal injuries, direct evaluation of major vessels and areas of bleeding, gauze packing of the bleeding area, and occlusion of internal iliac arteries.
- A formal exploratory trauma laparotomy is performed. Any associated intraperitoneal injuries are identified and treated.
- Sigmoid colon is reflected laterally to the patient's left to expose the retroperitoneal hematoma, distal aorta, iliac artery bifurcations, and ureters when the hematoma is decompressed and explored.

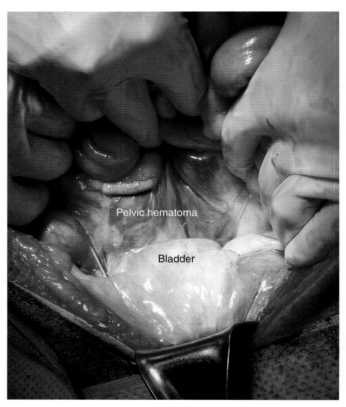

Pelvic hematoma

Bladder

Fig. 31.7. Operative photo depicting a pelvic hematoma associated with a pelvic fracture. The sigmoid colon is reflected laterally to facilitate exposure.

- The retroperitoneum is opened by medial mobilization of the left or the right colon or by incising the retroperitoneum directly over the common iliac artery bifurcation. The hematoma is evacuated and any obvious major bleeding from the large vessels is controlled with sutures, ligation, or repair.
- The common iliac arteries are dissected bilaterally and the internal iliac arteries are identified and isolated using right-angle clamps.
- Care must be taken to avoid injury to the ureters, which cross over the bifurcation of the common iliac artery into the external and internal iliac arteries.
- Vessel loops are applied to both internal iliac arteries and firm retraction is applied to occlude the pelvic arterial inflow.
- Surgical clips are placed on the retracted vessel loops to facilitate the temporary vessel–loop–clip occlusion of the internal iliac artery. The procedure is performed bilaterally for effective inflow occlusion.

(a)

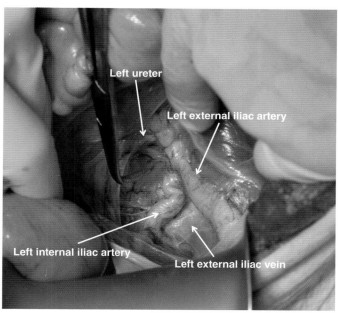

Fig. 31.8(a). The sigmoid colon has been reflected medially and the retroperitoneum has been opened exposing the left external and internal iliac arteries. The left external iliac vein is seen posterior and medial to the left external iliac artery.

(b)

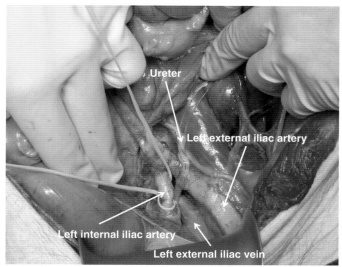

Fig. 31.8(b). The left internal iliac artery is isolated with a vessel loop. Note the ureter crossing over the external iliac artery.

- The use of the vessel–loop–clip occlusion technique allows vessel loop removal in the subsequent angiography setting for embolization following the surgical damage control.
- Alternatively, the internal iliac arteries can be bilaterally ligated or occluded using surgical clips. Surgical clip placement allows clip removal and angioembolization in the postoperative phase of care when warranted.

- Following the vascular control and application of local hemostatic sealants, pelvic packing, and temporary abdominal closure are performed.

(a)

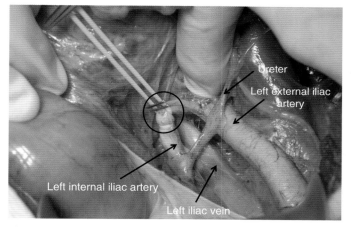

Fig. 31.9(a). Two clips (black circle) are placed on the vessel loop to facilitate temporary occlusion of the internal iliac artery.

(b)

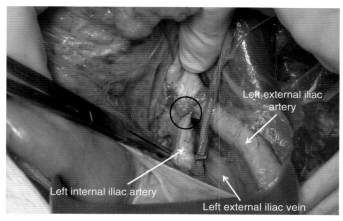

Fig. 31.9(b). A single clip (black circle) is placed across the internal iliac artery to facilitate temporary occlusion.

- Catheter-based angiogram of the aorta, lumbar arteries, and the external iliac branches should be considered in appropriate cases.

Tips and pitfalls

- In the presence of a pelvic hematoma the FAST examination may be unreliable in the diagnosis of intra-abdominal hemorrhage. If the condition of the patient does allow CT scan evaluation, consider diagnostic peritoneal aspirate.

- Failure to activate massive transfusion protocol early in the management of the hemodynamically compromised patient.
- Failure to appreciate the high incidence of intra-abdominal associated injuries.
- Failure to take the severely hemodynamically compromised patient to the operating room for abdominal exploration for associated injuries and possible damage control in the pelvis.

- Avoid ligation of the internal iliac artery in cases with acetabular fractures because it may interfere with subsequent surgical exposure and repair of the fracture.
- Inadequate knowledge of the anatomy of the iliac vessels and their relationship to the ureter may result in iatrogenic injury to the ureter.

Brachial artery injury

32

Peep Talving and Elizabeth R. Benjamin

Surgical anatomy

- The brachial artery lies in the groove between the biceps and triceps muscles. The proximal brachial artery lies medial to the humerus and gradually travels lateral to lie anterior to the humerus distally. At the antecubital fossa, it runs deep to the bicipital aponeurosis and bifurcates into the radial and ulnar arteries, just below the elbow. The artery is surrounded by the two brachial veins, which run on either side of the artery. At the upper part of the arm, they join to form the axillary vein.

- The profunda brachial artery is a large branch arising from the medial and posterior part of the proximal brachial artery and follows the radial nerve closely. It provides collateral circulation to the lower arm.

- The basilic vein courses in the subcutaneous tissue in the medial aspect of the lower arm. At the mid arm, it penetrates the fascia to join one of the brachial veins.

- The cephalic vein is entirely in the subcutaneous tissues, courses in the deltopectoral groove, and empties at the junction of the brachial and axillary veins.

- In the upper arm, the median nerve is in front of the brachial artery. It then crosses over the artery mid upper arm and distally it lies behind the artery.

- The ulnar nerve is behind the artery in the upper half of the arm. At about the middle, it pierces the intermuscular septum and courses more posteriorly, away from the artery, behind the medial epicondyle.

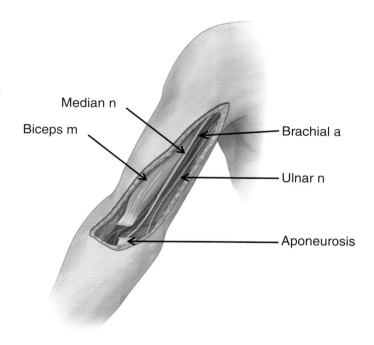

Fig. 32.1. The brachial artery lies in the groove between the biceps and triceps muscles. Note the close anatomical relationship with the median and ulnar nerves. In the upper arm the median nerve is anterolateral to the artery and at the middle it crosses over to course posteromedial to the artery. The artery bifurcates into the ulnar and radial arteries under the bicipital aponeurosis, at the antecubital fossa.

Atlas of Surgical Techniques in Trauma, ed. Demetrios Demetriades, Kenji Inaba, and George Velmahos. Published by Cambridge University Press. © Cambridge University Press 2015.

(a)

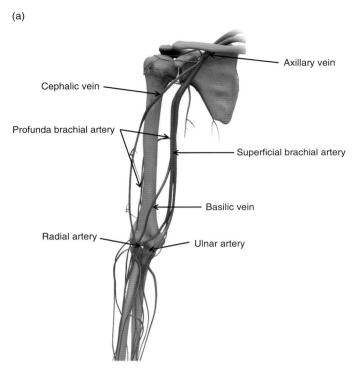

Axillary vein

Cephalic vein

Profunda brachial artery

Superficial brachial artery

Basilic vein

Radial artery

Ulnar artery

Fig. 32.2(a). Anatomy of the major branches of the brachial artery and the superficial and deep veins in the arm.

(b)

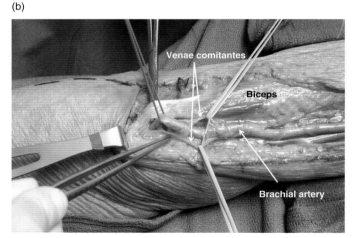

Venae comitantes

Biceps

Brachial artery

Fig. 32.2(b). Paired venae comitantes run on either side of the brachial artery.

General principles

- "Hard signs" of extremity vascular injury, including pulsatile bleeding, expanding or pulsatile hematoma, palpable thrill, audible bruit, absent peripheral pulse, and/or distal ischemia are a strong indication for immediate operative exploration. Patients with multiple level

penetrating injuries or shotgun injuries may benefit from preoperative imaging. "Soft signs" of vascular injury include minor bleeding, stable small hematoma, and an abnormal pulse index. In these cases arterial evaluation by CT angiogram should be performed.

- Hemorrhage from the brachial artery can be temporarily controlled using direct digital compression or a proximal tourniquet.
- Ligation of the brachial artery is associated with a high incidence of limb loss and should not be done. In patients in extremis a temporary shunt and delayed reconstruction should be considered.
- In the event of a mangled extremity, the priority is restoration of distal blood flow. This can be accomplished with shunt placement, external fracture fixation as needed, followed by debridement and definitive vascular repair.
- Brachial artery injury is treated with primary repair or autologous vein graft reconstruction. Synthetic grafts below the shoulder have poor long-term patency.
- Completion angiogram is indicated if there is any concern regarding distal flow.
- Intra- and postoperatively, patients with brachial artery injuries should be monitored for compartment syndrome with serial clinical examinations, compartment pressure monitoring, and serial blood creatine kinase (CK) levels. Fasciotomy should be considered in appropriate cases.

Special surgical instruments

- In patients with suspected brachial artery injury, a vascular tray is necessary.
- A sterile tourniquet should be in the field for proximal control.
- A sterile Doppler probe should be available for perfusion monitoring and an ultrasound for saphenous vein mapping.
- Fogarty catheters, 3 and 4Fr should be available to clear the vessel of clots.
- Heparin solution for local use consisting of 5000 units of heparin in 100 mL of normal saline.
- An array of shunt sizes should be available to restore blood flow in case immediate repair or reconstruction are not possible. 15 cm Argyle shunts ranging from 8–14Fr should be adequate for most injuries.
- If an angiogram is to be performed, C-arm fluoroscopy, 18G butterfly needle, and water-soluble contrast should be available.

Positioning

- For a brachial artery injury, the patient is positioned in the supine position with the injured arm abducted 90 degrees, externally rotated to face palm up with an arm table board. Skin preparation should include the hand, circumferential arm to the axilla, shoulder, neck and chest. The patient's prepped hand should be covered with a sterile stockinette or blue towel.

- Potential operative needs to be considered during skin preparation include access to the wrist and hand for perfusion monitoring, forearm for compartment pressure monitoring, and the axilla and chest for emergent proximal vascular control.
- The bilateral groins should be prepared for possible vein harvest.

Incision

- The skin incision to expose the brachial artery is made between the biceps and triceps brachii bellies that can be extended proximally to the delto-pectoral groove for axillary artery exposure. The incision can be extended distally, curving towards the radius in the antecubital fossa to expose the brachial bifurcation. The basilic vein is identified and protected in the subcutaneous tissue in the lower part of the arm.

(a)

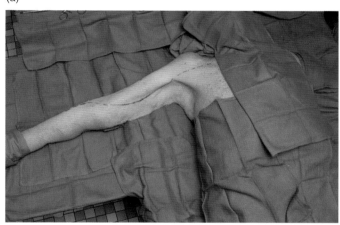

(b)

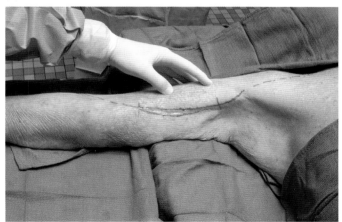

Fig. 32.3(a),(b). The skin incision for brachial artery exposure extends proximally from the deltopectoral groove, along the groove between the biceps and triceps muscles, curving radially over the antecubital fossa (solid line). For more proximal control at the axillary artery level, the incision is extended into the deltopectoral groove (interrupted line). The incision can be extended distally curving toward the radius in the antecubital fossa to expose the brachial bifurcation (interrupted line).

Exposure

- Access to the brachial artery requires superior retraction of the biceps and inferior retraction of the triceps muscles in order to expose the neurovascular structures.
- The brachial artery is covered by a fascial sheath within the groove between the biceps and triceps muscles.

(a)

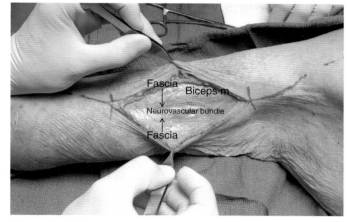

Fig. 32.4(a). The neurovascular bundle runs between the biceps and triceps brachii muscles, under the fascia.

(b)

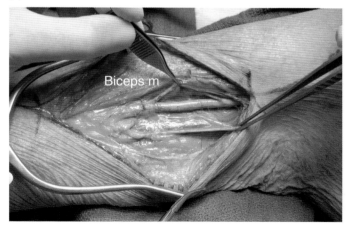

Fig. 32.4(b). Exposed neurovascular bundle.

- In the proximal arm, the brachial artery lies just posterior and medial to the median nerve and anterior and lateral to the ulnar nerve. The basilic vein lies medial, outside the brachial artery sheath. Once the muscle bellies are retracted, the ulnar nerve and basilic vein should fall posteriorly with the triceps muscle and be out of the operating field.

- The profunda brachial artery is a medial branch of the brachial artery in the proximal third of the upper arm and is accompanied by the radial nerve. It is important to preserve this branch if not injured as it provides collateral circulation to the lower arm.

- Mid arm, the median nerve crosses over the brachial artery and then courses medial to the artery as it bifurcates into the radial and ulnar arteries at the antecubital fossa.
- In order to access the brachial artery bifurcation, the bicipital aponeurosis must be divided. Division of this aponeurosis has no clinical consequence and it does not require reconstruction.

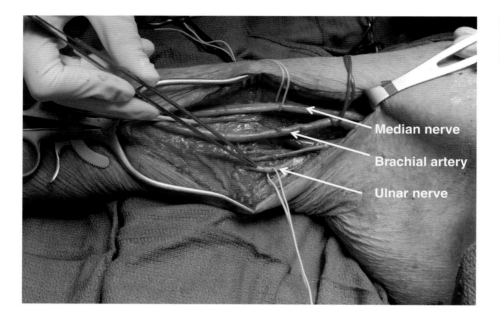

Fig. 32.5. Exposure of the brachial artery. The median nerve is anterolaterally and the ulnar nerve posteromedially. The ulnar nerve courses posteriorly.

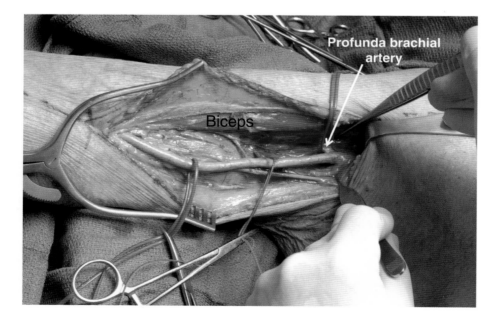

Fig. 32.6. The proximal brachial artery gives off a profunda branch. This branch should be preserved, whenever possible, because it may provide important collateral circulation to the lower arm.

(a)

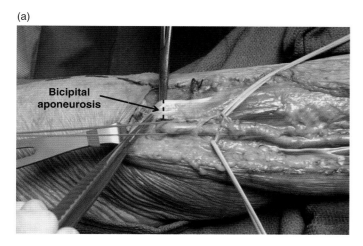

Bicipital
aponeurosis

(b)

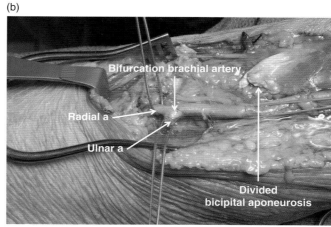

Bifurcation brachial artery

Radial a

Ulnar a

Divided
bicipital aponeurosis

Fig. 32.7(a),(b). Division of the bicipital aponeurosis at the antecubital fossa exposes the bifurcation of the brachial artery into the radial and ulnar arteries.

Vascular repair

- Once the injury is identified, proximal and distal control are obtained using bulldog clamps.

- When definitive repair is feasible, debridement of the injured segment to a healthy vessel is performed. If a temporary shunt is utilized, debridement of the injured vessel is delayed until the time of definitive repair.

Fig. 32.8. Proximal and distal control of the arterial injury (circle).

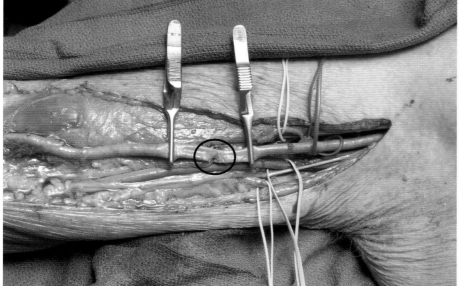

- A 3Fr Fogarty catheter is passed proximally and distally to clear the vessel of clots.
- Regional heparinization is achieved using heparinized saline solution (5000 units in 100 mL normal saline), 50 mL proximally, and 50 mL distally followed by reapplication of the vessel clamps.

(a)

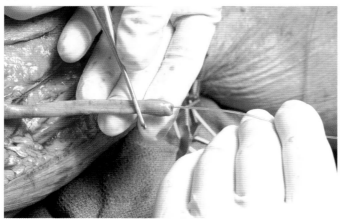

(b)

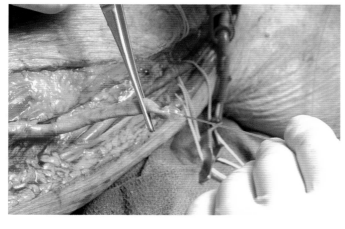

Fig. 32.9(a),(b). Prior to shunt placement, repair, or graft, the artery is cleared of clot by proximal and distal passage of a 3Fr Fogarty catheter.

- Prior to definitive repair, the proximal and distal ends of the artery are trimmed using Potts scissors. The ends can be beveled as needed for repair.
- Small caliber arteries and the vein graft can be dilated using a Fogarty catheter. Local anesthetic or papaverin can be used regionally to counteract vasospasm.
- Repair is achieved by primary repair or by utilizing a reversed autologous vein graft as the conduit. A PTFE interposition graft remains the last resort.
- The vascular anastomosis is performed using a running or interrupted monofilament suture with the needle passing from the intima to adventitia on the artery side in order to

minimize the risk of intimal flaps and dissection. The more technically complex anastomosis is created first, and the artery is vented to release air bubbles prior to securing the final suture line.
- After restoration of blood flow, distal pulses should be documented and the surgeon should consider an on-table angiogram prior to leaving the operating room if there is any question regarding flow.

Temporary shunt

- When a temporary shunt is utilized as part of damage control, a 0 silk tie is used to secure the shunt proximally and distally. These ties are then tied together around the center of the shunt.
- The presence of distal flow must be confirmed after shunt placement with Doppler ultrasound.

(a)

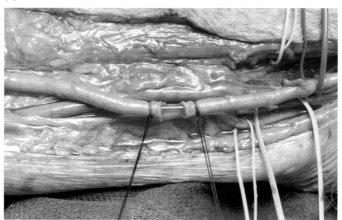

(b)

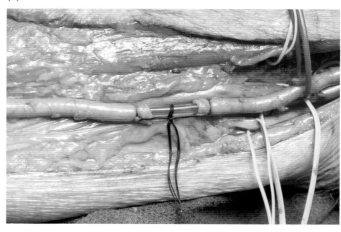

Fig. 32.10(a),(b). A temporary shunt is placed to restore distal blood flow. A 0 silk tie is used to secure the shunt proximally and distally in order to prevent accidental dislodgement. The profunda brachial artery is a proximal branch that provides collateral circulation to the lower arm.

Tips and pitfalls

- The median and ulnar nerves are in close proximity to the brachial artery and it is important to prevent iatrogenic nerve injury. High risk areas for injury include ulnar nerve injury with initial exposure prior to inferior retraction of the nerve with the triceps brachii and injury to the median nerve as it crosses anteriorly over the brachial artery as they course down the arm.
- During proximal brachial artery dissection, whenever possible, preserve the profunda brachial artery as it provides significant collateral circulation to the lower arm.
- A single individual should perform the Fogarty catheter passage. The resistance placed on the balloon during thrombus extraction is a dynamic process, and care must be taken not to exert excessive force on the intima and create iatrogenic injury.
- After thrombus extraction, there should be generous forward and adequate backflow. If there is not adequate flow prior to creation of the anastomosis, there is a risk of a distal clot or missed injury.
- In the event of a destructive injury, it is important to adequately prepare the anastomotic bed by debridement of all devitalized tissues. Failure to do so can interfere with graft and wound healing and lead to secondary infection.
- When sizing the length of the saphenous vein graft, it is important to place the arm in gentle flexion of 10–20 degrees. A common mistake is redundant graft length, which will lead to kinking of the graft.
- Arterial repair or anastomosis must be performed without tension. In select cases, such as in knife wounds, gentle mobilization of the proximal and distal ends of the artery can allow primary anastomosis. In most cases with gunshot wounds or blunt trauma, a reversed interposition vein graft is required.
- During shunt placement, avoid debridement of the injured vessel. This should be performed at the time of definitive reconstruction, in order to preserve as much normal artery as possible.
- Compartment syndrome of the forearm is a common complication after brachial artery injury, especially with associated extensive soft tissue trauma or prolonged ischemia. Evaluate intraoperatively and postoperatively for clinical signs of compartment syndrome. In appropriate cases measure the compartment pressures. Postoperatively routine monitoring of CK levels is important. Consider early fasciotomy in appropriate cases (see Chapter 33).

Upper extremity fasciotomies

Jennifer Smith and Mark W. Bowyer

Surgical anatomy

- The arm is divided into two muscle compartments:

  o The anterior compartment, which contains the biceps, the brachialis and coracobrachialis, all innervated by the musculocutaneous nerve.

  o The posterior compartment, which contains the triceps, is innervated by the radial nerve.

- The forearm is divided into three anatomic compartments.

  o The anterior or flexor compartment, which contains the muscles responsible for wrist flexion and pronation of the forearm. There are a total of eight muscles innervated by the median and ulnar nerves, all receiving blood supply from the ulnar artery. The posterior or extensor compartment, which contains the muscles responsible for wrist extension, is innervated by the radial nerve. The blood supply is provided by the radial artery.

  o The mobile wad is a group of three muscles on the radial aspect of the forearm that act as flexors at the elbow joint. These muscles are occasionally grouped together with the dorsal compartment. The blood supply is provided by the radial artery and the innervation by branches of the radial nerve.

- The hand includes ten separate osteofascial compartments.

  o The transverse carpal ligament, over the carpal tunnel, is a strong and broad ligament. The tunnel contains the median nerve and the finger flexor tendons.

General principles

- Compartment syndrome is a limb- and life-threatening condition. Renal failure due to myoglobinemia and myoglobinuria is a common serious systemic complication due to delayed diagnosis. Volkmann's ischemic contracture is another complication resulting in permanent disability.

- Common causes of forearm compartment syndrome include vascular injuries, severe fractures, crush injuries, extrinsic compression devices such as casts and dressings, extravasation of intravenous infusions, burns, edema from infection, and snakebites.

- The diagnosis of compartment syndrome is made by a constellation of clinical findings including tense compartments and pain (usually out of proportion to that expected from the existing injury) with passive stretch of the fingers. When conclusive evidence is not present, or patients are not evaluable, compartment pressures may be measured.

- An absolute compartment pressure of >30 mm Hg or a delta pressure less than 30 mm Hg (diastolic blood pressure minus tissue pressure) should prompt surgical decompression.

- Systemic blood pressure may have an effect on extremity perfusion, so a lower absolute threshold for fasciotomy should be considered in patients who are hypotensive.

- Reversible muscle ischemia and neuropraxia occur in up to 4–6 hours of ischemia time. Irreversible muscle ischemia and axonotmesis occur beyond 6 hours of ischemia time.

- The prognosis of acute compartment syndrome depends upon the extent and duration of the pressure maintained in the compartment. Failure to decompress compartment syndrome will result in progressive muscle and nerve ischemia, leading to paresthesia, paralysis, pulselessness, and ultimately amputation.

- The most common muscle compartment in the upper extremity affected by compartment syndrome is the anterior (flexor) compartment of the forearm. The upper arm is the least commonly affected, because it has a greater capacity to swell before the compartment pressures increase.

Atlas of Surgical Techniques in Trauma, ed. Demetrios Demetriades, Kenji Inaba, and George Velmahos. Published by Cambridge University Press. © Cambridge University Press 2015.

Special surgical instruments

- Basic orthopedic tray.
- Stryker® intra-compartmental pressure measuring system using an 18-gauge side-ported needle is a readily available method for measuring compartment pressures (see technique in Chapter 38).
- For vessel–loop shoelace wound closure: vessel loops and skin staples.
- Negative pressure dressing system (NPDS).

Positioning

The affected arm is placed 90 degrees from the body on an arm board. The entire chest, arm, forearm, and hand are prepped into the surgical field.

Upper arm fasciotomy

- The two upper arm muscle compartments can be released through a single lateral skin incision from deltoid insertion to lateral epicondyle.
  - At the fascial level two skin flaps are mobilized anteriorly and posteriorly.
  - The intermuscular septum between the anterior and posterior compartment is identified and the fascia over each compartment is incised longitudinally.
  - Protect the radial nerve as it passes through the intermuscular septum from the posterior compartment to the anterior compartment just under the fascia.

(a)

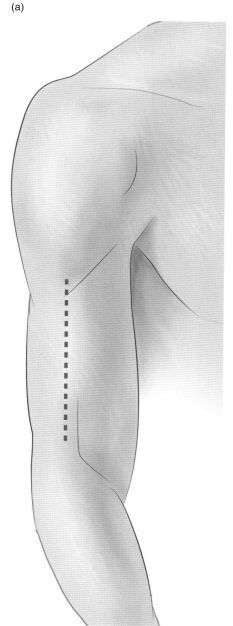

Fig. 33.1(a). The two upper arm muscle compartments can be released through a single lateral skin incision from deltoid insertion to lateral epicondyle.

(b)

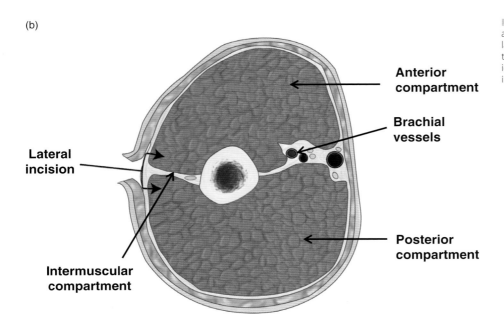

Anterior compartment

Brachial vessels

Lateral incision

Posterior compartment

Intermuscular compartment

Fig. 33.1(b). Decompression of the two upper arm compartments of the right arm, through a lateral incision. The intermuscular septum between the anterior and posterior compartments is identified and the fascia over each compartment is incised longitudinally.

Forearm and hand fasciotomies

Incisions

- A variety of incisions are described to decompress the three compartments of the forearm. The most common approach utilizes two incisions (a dorsal and a volar incision) to decompress the three compartments.

- The most commonly described volar or anterior incision is the so-called "Lazy S." The incision begins just proximal to the antecubital fossa on the medial aspect of the forearm

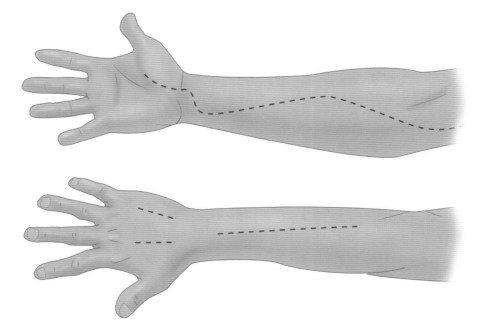

Fig. 33.2. The standard volar and dorsal incisions used to perform fasciotomy of the forearm and the hand.

in the groove between the biceps and triceps. It is extended in a curvilinear fashion toward the radial aspect of the mid forearm and then curved back toward the ulnar aspect of

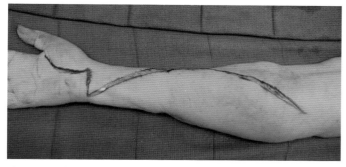

Fig. 33.3. The Lazy S incision used to open the volar (anterior) and mobile wad (lateral) compartments demonstrated on the right arm.

the forearm at the wrist. The incision is then carried transversely to the center of the wrist and then carried on to the hand curving up on to the thenar eminence.

- The skin flap of the forearm is then elevated and the underlying fascia encasing the flexor muscle bellies are exposed and opened with scissors.
- At the wrist, the carpal tunnel is completely decompressed, taking care to prevent injury to the median nerve found just deep to the divided flexor retinaculum (transverse carpal ligament).
  - Adequate decompression of the volar forearm and palmar hand requires wide epimysiotomy (sectioning of the muscle sheath) over all muscle bellies of the volar forearm as well as carrying the incision well on to the thenar aspect of the palm to completely decompress the flexor retinaculum, which extends well beyond the wrist.

(a)

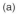
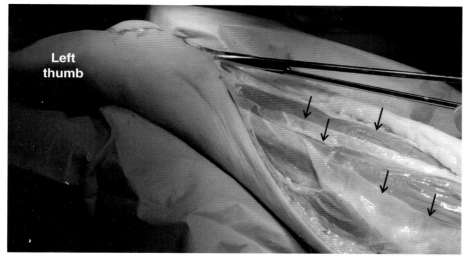

Fig. 33.4(a). Scissors are used to open the fascial layers (arrows) (epimysiotomy) overlying the muscle bellies of the volar (anterior) and mobile wad (lateral) compartments as shown on the left arm.

(b)

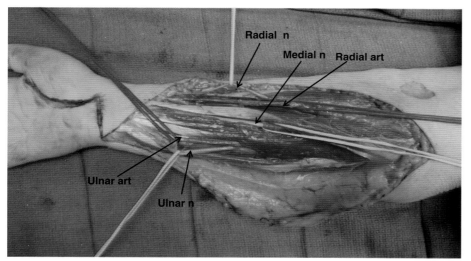

Fig. 33.4(b). Complete opening of all fascial layers and decompression of all flexor muscles of the left arm. The nerves should be protected.

(a)

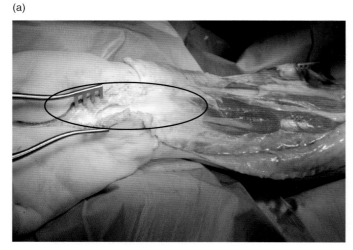

Fig. 33.5(a). A completed fasciotomy of the left forearm demonstrating complete epimysiotomy of the flexor muscles. The transverse carpal ligament (circle), over the carpal tunnel, is a strong and broad ligament and extends well beyond the wrist. Adequate decompression requires division of this ligament.

(b)

Median n

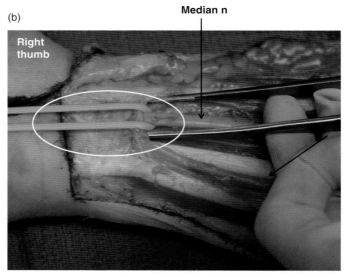

Fig. 33.5(b). The transverse carpal ligament (circle) with the underlying median nerve.

(c)

Divided transverse ligament

Median n

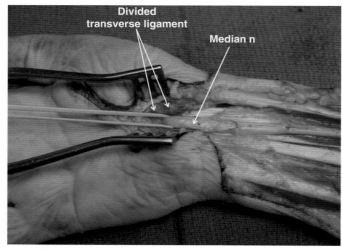
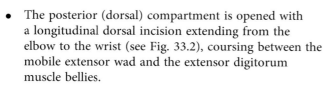

Fig. 33.5(c). Division of the transverse carpal ligament and decompression of the median nerve.

(a)

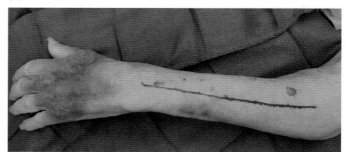

Fig. 33.6(a). The incision for the decompression of the dorsal compartment of the forearm extends from the elbow to proximal to the wrist.

(b)

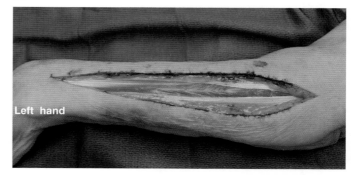

Fig. 33.6(b). Decompression of the dorsal compartment of the left forearm: the fascia over each of the muscle bellies is opened.

- The posterior (dorsal) compartment is opened with a longitudinal dorsal incision extending from the elbow to the wrist (see Fig. 33.2), coursing between the mobile extensor wad and the extensor digitorum muscle bellies.
- The hand includes ten separate osteofascial compartments, which can be released with carpal tunnel release and two dorsal incisions. For complete hand fasciotomies, in addition to the division of the transverse ligament over the carpal tunnel described above, two incisions are made on the dorsum of the hand over the

(a)

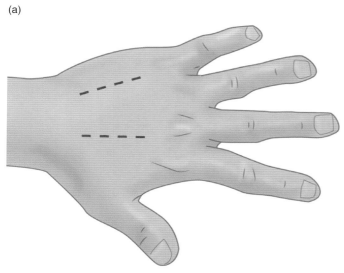

Fig. 33.7(a). The interosseous compartments of the left hand are decompressed via two incisions placed on the dorsum over the second and fourth metacarpal spaces.

(b)

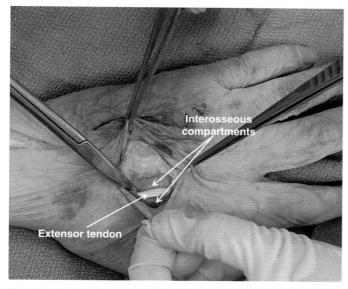

Interosseous compartments

Extensor tendon

Fig. 33.7(b). Dorsal fasciotomy of the left hand: the fascia over the interosseous compartments are opened sharply, on either side of the tendons.

second and fourth metacarpal spaces (see Fig. 33.2). The extensor tendons are retracted, and the underlying compartments are opened with longitudinal slits on either side of each tendon.

Fasciotomy wound management

- The wound should initially be left open to prevent recurrence of compartment syndrome while the edema decreases. A moist dressing should be placed on the muscle bellies to prevent desiccation.
- Negative pressure therapy dressing (VAC) is a useful modality to manage the fasciotomy sites. It prevents wound retraction, removes excessive soft tissue edema, and facilitates delayed primary skin closure. However, its application in the presence of incomplete hemostasis may result in an increase in bleeding. It is advisable that this dressing be used after the second look operation, when hemostasis is complete.
- Vessel–loop shoelace wound closure is a useful technique to achieve delayed primary skin closure.
- Split-thickness skin grafting may be necessary for wound closure, if delayed primary closure is not possible.

Tips and pitfalls

- Delayed diagnosis is the most common problem in the management of compartment syndrome. A high index of suspicion, serial clinical examinations, compartment pressure measurements, and serial creatine phosphokinase (CK) levels remain the cornerstone of early diagnosis and timely fasciotomy. (The CK levels may be normal in cases where delayed recognition of the compartment syndrome results in completely dead muscle.)
- In suspected compartment syndrome the pressures should be measured in all muscle compartments. The pressures may be normal in one compartment and abnormal in the adjacent one.
- Poor knowledge of the anatomy of the extremity muscle compartments is the most common cause of incomplete fasciotomy or iatrogenic damage to the neurovascular bundle.
- The muscle compartment responsible for the compartment syndrome is usually obvious once the skin and fascia are opened, and care should be taken to completely open the fascia over any bulging and tense compartments.
  - The transverse carpal ligament is broader than most surgeons realize, and adequate decompression of the carpal tunnel requires full division of the ligament well up on to the thenar eminence of the hand.

Chapter

34

Upper extremity amputations

Peep Talving and Scott Zakaluzny

Surgical anatomy

- The upper arm has two muscle compartments, the anterior which includes the biceps muscle, and the posterior, which includes the triceps muscle.
- The forearm has two major compartments, the anterior containing the flexor muscles, and the posterior containing the extensor muscles.
- The upper extremity is perfused by branches from the deep and superficial brachial artery. The proximal brachial artery lies in the groove between the biceps and triceps muscles. Distally, it courses in front of the humerus. At the antecubital fossa, it runs deep to the bicipital aponeurosis and bifurcates into the radial and ulnar arteries, just below the elbow. The artery is surrounded by the two brachial veins, which run on either side of the artery.
- The profunda brachial artery is a large branch arising from the proximal brachial artery and follows the radial nerve closely. It provides collateral circulation to the lower arm.
- The basilic vein courses in the subcutaneous tissue in the medial aspect of the lower arm. At the midpoint, it penetrates the fascia to join one of the brachial veins.
- The cephalic vein is entirely in the subcutaneous tissues, courses in the deltopectoral groove, and empties into the junction of the brachial and axillary veins.
- In the upper arm, the median nerve lies in front of the brachial artery. It then crosses over the artery midway down the upper arm, where distally it lies behind the artery.
- The ulnar nerve is behind the artery in the upper half of the arm. Midway down the arm, it pierces the intermuscular septum and courses more posteriorly, away from the artery, behind the medial epicondyle.

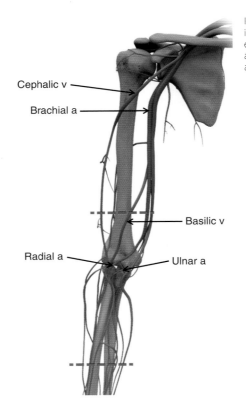

Fig. 34.1. Anatomic illustration of the upper extremity with typical arm and forearm amputation sites.

Cephalic v

Brachial a

Basilic v

Radial a

Ulnar a

General principles

- In many trauma cases with a mangled extremity, primary amputation may be preferable to multiple and often futile, salvage attempts.
- The level and type of amputation should be determined by the general condition of the patient, the functional status of the limb, the type and severity of associated fractures, the extent of soft tissue damage, the adequacy of blood supply, and the availability of healthy skin flaps to cover the stump.

Atlas of Surgical Techniques in Trauma, ed. Demetrios Demetriades, Kenji Inaba, and George Velmahos. Published by Cambridge University Press. © Cambridge University Press 2015.

- Preserve as much functional length as possible to improve prosthesis fitting and functionality of the remaining limb.
- Use tourniquets to minimize blood loss. Elevation of the arm and the use of bandage or tourniquet exsanguinators should be considered. The inflation pressure is usually set at approximately 250 mmHg in adults or about 100 mmHg above the systolic pressure.
- All non-viable tissues must be removed.
- Nerves should be sharply divided as high as possible and allowed to retract. The ends of the nerves should be away from areas of pressure.
- Preserve sufficient soft tissues to cover the end of the bone without tension. However, avoid excessive amount of soft tissues because it may interfere with skin closure and prosthesis fitting.
- Bone edges should be filed to remove any sharp edges.
- Wounds should be closed without tension and suture lines should be placed away from weight-bearing surfaces when possible.
- In the multiply injured patient in extremis, a guillotine amputation should be considered. The definitive stump closure may be performed once the condition of the patient stabilizes.

Special instruments

- Use a wide arm table board to rest the injured extremity.
- Pneumatic tourniquet and bandage or tourniquet exsanguinator.
- Power saw or Gigli saw.
- Bone files or rasps.

- Compression wraps for postoperative dressings are helpful to decrease edema and to shape the stump for early fitting of prosthetics.

Patient positioning

- Supine position with the injured arm abducted 90 degrees on an arm table board.
- Skin preparation should include the hand, and the entire arm circumferentially, including the axilla and shoulder. The hand should be covered with a sterile stockinette. A Doppler probe should be in the sterile field to assess arterial supply.
- Apply a sterile pneumatic tourniquet if possible.

Above-elbow amputation

Incision

- Perform a fish-mouth incision and create symmetrical anterior and posterior flaps. The medial and lateral apexes of the incision should be distal to the level of the planned osteotomy.
- For amputations proximal to the middle of the humerus, preserve as much bone length as possible.
- For distal above-elbow amputation, preserve part of the humerus condyles to create a solid bone base for interaction with the prosthesis. If the condyles cannot be spared, remove at least 4 cm of the distal humerus to facilitate prosthesis fitting with an elbow-lock mechanism that is equal in length to the contralateral arm.

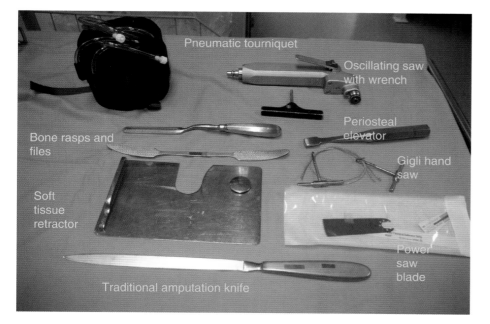

Fig. 34.2. Essential instruments for amputations in trauma: pneumatic tourniquet, bandage or tourniquet exsanguinators, power saw or Gigli saw, bone files, or rasps.

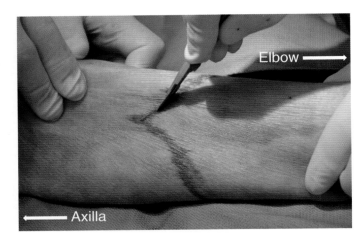

Fig. 34.3. Left arm amputation: fish-mouth incision with equal anterior and posterior musculocutaneous flaps.

Procedure

- The skin incision should be carried through the subcutaneous tissue and fascia.
- The brachial artery should be identified in the groove between the biceps and triceps muscles with the median nerve located medially. The brachial artery is identified and ligated.
- The median nerve is retracted gently and sharply divided. This allows retraction of the nerve end into the soft tissues, away from the load-bearing surface.

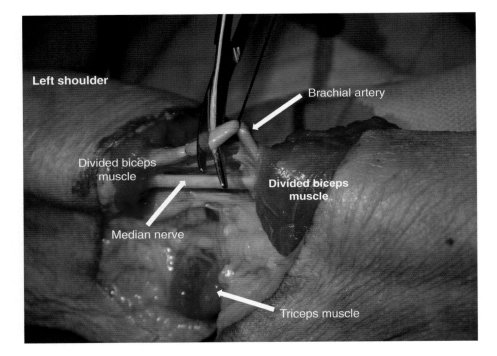

Fig. 34.4. Division of the left brachial artery. Note its close proximity to the median nerve.

- The ulnar nerve is located an inch posterior to the median nerve on the medial aspect of the triceps muscle. Likewise, the radial nerve is identified as it courses on the posterior aspect of the humerus deep to the triceps muscle. These nerves are divided, as described above.

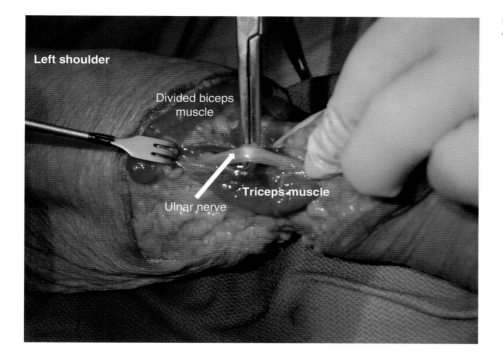

Fig. 34.5. In the arm, the ulnar nerve is located on the anteromedial aspect of the triceps muscle.

- The muscles are divided sharply to create the soft tissue flaps. The posterior (triceps) muscle flap should be longer to allow coverage of the bone upon closure.

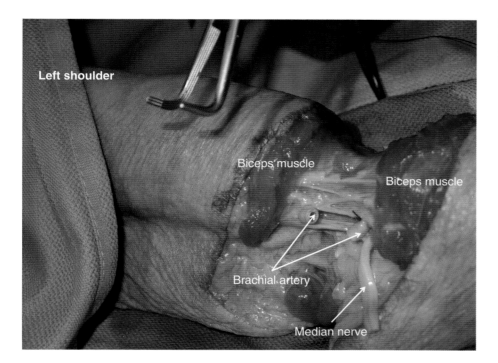

Fig. 34.6. Photograph showing divided biceps muscle, brachial artery, and median nerve. The proximal median nerve has retracted under the divided biceps muscle.

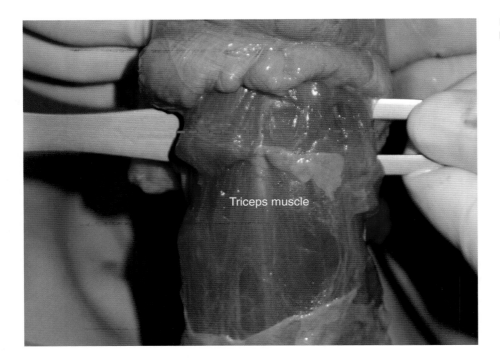

Triceps muscle

- The periosteum is elevated proximal to the skin and muscle flap up to the point of planned bone division. The humerus is then divided with the power saw or Gigli saw.

- The divided end of the humerus is then smoothed with a rasp.

(a)

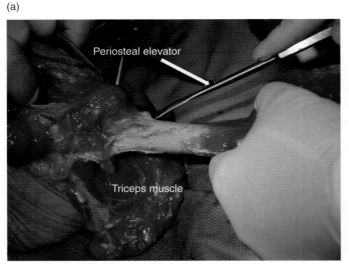

Periosteal elevator

Triceps muscle

Fig. 34.8(a). Cobb's periosteal elevator is used to clear the osteotomy site from the periosteum and soft tissues.

(b)

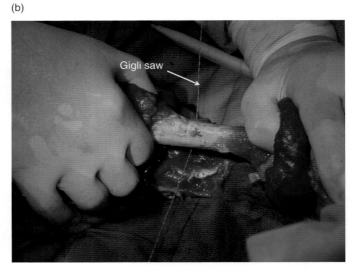

Gigli saw

Fig. 34.8(b). Division of the humerus with the Gigli saw.

(c)

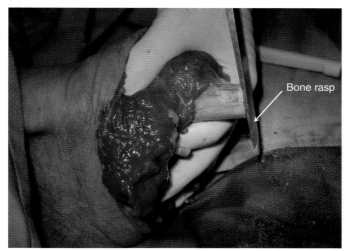

Fig. 34.8(c). Bone rasp is utilized to smooth the edges of osteotomy.

- The triceps tendon is removed from the olecranon process; the posterior fascia of the triceps muscle is brought from posterior, over the bone, and secured to the anterior fascia of the biceps fascia anteriorly.
- The skin is then closed over the fascial closure.

(a)

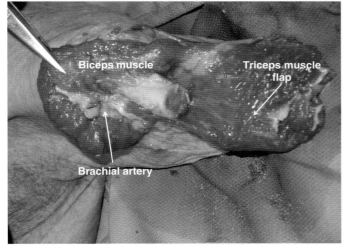

Fig. 34.9(a). The triceps flap is used to cover the bone stump.

(b)

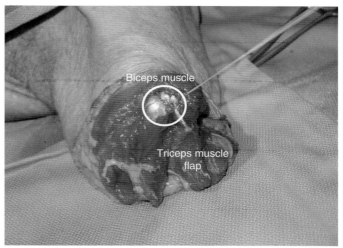

Fig. 34.9(b). Myoplasty (circle) using biceps and triceps muscles over the humerus stump.

(a)

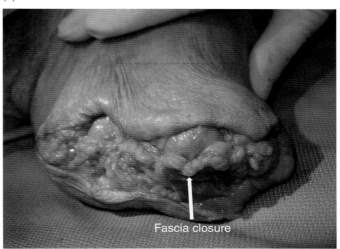

Fig. 34.10(a). Closure of the fascia over the myoplasty.

(b)

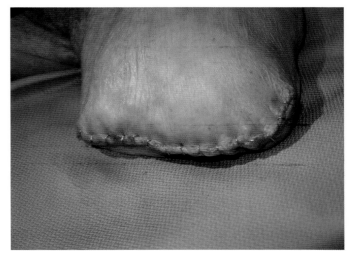

Fig. 34.10(b). A tension free skin closure completes the amputation.

Below-elbow amputation

Incision

- Perform a fish-mouth incision, with symmetrical anterior and posterior flaps. The medial and lateral apexes of the incision should be distal to the level of planned bone division.

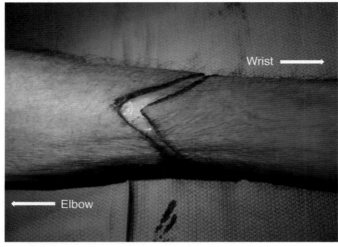

Fig. 34.11. Left below-forearm amputation: fish-mouth incision with equal anterior and posterior musculocutaneous flaps.

Procedure

- The skin incision is carried through the subcutaneous tissue and fascia.
- The radial and ulnar arteries should be identified laterally and medially, respectively, and ligated.
- Similarly, the radial and ulnar nerves should be identified. Traction should be applied to the nerves prior to sharp division and ligation as described above.
- The muscles are then divided. Adequate soft tissue should be preserved to allow coverage of the bone. Avoid excess

(a)

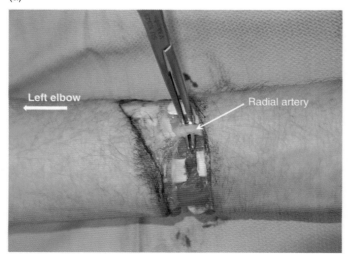

Fig. 34.12(a). The radial artery is identified under the brachioradial muscle and ligated.

(b)

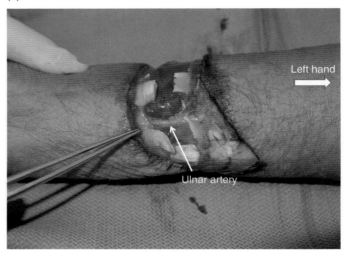

Fig. 34.12(b). The ulnar artery is identified between the flexor digitorum profundus and flexor carpi ulnaris muscles and ligated.

(c)

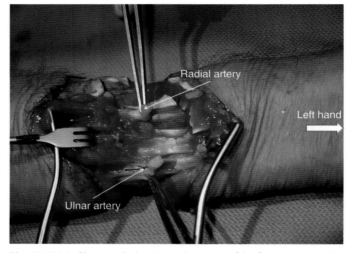

Fig. 34.12(c). Photograph depicting volar aspect of the forearm amputation with ligated radial and ulnar arteries.

(d)

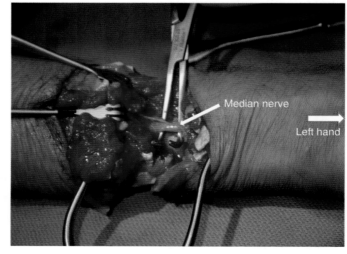

Fig. 34.12(d). Photograph showing the median nerve located on the interosseous membrane in a deep aspect of the forearm.

muscle bulk, as it creates problems with skin coverage and the subsequent application of the prosthesis.

- The median nerve lies deep, on top of the interosseous membrane between the radius and ulna. The nerve is sharply divided and ligated, as described above.
- The periosteum is elevated proximal to the skin and muscle flap, up to the point of planned bone division. The radius

(a)

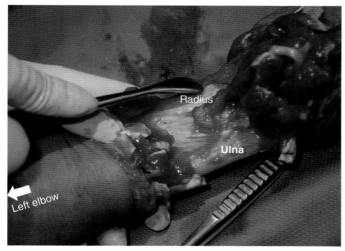

Fig. 34.13(a). Cobb's periosteal elevator is used to clear the radius and ulna of the periosteum and soft tissues.

(b)

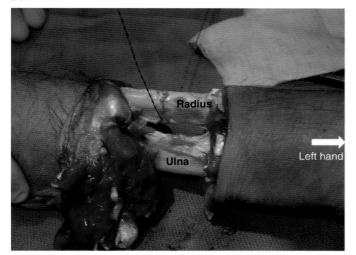

Fig. 34.13(b). Division of the radius with the Gigli saw.

(c)

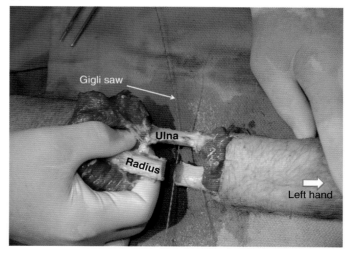

Fig. 34.13(c). Division of the ulna with the Gigli saw.

and ulna are divided separately at the same length with the use of a power saw or Gigli saw.

- Sharp ends of bone should be smoothed with a rasp.
- The anterior and posterior deep fascia are re-approximated and closed over the divided bones.
- The skin is closed over the muscle.

(a)

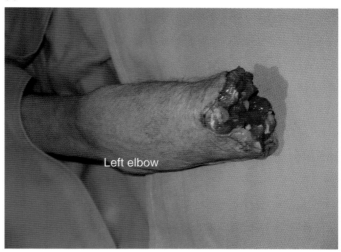

Fig. 34.14(a). Photograph showing equal musculocutaneous flaps for closure of the forearm amputation.

(b)

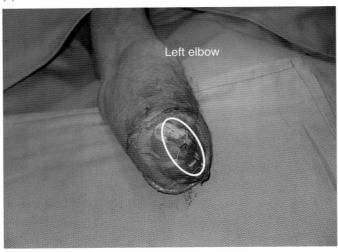

Left elbow

Fig. 34.14(b). Fascia closure (circle) is achieved using absorbable sutures.

(c)

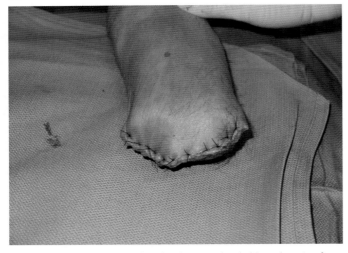

Fig. 34.14(c). The stump is closed with a non-absorbable and tension-free suture line.

Tips and pitfalls

- In many cases with a mangled extremity, primary amputation may be preferable to multiple and often futile salvage attempts.
- Guillotine amputation with delayed reconstruction should be considered in patients in extremis.
- Preserve length to improve functional outcome, even if it requires a skin graft or other plastics procedure for coverage.
- There is no difference in neuroma formation whether or not the divided nerve is ligated. However, the transected nerve ends should be retracted and located in a well-cushioned tissue bed away from the load-bearing surface.

Femoral artery injuries

George Velmahos and Rondi Gelbard

Surgical anatomy

- The common femoral artery is a continuation of the external iliac artery and is approximately 4 cm long. It begins directly behind the inguinal ligament, midway between the anterior superior iliac spine and the symphysis pubis.
- The profunda femoris artery arises from the lateral aspect of the common femoral artery, towards the femur, approximately 3 to 4 cm below the inguinal ligament. The common femoral artery continues obliquely down the anteromedial aspect of the thigh as the superficial femoral artery.
- The superficial femoral artery exits the femoral triangle to enter the subsartorial canal and ends by passing through an opening in the adductor magnus to become the popliteal artery.
- In the upper third of the thigh the femoral vessels are contained within the femoral triangle (Scarpa's triangle).
  - The femoral triangle is formed laterally by the medial border of the sartorius muscle, medially by the adductor longus and superiorly by the inguinal ligament.
  - In the femoral triangle the femoral vein lies medial to the femoral artery. The long saphenous vein drains into the femoral vein about 3–4 cm below the inguinal ligament. Further distally, the femoral vein lies posterior to the artery and maintains this relationship in the popliteal fossa. The femoral nerve and its branches are found lateral to the common femoral artery.
- In the middle third of the thigh the femoral artery lies within the adductor canal (Hunter's canal), an aponeurotic tunnel that extends from the apex of the femoral triangle to the opening in the adductor magnus.
  - The adductor canal is bounded by the sartorius muscle anteriorly, the vastus medialis laterally, and the adductor longus and magnus posteromedially. A fascial

plane between the vastus medialis and adductor longus and the adductor magnus covers the canal (see Fig. 35.7).
  - The canal contains the femoral artery and vein, the saphenous nerve which crosses from lateral to medial, and branches of the femoral nerve.
  - The femoral vein courses from a medial position in the groin to a posterior and then to a lateral position with respect to the artery as it moves distally towards the knee.
  - The greater saphenous vein courses medially to lie on the anterior surface of the thigh before entering the fascia lata and joining the common femoral vein at the sapheno-femoral junction near the femoral triangle.

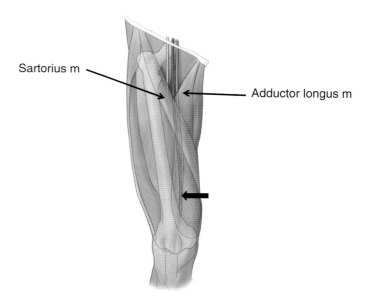

Sartorius m

Adductor longus m

Fig. 35.1. Anatomical relationship of the femoral artery and vein as they course down the anteromedial aspect of the thigh. Note the femoral vein coursing from a medial position to a posterior and then lateral position with respect to the artery as it moves distally towards the knee (thick arrow).

Atlas of Surgical Techniques in Trauma, ed. Demetrios Demetriades, Kenji Inaba, and George Velmahos. Published by Cambridge University Press. © Cambridge University Press 2015.

(a)

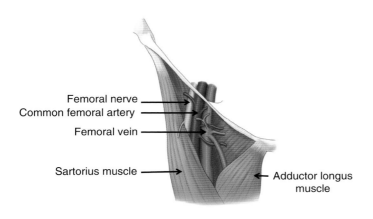

Femoral nerve
Common femoral artery
Femoral vein
Sartorius muscle
Adductor longus muscle

(b)

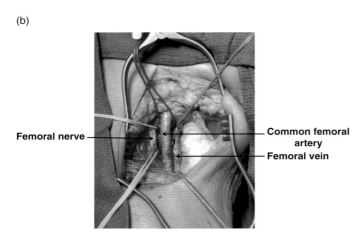

Femoral nerve
Common femoral artery
Femoral vein

Fig. 35.2. Schematic (a) and photograph (b) showing the anatomy of the right femoral triangle. The femoral vein lies medial to the femoral artery, while the femoral nerve and its branches are found lateral to the femoral artery.

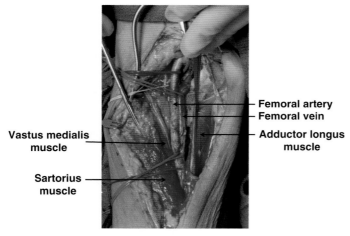

Femoral artery
Femoral vein
Vastus medialis muscle
Adductor longus muscle
Sartorius muscle

Fig. 35.3. The adductor canal is bounded by the sartorius muscle anteriorly, the vastus medialis laterally, and the adductor longus and magnus posteromedially; a fascia between the vastus medialis and adductor longus and magnus covers the canal.

General principles

- The profunda femoris can be ligated without any problems. However, ligation of the common or the superficial femoral artery results in ischemia and loss of limb in most patients. For patients requiring damage control, shunting is always preferable to ligation.
- Arterial reconstruction above the knee can safely be performed with a prosthetic or autologous graft. Injuries at the popliteal fossa should always be repaired with autologous vein.
- A Fogarty catheter should always be passed proximally and distally to remove any clots. Systemic heparinization can be considered, but is not necessary if the patient is coagulopathic or has multisystem injuries at risk of bleeding. Local proximal and distal infusion of heparin solution (5000 units in 100 mL of normal saline), however, is recommended for routine use.
- At the completion of the arterial repair, examine for a palpable peripheral pulse. On-table angiography should be considered in cases where only a Doppler signal is detected.
- The extremity compartments should always be monitored peri-operatively. Routine prophylactic fasciotomies are not indicated. However, therapeutic fasciotomies should be performed without delay.
- Continued postoperative monitoring with serial clinical examinations and serial serum creatine kinase (CK) levels should be performed. Fasciotomy should be considered in appropriate cases.
- The femoral vein can usually be ligated with impunity. Application of a compression bandage or elastic stocking may reduce the degree of postoperative edema.

Positioning

- The patient should be placed in the supine position with the hip and knee slightly flexed and externally rotated. A bolster can be placed under the thigh and the knee.

Incision(s)

A vertical incision is made approximately halfway between the pubic tubercle and the anterior iliac spine, directed towards the medial femoral condyle. The length of the incision is determined by the site of the vascular injury.

- For proximal common femoral vascular injuries, the incision may have to be extended proximally through the inguinal ligament to gain adequate proximal control at the external iliac artery level. It can also be curved superiorly and laterally, parallel to the inguinal ligament, to allow for retroperitoneal exposure of the iliac vessels.
- For injuries to the superficial femoral artery, a longitudinal incision is extended over the anterior border of the sartorius muscle. A useful external landmark is a line

joining the middle of the inguinal ligament with the medial femoral condyle.

- Care must be taken to avoid injuring the greater saphenous vein in its superficial location in the subcutaneous tissues, along the medial edge of the incision.

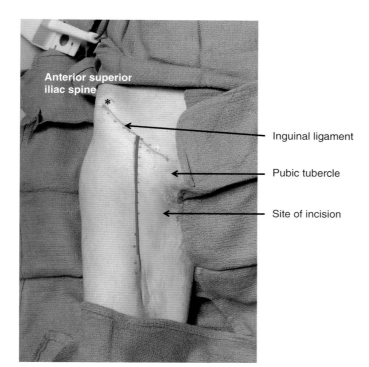

Fig. 35.4. Exposure of the common femoral vessels: a vertical incision is made, starting approximately halfway between the pubic tubercle and anterior superior iliac spine, and with a direction towards the medial femoral condyle.

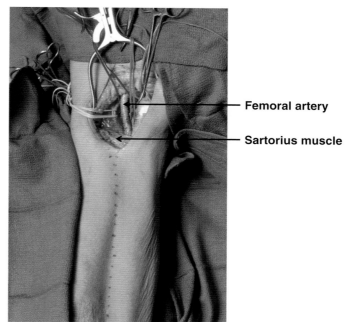

Fig. 35.5. Exposure of the common femoral artery through a standard vertical incision. In order to expose the superficial femoral artery, the longitudinal incision is extended over the anterior border of the sartorius muscle, along a line extending from the anterior superior iliac spine to the medial femoral condyle (interrupted line).

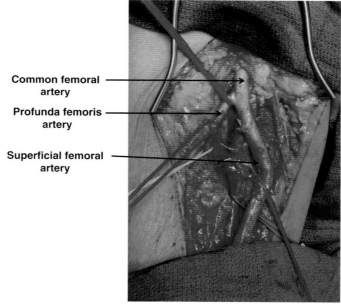

Fig. 35.6. Medial and upward retraction of the common and superficial femoral arteries allows exposure of the profunda femoris artery.

Exposure and procedure

- Following the skin incision and dissection of the subcutaneous tissue and superficial and deep fascia, the femoral sheath is opened directly over the femoral artery, using a combination of cautery and sharp dissection. The femoral vein and the lymph nodes are medial to the artery. A self-retaining Weitlaner or cerebellar retractor is placed.
- The long saphenous vein is identified along the medial edge of the incision, and preserved in case it is needed as an autologous graft.
- The common femoral artery is dissected circumferentially, and a vessel loop is placed around it for proximal control. The same approach is followed for the superficial femoral artery.
- The vessel loops around the common and superficial femoral arteries are retracted upwards and medially to expose the profunda femoris artery, and a vessel loop is placed around it.
- Exposure of the superficial femoral artery in the mid thigh requires opening of the adductor canal by incising the

aponeurosis, which forms its roof, and retracting the sartorius and vastus medialis muscles laterally and the adductor longus medially.

- Distally, the superficial femoral artery is exposed by opening the aponeurotic roof of the adductor magnus canal. The very distal part of the artery exits from the adductor canal through the adductor magnus hiatus.

305

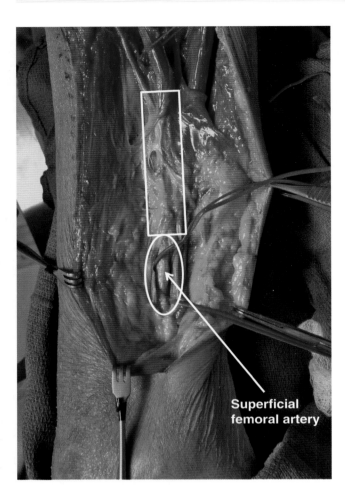

Fig. 35.7. Exposure of the distal superficial femoral artery requires opening of the aponeurotic roof of the adductor canal (white box). The artery exits from the adductor canal through the adductor magnus hiatus (white circle).

Superficial femoral artery

- In severely injured or unstable patients, or if the skillset of the surgeon precludes definitive repair, blood flow can be restored temporarily using a shunt. Injuries to the common femoral and superficial femoral arteries must eventually undergo definitive reconstruction.
- The femoral vein can be ligated without any significant problems. Repair should be considered only if it can be performed with simple techniques and without producing significant stenosis. Stenosis greater than 50% increases the risk of thrombosis and pulmonary embolism.
- At the completion of operation, the muscle compartments of the lower leg should be evaluated and in appropriate cases fasciotomies should be performed.

Tips and pitfalls

- Patients with combined venous and arterial injuries are at particularly high risk of developing compartment syndrome.

- Although prophylactic fasciotomies are not recommended, the patient must be closely monitored postoperatively for the development of compartment syndrome.
- In hemodynamically stable patients, mannitol may be given intra- and postoperatively to decrease the risk of developing compartment syndrome.
- Because lymphatics are abundant in this area, lymph vessels should be ligated or controlled with small hemoclips to prevent formation of a lymphocele or lymph fistula. The saphenous vein and lymph nodes are medial to the artery.
- Identification of the common and proximal superficial femoral artery may be difficult in cases with thrombosis and no pulse. Remember the external landmark, a line drawn from the middle of the inguinal ligament to the medial femoral condyle.

Lower Extremities

Popliteal artery

Peep Talving and Nicholas Nash

Surgical anatomy

- The popliteal fossa is diamond-shaped and its borders are formed by the semi-membranosus and semi-tendinosus muscles superiomedially, the biceps femoris superolaterally, the medial head of the gastrocnemius inferomedially, and the lateral head of the gastrocnemius inferolaterally. It contains the popliteal vessels, the tibial and common peroneal nerves and is covered only by subcutaneous tissue and skin.
- The popliteal artery is the continuation of the superficial femoral artery. It starts at the opening in the adductor magnus muscle, at the junction of the middle and lower thirds of the thigh, and courses downward and laterally, between the two condyles of the femur, into the popliteal fossa.

- The popliteal artery gives the superior and inferior genicular branches, which provide blood supply to the knee joint and the surrounding tissues.
- Popliteal artery below the knee gives the anterior tibial artery and becomes the tibioperoneal trunk. The tibioperoneal trunk gives the fibular artery about 2–3 cm distally, and ultimately continues as the posterior tibial artery.
- The anterior tibial artery pierces the upper part of the interosseous membrane, courses in front of the membrane, under the extensor muscles of the anterior muscle compartment, and becomes distally the dorsalis pedis artery.
- The posterior tibial artery is the continuation of the popliteal artery, and is located under the gastrocnemius and

(a)

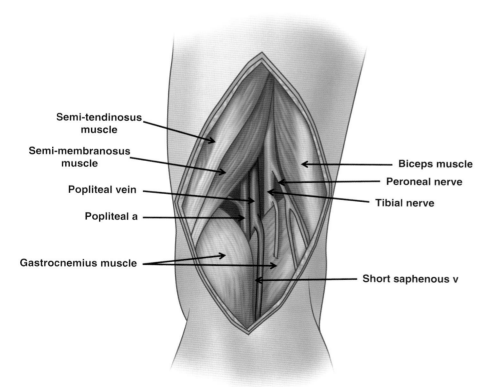

Fig. 36.1(a). Anatomy of the right popliteal fossa: the popliteal vein and tibial nerve are more superficial and are lateral to the popliteal artery.

Semi-tendinosus muscle

Semi-membranosus muscle

Popliteal vein

Popliteal a

Gastrocnemius muscle

Biceps muscle

Peroneal nerve

Tibial nerve

Short saphenous v

Atlas of Surgical Techniques in Trauma, ed. Demetrios Demetriades, Kenji Inaba, and George Velmahos. Published by Cambridge University Press. © Cambridge University Press 2015.

(b)

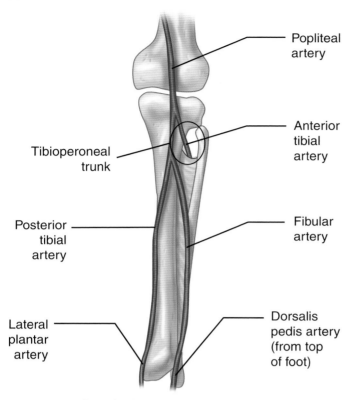

Popliteal
artery

Anterior
tibial
artery

Tibioperoneal
trunk

Posterior
tibial
artery

Fibular
artery

Lateral
plantar
artery

Dorsalis
pedis artery
(from top
of foot)

Fig. 36.1(b). Right popliteal artery posterior view: the anterior tibial artery pierces the upper part of the interosseous membrane (circle) and courses in front of the membrane, in the anterior muscle compartment. The popliteal artery then gives the peroneal branch, and continues as the posterior tibial artery.

soleus muscles and becomes superficial behind the medial malleolus.

- The popliteal vein and tibial nerve are more superficial and lateral in relation to the popliteal artery.

General principles

- Injury to the popliteal artery is recognized as the most limb-threatening of peripheral vascular injuries in trauma and is associated with a high incidence of amputation.
- Popliteal artery occlusion or ligation results in a limb amputation rate of approximately 75%.
- Prognostic factors affecting limb salvage include the time interval between injury and treatment with a goal of less than 6 hours, mechanism, associated soft tissue injuries, and chronic vascular disease.
- Posterior dislocation of the knee is associated with a high incidence of popliteal arterial injury. Reduce the

dislocation without any delay and always evaluate clinically, measuring the ankle brachial index and in the appropriate cases perform a CT angiogram or color flow Doppler.

- "Hard signs" of vascular trauma include active hemorrhage, expanding or pulsatile hematoma, bruit or thrill, absent pulses, and distal ischemia.
- Most popliteal artery injuries due to firearm injuries or blunt trauma require resectional debridement and reconstruction with interposition vein graft. In rare occasions after a stab wound, an end-to-end primary anastomosis may be possible.
- In the presence of associated major orthopedic injuries, the blood flow is restored with a temporary shunt, followed by the orthopedic fixation. The definitive vascular reconstruction is performed last.
- For patients requiring damage control or where the surgeon skillset is insufficient to perform definitive reconstruction, vascular shunting is the preferred method of restoring flow. Ligation should not be performed due to the high limb loss rate.
- On-table completion angiogram should be considered liberally if no good palpable pulse is obtained at the end of the operation.
- Always evaluate the lower leg for muscle compartment syndrome, clinically and with pressure measurements. Four-compartment fasciotomy should be performed in the appropriate cases (see Chapter 38).

Special instruments

- Head light, magnifying loupes.
- Major vascular tray, vessel loops, Fogarty catheter (usually 3 Fr), sterile Doppler probe, Argyle shunts.
- Device to measure muscle compartment pressures.
- Heparinized saline for regional heparinization (5000 units heparin in 100 mL saline solution), papaverin solution, and water-soluble contrast solution.

Positioning

- Supine position, the leg is positioned with slight flexion of the knee supported with a bump, with the hip abducted and externally rotated.
- Full skin preparation of the injured leg and the contralateral groin, in case autogenous vein harvesting is required.
- If an external bone fixator is needed, it should be placed after a temporary arterial shunt has restored distal flow, with the knee in a slightly flexed position.

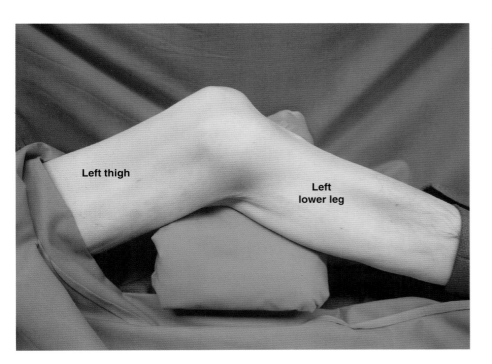

Fig. 36.2. Position for exposure of the left popliteal vessels: supine position, the leg in slight flexion and external rotation of the knee, which is supported with a bump.

Incision

- Mark the skin incision with marking pen. The incision starts proximally above the tubercle of the femur, about 1 cm posterior to the femur, between the sartorius muscle and the vastus medialis muscles.

It continues distally, across the knee fold onto the distal lower extremity, approximately 1 cm posterior to the tibia. The extent of the incision can be adapted to the portion of the popliteal artery requiring intervention.

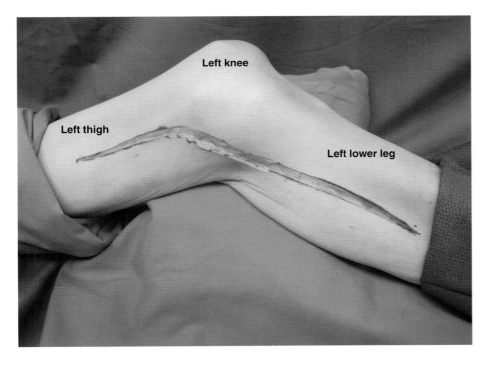

Fig. 36.3. The incision starts about 1 cm posterior to the femur, continues distally, across the knee fold onto the distal lower extremity, approximately 1 cm posterior to the tibia.

- During the skin incision, care should be taken to identify and preserve the saphenous vein, because it improves venous drainage of the extremity, especially in the presence of a concomitant popliteal venous injury.

Exposure

- The dissection is carried on through the subcutaneous tissues to the fascia, with care taken to avoid injury to the saphenous vein, which should remain in the posterior flap.

- In the superior part of the incision, the groove between the vastus medialis of the anterior thigh and the sartorius muscle is entered, with the sartorius being retracted posteriorly. The popliteal vessels are located in the fat tissue right under the distal shaft of the femur in the suprageniculate position.

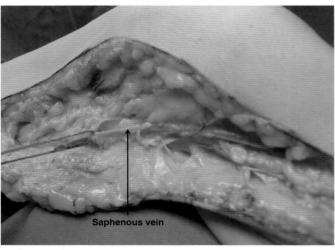

Fig. 36.4. Isolation and preservation of the saphenous vein are essential for venous drainage of the extremity, in suspected cases with popliteal venous injury.

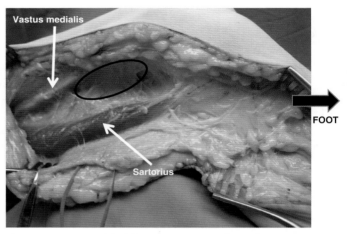

Fig. 36.5. Exposure of the left popliteal artery: the fascia of the thigh has been entered and the sartorius (inferiorly) and the vastus medialis muscle (superiorly) have been exposed. The popliteal vessels are located in the fat tissue right under the distal shaft of the femur in the suprageniculate position (circle).

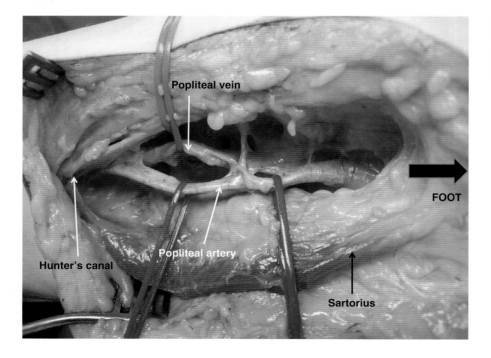

Fig. 36.6. The suprageniculate popliteal artery (encircled by red vessel loops) and popliteal vein exposed (blue vessel loop) with their accompanying geniculate branches. Note the anatomical relationship of the two vessels, with the artery being medial to the vein above the knee.

- The sartorius muscles covering the medial portion of the knee fold can be divided in sequential fashion, including the semi-membranosus, the semi-tendinosus, and the gracilis muscles (pes anserinus). They should be tagged proximally and distally with different color sutures to allow their reapproximation during closure of the wound for optimal functional results.
- The femur is palpated, and the dissection continues to expose the neurovascular bundle directly behind the femur, with the popliteal artery being the most medial structure first encountered, followed by the popliteal vein, and then the tibial nerve as the dissection continues laterally.
- The dissection can be carried more proximally towards the popliteal artery's entry into the fossa through the Hunter's canal, if more proximal control is required.
- If more distal control is necessary, the remainder of the popliteal fossa can be opened by retracting the head of the gastrocnemius posteriorly, and detaching tibial attachments of the soleus muscle.

Management of the injured vessel

- After appropriate proximal and distal control is gained, the injured portion of the vessel is resected back to healthy edges.

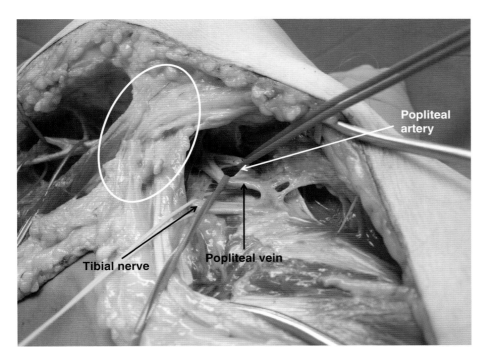

Fig. 36.7. Exposure of the infrageniculate popliteal artery. The pes anserinus (composed of the sartorius, gracilis, and semi-tendinosus tendons) (circle) has been left in place to provide orientation. The soleus muscle has been taken down from the tibia to allow exposure of the popliteal vein (blue vessel loop), the popliteal artery (red vessel loop), and the tibial nerve (yellow vessel loop). This is the exact order in which each are encountered during the dissection from medial to lateral.

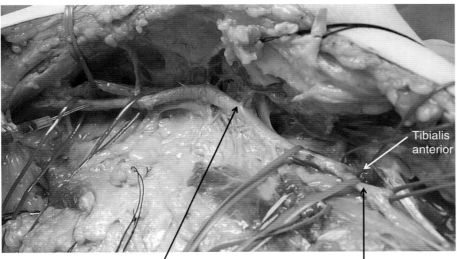

Fig. 36.8. Exposure of the entire popliteal artery. The pes anserinus has been divided, with each of the ends marked after division with silk ties to allow their reapproximation after the vascular repair. The divisions of the popliteal artery into the tibioperoneal trunk and the tibialis anterior artery below the knee are marked with red vessel loops.

- A Fogarty balloon (3Fr) is then advanced both proximally and distally to clear clots, followed by the injection of heparinized saline into the two ends.
- Depending on the extent of the vascular injury, a reverse saphenous vein interposition graft for definitive repair or a temporary shunt followed by an interposition graft is performed.
- Prior to definitive repair, the proximal and distal ends of the artery are trimmed using Potts scissors to healthy vessel ensuring that intima is intact at the free edge. The ends can be spatulated as warranted for repair.

- The tension-free anastomosis is performed using a running or interrupted monofilament 5–0 or 6–0 polypropylene suture, with the needle passing from the intima to adventitia on the artery side, in order to minimize the risk of intimal flaps and dissection. The more technically complex anastomosis is performed first.
- Small caliber arteries can be dilated using a Fogarty catheter. Local anesthetic or papaverin can be used locally to counteract vasospasm.
- Distal flow is confirmed by a combination of physical examination and an on-table Doppler.

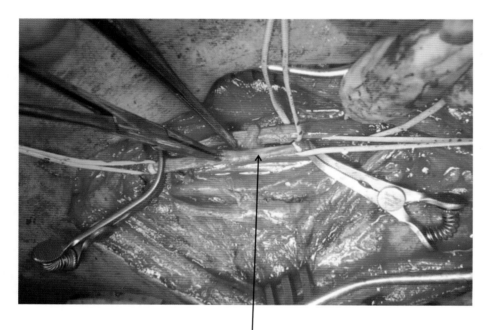

Popliteal artery

Fig. 36.9. Proximal and distal control of the arterial injury with bulldog clamps.

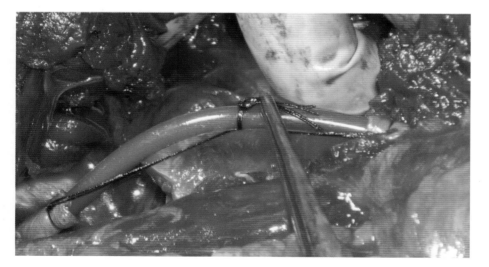

Fig. 36.10. A temporary shunt can be utilized in damage control setting or to restore perfusion during the vein graft harvest.

- If a temporary shunt has been utilized, a 0 silk tie is used to secure the shunt proximally and distally. These ties are then tied together around the center of the shunt to prevent dislodgement of the shunt. Prior to shunting, no debridement of the arterial edges should be performed.

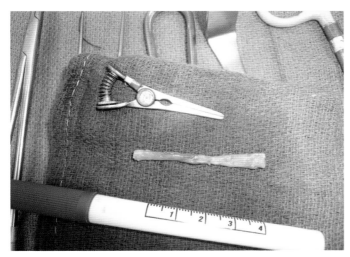

Fig. 36.11. For popliteal artery repair, the reversed autologous venous graft is the only conduit utilized.

Other considerations

- A completion angiogram should be considered liberally, especially in patients without the return of palpable pulses post procedure.
- The four muscle compartments of the leg should be examined clinically, and if in doubt the compartment pressures should be measured. Fasciotomies should be performed in the appropriate cases. Postoperatively, monitor serum CK levels.

- In the presence of associated extensive soft tissue damage, the devitalized tissues should be excised and the vascular repair should be covered with surrounding healthy tissues.

Tips and pitfalls

- Failure to allow a 30-degree flexion when applying an external fixator for fracture stabilization makes access to the popliteal vessel very difficult.
- Preservation of the saphenous vein during exposure of the popliteal vessels is important in cases with suspected popliteal vein injury, in order to preserve a good venous drainage of the extremity.
- In exposing the suprageniculate popliteal artery, the sartorius muscle must remain inferior to the dissection plane while gaining access to the Hunter's canal.
- Failure to debride the anastomotic bed of all devitalized tissues and cover the anastomosis at the end of the procedure may result in graft infection and graft failure.
- Arterial repair or anastomosis must be performed in the absence of tension. In select cases, gentle mobilization of the proximal and distal segments of the artery can allow primary anastomosis. In most cases, however, a reversed interposition vein graft is required.
- Failure to reapproximate the divided tendons may result in knee instability.
- Perform routine postoperative monitoring of serum CK levels. Persistently elevated CK levels in patients without fasciotomies are highly suspicious for compartment syndrome, and emergency fasciotomies should be performed. Persistently elevated CK levels in patients with fasciotomies suggest incomplete fasciotomies or missed muscle compartments and these patients should be returned to the operating room.

Chapter 3

Lower extremity amputations

Peep Talving, Stephen Varga, and Jackson Lee

Surgical anatomy

- Above and below the knee amputations require basic anatomy knowledge of the muscle compartments, nerves, and arteries of the lower extremity.
- The thigh has three compartments: anterior, posterior, and medial. The calf has four compartments: anterior, lateral, and posterior superficial and deep.
- The lower extremity is perfused by the superficial and deep femoral artery. The superficial femoral artery continues as the popliteal artery after exiting the Hunter's canal. The popliteal artery bifurcates into the tibialis anterior artery and the tibioperoneal trunk that in the second order branches into the tibialis anterior and tibialis posterior arteries. The femoral and sciatic nerves provide innervation to the lower extremity.

General principles

- The goal with amputation surgery is a functional extremity with a residual limb that successfully interacts with the patient's future prosthetic and external environment.
- The rule of preserving as much length as possible is not always applicable in the lower leg. Long leg stumps often do not heal well because of poor blood supply and do not tolerate prosthesis well.
- A short below-knee stump is preferable to knee dislocation, but a stump shorter than 6 cm may not be functional.
- Optimal above the knee amputation level is between 12–18 cm below the trochanter major.
- Use tourniquets to minimize blood loss. The cuff should not be placed directly over bony prominences, such as the head of the fibula or malleoli, to avoid the risk of direct nerve compression and damage. Elevation of the leg to empty the venous blood and reduce blood loss should be done before inflation of the tourniquet cuff. This process may be facilitated with the use of bandage or tourniquet

exsanguinators. The inflation pressure is often set at about 250 mmHg in adults or about 100 mmHg above the systolic pressure.
- All non-viable or contaminated tissue must be removed and there must be sufficient arterial perfusion to allow healing.
- Sufficient soft tissues should be preserved to cover the end of the bone without tension. However, an excessive amount of soft tissues may interfere with prosthesis fitting.
- The scars of weight-bearing stumps should preferably be posteriorly to the edge of the stump.
- Nerves are divided as high as possible and allowed to retract. They should be divided sharply and ligated with non-absorbable sutures to reduce the risk of formation of potentially painful neuromas. The ends of the nerves should be away from areas of pressure.
- Bone edges should be filed after transaction to remove any sharp edges, and all attempts should be made to maintain a myofascial layer between the bone and the skin.
- Wounds should be closed without tension, and suture lines should be placed away from weight-bearing surfaces when possible.
- Drains can be used to reduce dead space and to drain residual bleeding.

Special surgical instruments

- Pneumatic tourniquet and bandage or tourniquet exsanguinator.
- Power saw or Gigli saw for the division of the bone.
- Bone files or rasps are essential to smooth out bone edges.
- Compression wraps for postoperative dressings are helpful to decrease edema and to shape the stump for early fittings of prosthetics.

Atlas of Surgical Techniques in Trauma, ed. Demetrios Demetriades, Kenji Inaba, and George Velmahos. Published by Cambridge University Press. © Cambridge University Press 2015.

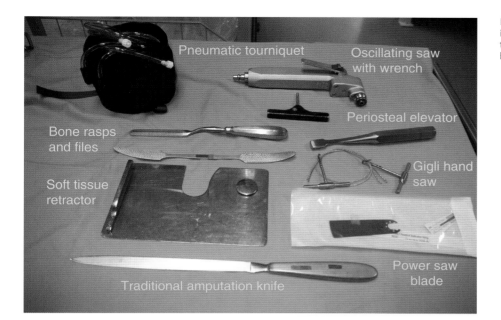

Fig. 37.1. Essential instruments for amputations in trauma: pneumatic tourniquet, bandage or tourniquet exsanguinators, power saw or Gigli saw, bone files or rasps.

Patient positioning

- The patient is placed in the standard supine trauma position with both arms at 90 degrees to allow anesthesia access to the upper extremities.
- The leg should be prepped circumferentially and a pneumatic tourniquet applied proximal to the injury to minimize blood loss during the procedure. Padding or surgical towels can be placed under the thigh to allow for elevation of the extremity.
- The surgeon stands on the inner side of the leg for a better view of the vessels and nerves.

Above-knee amputation (AKA)

- The femur can be divided at any length necessary; most commonly this is at the junction of the middle and distal third of the femur shaft for optimal functional interaction with the prosthetic limb (12–18 cm below the trochanter major).

(a)

- Start with applying a pneumatic tourniquet if there is enough femur length.
- Mark with a marking pen a transversely oriented fish-mouth incision. The anterior and posterior tissue flaps may be equal or the anterior flap may be longer. The skin incision should be about 15 cm below the planned division of the bone.
- The skin and subcutaneous tissue should be divided circumferentially. The saphenous vein is identified in the medial aspect of the thigh and ligated.

(b)

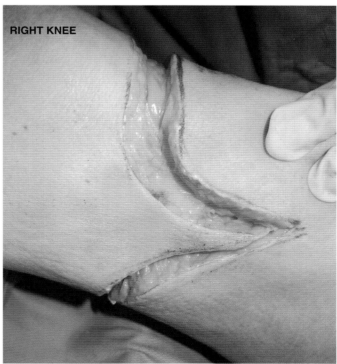

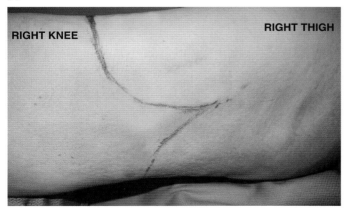

Fig. 37.2(a). Incision for right above-knee amputation: transversely oriented fish-mouth incision. The anterior and posterior tissue flaps may be equal or the anterior flap may be longer.

Fig. 37.2(b). Circumferential sharp dissection of the skin and subcutaneous tissue of the fish-mouth incision.

- The anterior thigh compartment muscles are sharply divided to the bone about 3–5 cm distal to the planned femoral osteotomy. The divided muscles are reflected proximally.
- The femoral artery and vein are identified deep to the sartorius muscle and individually ligated and divided.
- The transverse osteotomy is performed with a Gigli or power saw and sharp edges should be filed down with the bone rasp.

(a)

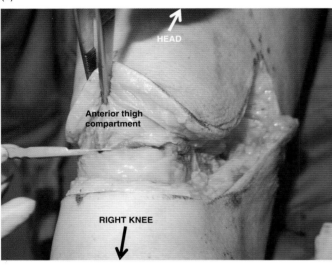

Fig. 37.3(a). The anterior thigh compartment muscles are sharply divided to the bone.

(b)

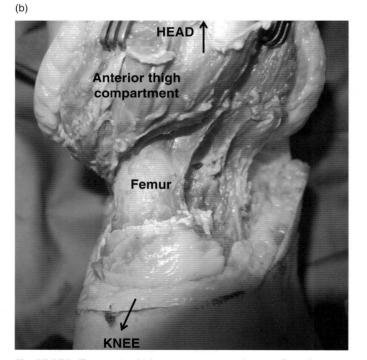

Fig. 37.3(b). The anterior thigh compartment muscles are reflected proximally to expose the femur.

(a)

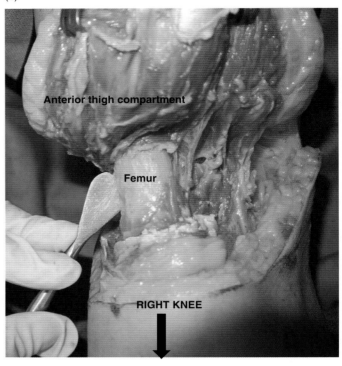

Fig. 37.4(a). Periosteal elevator is used to clear the femur circumferentially of soft tissue attachments.

(b)

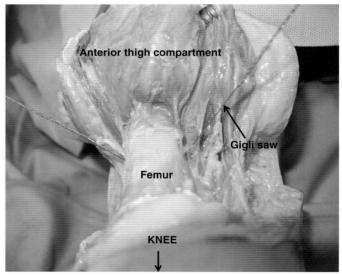

Fig. 37.4(b). A Gigli saw is used to divide the femur transversely.

- The posterior thigh compartment muscles are sharply divided an inch distally to the femoral osteotomy site. The deep femoral artery is ligated when encountered, depending on the level of AKA. The sciatic nerve is identified, divided sharply, and ligated as high as possible.

(a)

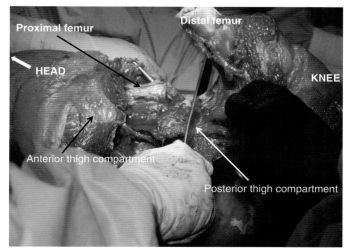

Fig. 37.5(a). Sharp division of the posterior thigh compartment muscles.

(b)

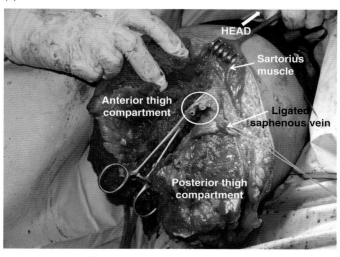

Fig. 37.5(b). Identification and ligation of the femoral artery and vein (white circle).

(c)

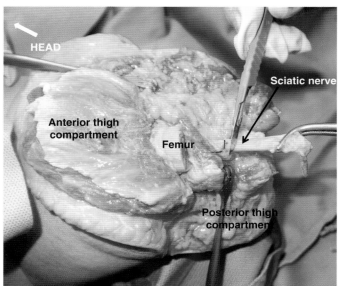

Fig. 37.5(c). Distal traction of the sciatic nerve with ligation and sharp division.

• A periosteal elevator is utilized to separate periosteum from the bone.

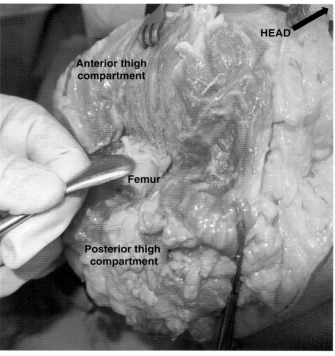

Fig. 37.6. Periosteal elevator is used to separate the periosteum from the femur in preparation for myodesis.

317

● Myodesis is performed to attach and stabilize muscles directly to bone, facilitating fixed resistance against which a muscle can move, to maintain function, and to provide distal padding of the osteotomy. Myodesis is performed by drilling four unicortical holes to the distal femur using a 2.5 mm drill screw to attach the adductor and medial hamstring muscles to the bone with three absorbable sutures.

(a)

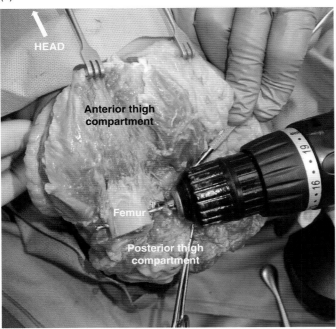

Fig. 37.7(a). Drilling of four unicortical holes to the distal femur using 2.5 mm drill screw for myodesis.

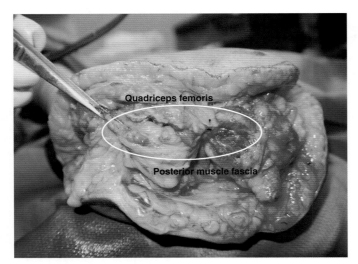

Fig. 37.8. Myoplasty over the femur. The quadriceps femoris is placed over the bone and sutured to the posterior fascia using interrupted absorbable sutures (white circle).

● Myoplasty is performed by bringing the quadriceps femoris over the bone and suturing to the posterior fascia using interrupted absorbable sutures over the drains.

(b)

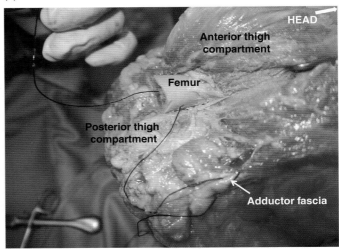

Fig. 37.7(b). Fascia of the adductor and medial hamstring muscles is attached to the femur through the four unicortical holes with three absorbable sutures.

● The skin is then closed with staples or interrupted 3–0 nylon vertical mattress sutures without tension.

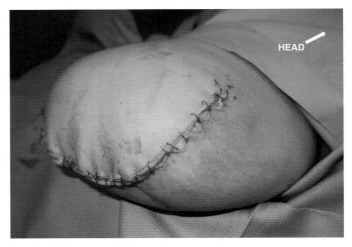

Fig. 37.9. Completed right above-knee amputation.

(a)

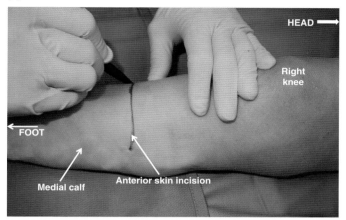

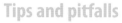

Fig. 37.10(a). Right below-knee amputation: the anterior skin incision is made transversely and located 10–12 cm or approximately one hand breadth below the tibial tuberosity and extended to both sides of the calf for a distance of about one-half of the calf circumference.

(b)

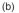

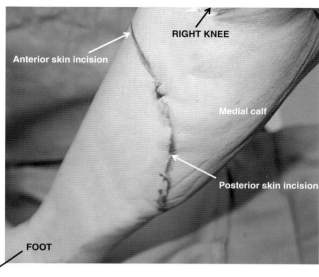

Fig. 37.10(b). The posterior skin incision is marked along the vertical axis of the leg for a length of one and a half times the transverse incision (12–15 cm). The incision should be gently curved to reduce dog-ears in the closure.

Tips and pitfalls

- Make sure to preserve as much femoral shaft length as possible to improve function and prosthetic fit.
- When making the anterior and posterior flaps, ensure there is enough tissue for adequate coverage of the femur and that the flaps are able to come together without tension.
- Be sure to flex the patient's hip to check for tension on the skin suture line. If tension is present, the femoral shaft requires further shortening.
- Make sure to myodese the adductor and medial hamstrings to the bone to prevent a non-functional and unstable femoral stump.

Below-knee amputation

- The most commonly used amputation involves the creation of a long posterior myocutaneous flap.
- Mark the skin incision with a marking pen.
- Inflate the pneumatic tourniquet.
- The anterior skin incision is made transversely and located 10–12 cm or approximately one hand breadth below the tibial tuberosity and extended to both sides of the calf for a distance of about one-half of the calf circumference. Ligate the saphenous vein when encountered in the medial aspect of the leg.
- To construct the posterior flap, extend the skin incision along the vertical axis of the extremity for a length of one and a half times the transverse incision (12–15 cm). The posterior flap should be gently curved to reduce dog-ears in the closure.

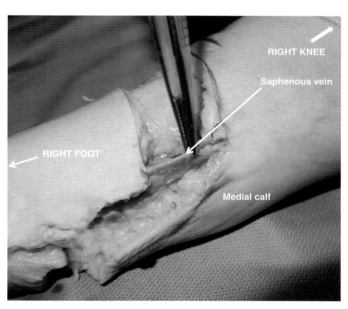

Fig. 37.11. Identification and division of the saphenous vein in the medial aspect of the calf.

- The anterior compartment muscles are divided sharply in the same plane as the transverse skin incision, and dissection is carried down until the anterior tibial artery and vein with the deep peroneal nerve are identified. The vessels are suture ligated with 2–0 silk sutures and the nerve is retracted and divided sharply.

- A periosteal elevator is used to clear muscular attachments to the tibia, and the interosseous membrane is divided sharply.
- The tibia is then divided using a power or Gigli saw proximal to the skin incision in a plane perpendicular to the long axis of the bone. The anterior lip of the tibia is then beveled and filed down to remove any sharp edges.

(a)

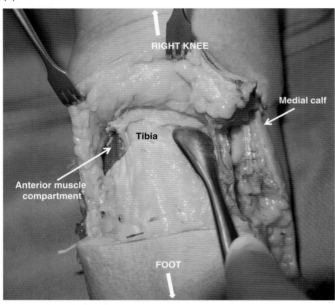

Fig. 37.12(a). Circumferential clearing of the tibia from the muscular attachments.

(b)

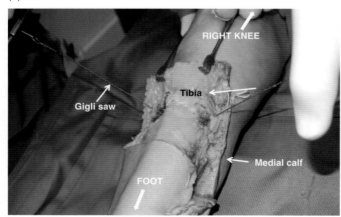

Fig. 37.12(b). Division of the tibia with a Gigli saw.

- The lateral compartment muscles are divided sharply in the same plane as the transverse skin incision. The fibula is identified and cleared of its muscular attachments circumferentially with a periosteal elevator. The fibula is transected with the power or Gigli saw 2–3 cm proximal to the tibia transaction; any sharp edges should be filed down. The fibula can be excised in young individuals.

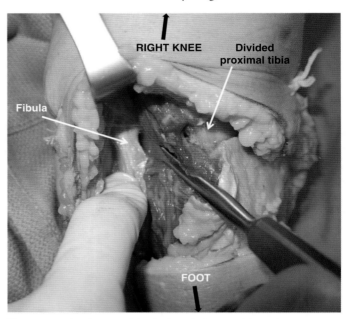

Fig. 37.13. Identification of the fibula with clearing of the soft tissue circumferentially with a periosteal elevator and division 2–3 cm above the level of the divided tibia.

- The posterior compartment muscles are divided in a plane below the distal tibia and fibula with a sharp amputation knife to create the posterior muscle flap. Remove enough of the soleus muscle to prevent excessive bulk or tension in the flap closure.
- The posterior tibial and peroneal vessels are identified and ligated with 2–0 silk sutures. The tibial and peroneal nerves should be divided sharply under tension and allowed to retract.
- The tourniquet should then be released and hemostasis checked and achieved with suture ligation, attempting to avoid electrocautery. The wound should then be irrigated, and the posterior flap rotated over a drain to cover the tibia and fibula.
- The deep fascia is approximated with interrupted 2–0 absorbable sutures, ensuring a tension-free closure.
- The skin is closed with staples or interrupted 3–0 nylon vertical mattress sutures.

Tips and pitfalls

- Failing to make the posterior flap long enough to cover the tibia will place the suture line under tension and will not provide adequate soft tissue coverage of the bones.
- Failure to make a gentle curve of the posterior incision will result in excessive skin and dog-ears during the closure.

(a)

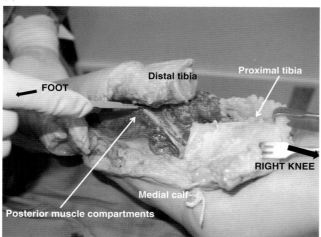

Fig. 37.14(a). Division of the posterior compartment muscles in a plane below the distal tibia and fibula with a sharp amputation knife to create the posterior muscle flap.

(b)

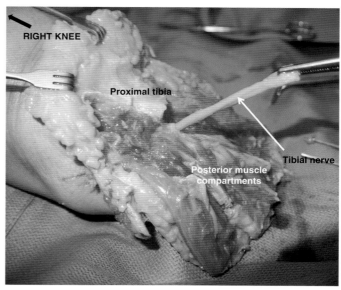

Fig. 37.14(b). Firm traction on the tibial nerve, followed by sharp division very proximally (red arrow). The nerve stump is then allowed to retract.

(c)

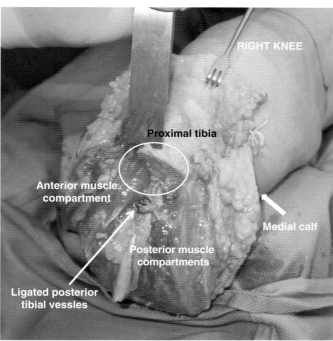

Fig. 37.14(c). Beveling the anterior lip of the tibia (circle) to remove any sharp edges.

• Failure to transect the fibula 1–2 cm proximal to tibial transaction will result in pain if left too long or if a conical stump is left too short, either of which will be difficult to fit with a prosthesis.

• Removing too much of the soleus muscle in the posterior flap will cause the soft tissue coverage of the bone to be too thin and may cause pain and irritation of the skin. Leaving too much of the soleus muscle will create a bulky stump and may add tension to the closure.

• Failure to place the nerves under tension and divide them sharply will prevent them from retracting and may result in neuroma formation.

(a)

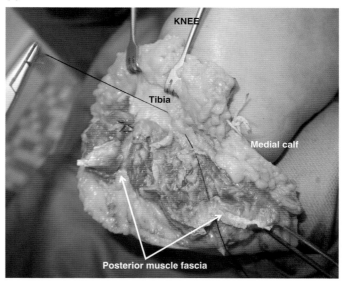

Fig. 37.15(a). Rotation of the posterior muscle flap with closure of the posterior muscle fascia over the tibia.

(b)

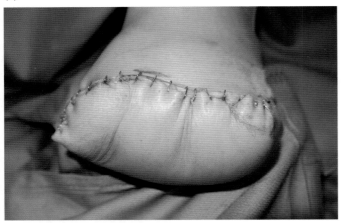

Fig. 37.15(b). Completed right below-knee amputation.

Guillotine amputation (below knee)

- The purpose of the guillotine amputation in the trauma setting is to quickly remove the mangled extremity in a damage control situation with the plan to return to the operating room in the future for a staged operation.
- The knife is used to make a circular incision in an area of viable tissue above the soft tissue requiring debridement. Sharp dissection is used to cut through the muscles and the power or Gigli saw is used to transect the tibia and fibula.

- The three major vascular bundles including the anterior tibial artery and vein, the posterior tibial artery and vein, and the peroneal artery and vein are ligated with 2–0 silk sutures. The peroneal vessels are the most difficult to control because of the difficult exposure between the tibia and fibula.
- If used, the tourniquet is released and hemostasis is checked and achieved. Local hemostatic agents may be used if necessary. Once hemostasis is achieved, a bulky moist dressing is applied and covered by an ice wrap; then the patient can be transported out of the operating room for further resuscitation.

Postoperative care

- Apply petroleum gauze over the skin incision and wrap the stump in a soft gauze dressing with a mild compression wrap to help reduce edema and protect the wound from trauma. If needed, a semi-rigid removable dressing may be applied to help prevent contractures.
- Postoperative care of amputation patients requires multidisciplinary cooperation with rehabilitation medicine, physical therapy, psychiatry services, and the surgical team. All must work coherently to get the patient ambulatory and fitted with a permanent prosthesis as soon as possible.

Lower extremity fasciotomies

Peep Talving, Elizabeth R. Benjamin, and Daniel J. Grabo

Surgical anatomy

- The lower extremity fascial compartments include three gluteal, three thigh, four calf, and nine compartments of the foot. These compartments contain muscles, nerves, and blood vessels.
- The compartments of the buttock include the gluteus maximus, the gluteus medius/minimus, and the extension of the fascia lata of the thigh into the gluteal region, which forms the third compartment, the tensor fascia lata. The sciatic nerve is the only major neurovascular structure in the compartments of the buttock.
- The thigh has three compartments: the anterior compartment (quadriceps femoris and sartorius muscle), the posterior compartment (biceps femoris, semi-tendinosus, and semi-membranosus), and the medial compartment (adductor muscle group and the gracilis muscle).
- The lower leg has four leg compartments:
  - *The anterior compartment*: contains the tibialis anterior muscle, extensor halluces muscle, extensor digitorum longus muscle, the anterior tibial artery, and the deep peroneal nerve.
  - *The lateral compartment*: contains the peroneus longus and brevis muscles and the superficial peroneal nerve.
  - *The superficial posterior compartment*: contains the gastrocnemius and soleus muscles and the sural nerve.
  - *The deep posterior compartment*: contains the flexor hallucis longus muscle, flexor digitorum longus muscle, tibialis posterior muscles, the posterior tibial artery, and the tibial nerve.
- The foot contains a total of nine compartments including four interosseous, the medial, lateral, deep and superficial central, and the adductor hallucis compartments that may require decompression in crush injuries to the foot. The medial, lateral, and superficial compartments pass through the entire length of the foot, while the interosseous compartments and the calcaneal compartments are confined to the forefoot and the hindfoot, respectively.

General principles

- The compartment syndrome is a limb- and life-threatening condition. Renal failure due to myoglobinemia and myoglobinuria is a common serious complication in delayed diagnosis.
- Extremity compartment syndrome may occur in patients with severe fractures, crush injury, ischemia due to vascular injury, venous outflow obstruction, circumferential burns, and constricting bandages or casts. On rare occasions, massive fluid resuscitation in trauma or burn patients may cause secondary compartment syndrome.
- The variables affecting the severity of the compartment syndrome include hypotension, compartment pressure, duration of elevated compartment pressure, perfusion pressure, and individual susceptibility. The compartmental perfusion pressure is defined as the difference in pressure (mmHg) between the patient's diastolic blood pressure and measured compartmental pressure. A perfusion pressure of 30 mmHg or less is associated with a high risk of compartment syndrome.
- Compartment pressures > 30 mmHg or perfusion pressures <30 mmHg should prompt an emergency fasciotomy.
- Reversible muscular ischemia and neuropraxia occur in up to 4–6 hours of ischemia. Irreversible muscular ischemia and axonotmesis occurs beyond 6 hours of ischemia.
- The anterior and lateral compartments of the calf are the most commonly affected by compartment syndrome.
- Limited skin incisions may result in inadequate decompression of the muscle compartments.
- The fasciotomy skin incisions should always be left open.
- After decompression of the compartments, the viability of the muscles is ensured with diathermy or forceps-induced contractions. Non-viable muscle mass is debrided and hemostasis is ensured.

Atlas of Surgical Techniques in Trauma, ed. Demetrios Demetriades, Kenji Inaba, and George Velmahos. Published by Cambridge University Press. © Cambridge University Press 2015.

Special instruments

- The Stryker® intracompartmental pressure measuring system using an 18-gauge side-ported needle is a readily available method for measuring compartment pressures.
- Basic orthopedic tray.
- For vessel–loop shoelace wound closure: vessel loops, skin staples.
- Negative pressure dressing system (NPDS).

Technique of compartment pressure measurement

- Excellent knowledge of the anatomy of the muscle compartments is critical! The pressure should be measured in all compartments individually! Adjacent compartments may have very different pressures.

- The most commonly used technique is with the hand-held Stryker® device. An alternative in the ICU is to set up a pressure transducer connected to a needle that may be inserted into the muscle compartment.
- Side-port needles are more accurate at measuring the compartment pressure than regular needles.
- Steps for compartment pressure measurement with a Stryker® device.

1. Connect the side-port needle (A) to the diaphragm chamber (B) and the diaphragm to the prefilled syringe (C). Insert the assembled system into the device and snap shut without forcing it (D). Turn unit on.
2. Press the zero button and wait for a few seconds until it shows zero.
3. Insert the needle perpendicular to the skin and insert into the muscle.
4. Slowly inject 0.3 mL into the compartment.

(a)

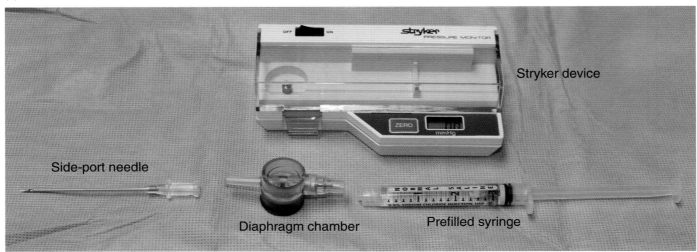

Fig. 38.1(a). Pieces of the Stryker® device for the measurement of muscle compartment pressures.

(b)

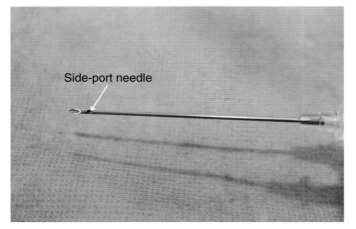

Fig. 38.1(b). Side-port needle provides more accurate measurements of the muscle compartment pressures.

(c)

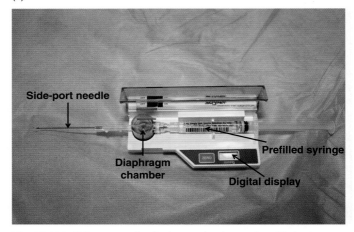

Fig. 38.1(c). Side-port needle, diaphragm chamber, and prefilled syringe assembled and placed in the device.

(d)

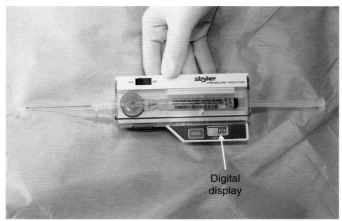

Fig. 38.1(d). The device is closed and is ready for use.

5. Wait for a few seconds for the display to reach equilibrium before reading the pressure.

Gluteal compartment fasciotomy

Patient positioning

- The gluteal compartment fasciotomies are performed in the prone or lateral decubitus position.

Incisions

- Gluteal compartment decompression can be achieved either through the traditional question mark incision or through a midaxial longitudinal incision.
- The question mark incision starts at the posterior superior iliac spine, courses along the iliac crest, turns medially over the greater trochanter, and below the buttock and it extends over the midline of the posterior upper thigh.

(a)

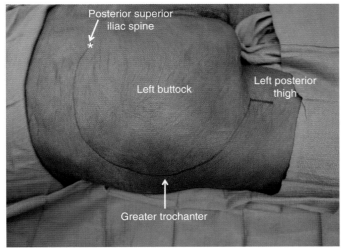

Fig. 38.2(a),(b). Left buttock question mark incision for gluteal fasciotomy.

(b)

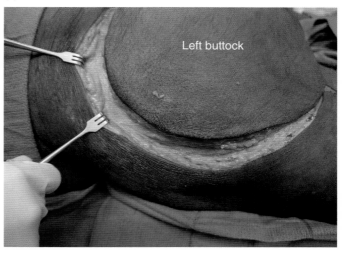

Fig. 38.2(a),(b). (cont.)

- The mid axial longitudinal incision begins just lateral to the posterior superior iliac spine and extends posterolaterally toward the lateral thigh. At the level of the trochanter, the incision turns inferiorly along the lateral aspect of the thigh to provide access to the fascia lata.

(a)

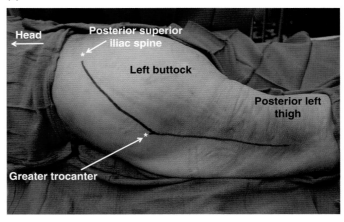

(b)

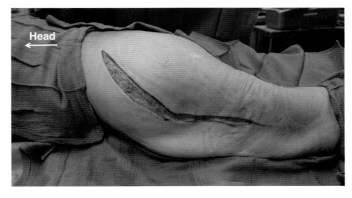

Fig. 38.3(a),(b). Left buttock mid axial longitudinal incision for gluteal fasciotomy. It begins just lateral to the posterior superior iliac spine and, at the level of the greater trochanter, it turns inferiorly along the lateral aspect of the thigh to provide access to the fascia lata.

Procedure

- The skin incision is carried through the subcutaneous tissue to the fascia. The gluteus maximus is directly encountered and the fascia is released.

(a)

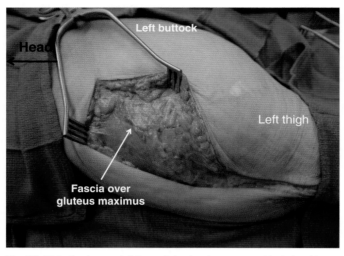

Fig. 38.4(a). Fasciotomy left buttock (patient in prone position): the skin incision is carried through the subcutaneous tissue and the fascia over the gluteus maximus is exposed.

(b)

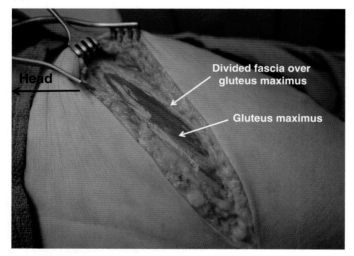

Fig. 38.4(b). The fascia overlying the gluteus maximus is incised to allow decompression of this compartment.

- The muscle fibers of the gluteus maximus are split to access the underlying gluteus medius/minimus compartment.
- The inferolateral portion of the incision is used to release the tensor fascia lata.
- Following fasciotomy, the viability of the muscles is ensured with diathermy or forceps-induced muscle contractions.

(a)

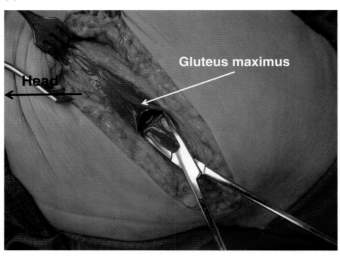

(b)

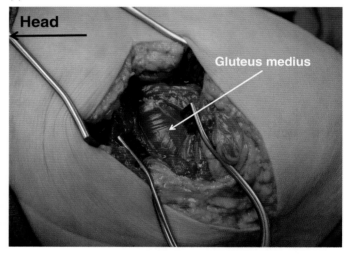

Fig. 38.5(a),(b). Using a muscle spreading technique, the gluteus maximus is divided along the lines of the fibers to access the underlying deep compartment.

- Non-viable muscle mass is debrided and hemostasis is ensured. The wound is covered with NPDS or wet-to-dry dressing.

Thigh fasciotomy

Incisions

- The entire extremity is prepared and draped from the iliac crest to the toenails.
- In most cases, one lateral incision is performed to decompress both the anterior and posterior thigh compartments. The medial compartment rarely needs decompression, but if needed it can be accomplished through a medial incision.

Procedure

Lateral incision

- The lateral incision decompresses both anterior and posterior thigh compartments.
- The skin incision extends from just below the greater trochanter to a few cm above the lateral femoral condyle. It is carried through the subcutaneous tissue and down to the fascia lata.

(a)

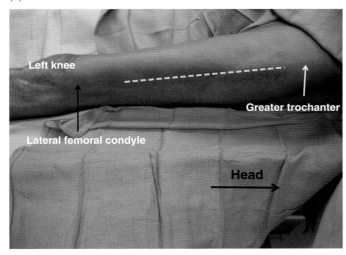

Fig. 38.6(a). Fasciotomy left thigh: the skin incision extends from just below the major trochanter to a few cm above the lateral femoral condyle.

(b)

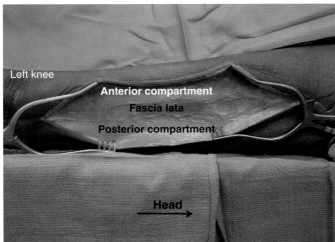

Fig. 38.6(b). The incision is carried through the subcutaneous tissue and down to the fascia lata.

- The fascia lata is divided with a longitudinal incision to decompress the anterior compartment.
- To decompress the posterior compartment, a posterior skin flap is mobilized and an incision is made in the fascia posterior to the intercompartmental septum.

(a)

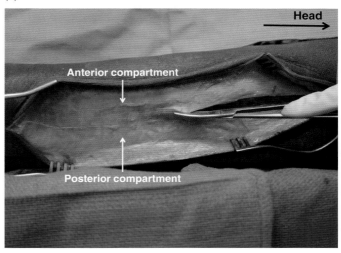

Fig. 38.7(a). The fascia lata is divided with a longitudinal incision to decompress the anterior compartment.

(b)

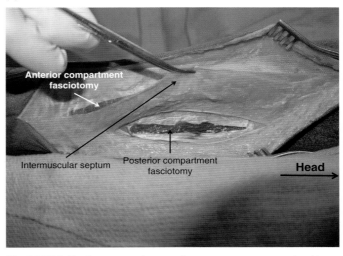

Fig. 38.7(b). To decompress the posterior compartment, a posterior skin flap is mobilized and an incision is made in the fascia posterior to the intercompartmental septum.

(c)

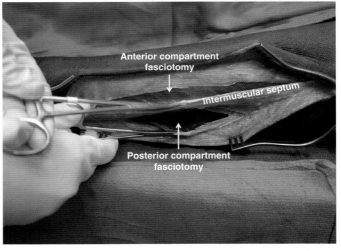

Fig. 38.7(c). Left thigh fasciotomy: decompression of the anterior and posterior compartments through fascial incisions in front of and behind the intermuscular septum.

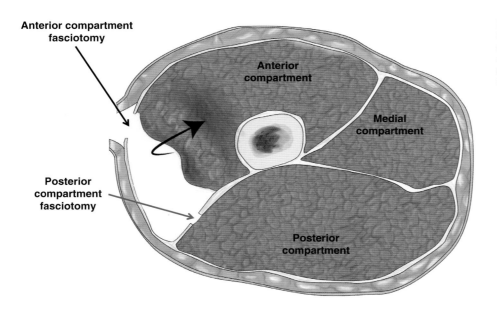

Anterior compartment fasciotomy

Anterior compartment

Medial compartment

Posterior compartment fasciotomy

Posterior compartment

Fig. 38.8. Left thigh fasciotomy through a lateral incision: the posterior compartment can be decompressed through the intercompartmental septum, which can be accessed and incised (red arrow) by retracting the exposed vastus lateralis muscle superiorly and medially.

- Alternatively, the intercompartmental septum can be accessed and incised by retracting the exposed vastus lateralis muscle superiorly and medially with large retractors.
- Subsequently, the lateral intermuscular septum between anterior and posterior compartments is incised for the length of the incision.

Medial incision

- This incision is rarely needed because the medial muscle compartment is rarely affected.
- By decompressing the anterior and posterior compartments, pressures in the medial compartment secondarily drop as well. Measure the medial compartment pressures before proceeding to fasciotomy.
- In the average size male, a 20- to 25-cm medial incision courses along the greater saphenous vein, extending to a few cm above the medial femoral condyle.
- If decompression of the medial compartment is warranted, the saphenous vein should be preserved.

(a)

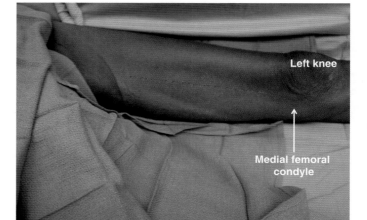

Left knee

Medial femoral condyle

Fig. 38.9(a). Left medial thigh fasciotomy incision: the incision courses along the greater saphenous vein extending to a few cm above the medial femoral condyle.

(b)

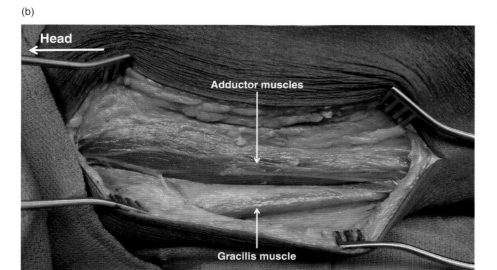

Fig. 38.9(b). Completed left medial thigh fasciotomy incision.

Lower leg fasciotomy

Incisions

- The standard four-compartment fasciotomy of the lower leg is achieved through two incisions.

- The lateral incision decompresses the anterior and lateral compartments.
- The medial incision decompresses the superficial and deep posterior compartments.

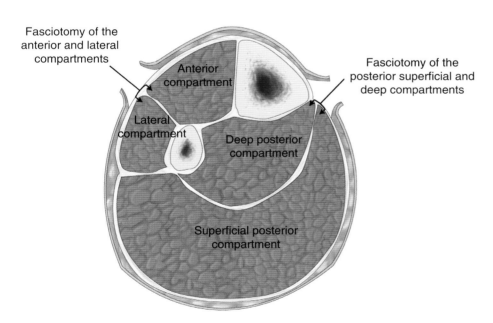

Fig. 38.10. Four-compartment fasciotomy of the right leg through two incisions. The lateral incision decompresses the anterior and lateral compartments and the medial incision decompresses the superficial and deep posterior compartments.

Lateral incision

- The lateral incision is performed midway between the fibula and the lateral tibial edge (or about two finger breadths in front of the fibula), starting two to three finger breadths below the tibial tuberosity and extending to two to three finger breadths above the ankle. This incision is approximately over the septum separating the anterior from the lateral compartments. A useful external landmark for the fibula is a line drawn from the head of the fibula to the lateral malleolus.
- The skin incision should be carried through the subcutaneous tissue and down to the investing leg fascia. Skin flaps are raised to expose the fascia covering the anterior and lateral compartments of the leg.

- The anterior compartment is decompressed through a fasciotomy, about two to three finger breadths lateral to the lateral tibial edge, anterior to the septum separating the anterior from the lateral compartments. As mentioned above, the septum is approximately under the skin incision. Perforating vessels entering the septum may facilitate identification of the septum. Another method to identify the septum is a transverse incision over the estimated site of the septum. Decompression of the anterior compartment is achieved through a longitudinal fasciotomy with long, blunt-pointed scissors. The scissor tips are always turned away from the septum. The fasciotomy is directed towards the big toe distally and the patella proximally.

(a)

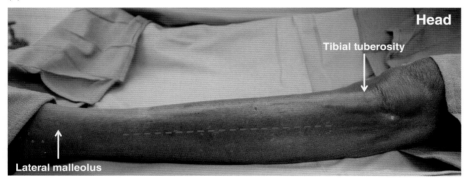

Fig. 38.11(a). Fasciotomy of the left lower leg. The lateral incision is made midway between the fibula and the lateral tibia edge starting two to three finger breadths below the tibial tuberosity and extending to two to three finger breadths above the ankle.

(b)

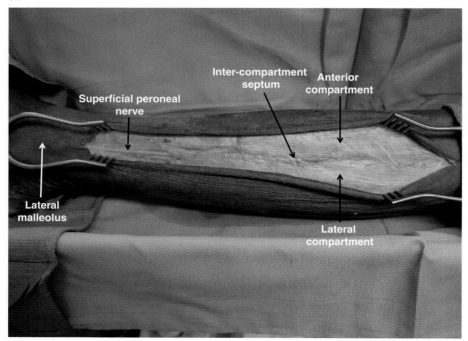

Fig. 38.11(b). Lateral incision for left leg fasciotomy. The skin incision is carried down to the investing leg fascia. Skin flaps are raised to expose the fascia covering the anterior and lateral compartments of the leg. Note the septum between the anterior and lateral compartments. Care should be taken to avoid injury to the superficial peroneal nerve, in the lower part of the leg.

- The lateral compartment is decompressed with a longitudinal incision behind the intercompartmental septum. The fascia is incised with a direction towards the lateral malleolus distally and the head of the fibula proximally. Directing the distal fasciotomy towards the

lateral malleolus is critical in order to avoid injury of the superficial peroneal nerve, as it pierces the septum in the distal third of the leg to take a subcutaneous course.

(a)

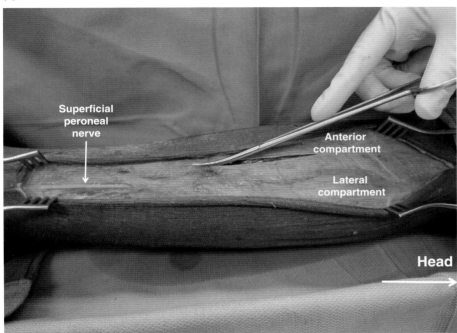

Fig. 38.12(a). Left leg fasciotomy, lateral incision. The anterior compartment is decompressed through a fasciotomy, about two to three finger breadths lateral to the lateral tibial edge, anterior to the septum separating the anterior from the lateral compartments.

(b)

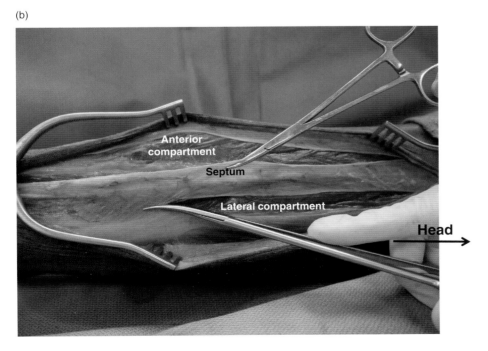

Fig. 38.12(b). Identification of the septum, which separates the anterior and lateral compartments. The lateral compartment is decompressed with long scissors.

Medial incision

- The medial incision is performed two finger breadths posterior to the medial edge of the tibia starting two to three finger breadths below the knee and extending to two to three finger breadths above the ankle.

- The skin incision is carried through the subcutaneous tissue and down to the investing fascia taking care to identify and preserve the saphenous vein facilitating venous outflow from the leg.

(a)

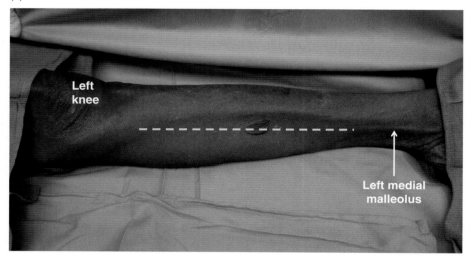

Fig. 38.13(a). The medial incision is placed approximately two finger breadths posterior to the medial border of the tibia, starting two to three finger breadths below the knee and extending to two to three finger breadths above the ankle.

(b)

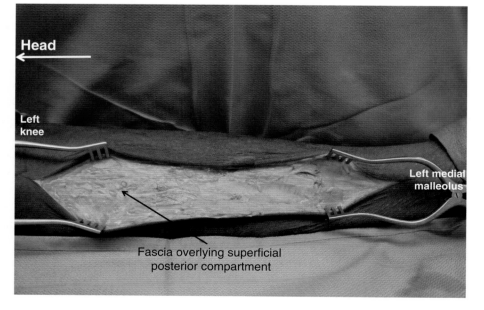

Fig. 38.13(b). Left leg fasciotomy, medial incision: The incision is carried down to the fascia and skin flaps are slightly mobilized.

- The superficial compartment is decompressed with a fascial incision, made about two finger breadths posterior and parallel to the medial fasciotomy.
- The deep posterior compartment is decompressed with a fascial incision just behind the edge of the tibia. Identification of the posterior tibial neurovascular bundle ensures that the deep compartment has been properly identified.

(a)

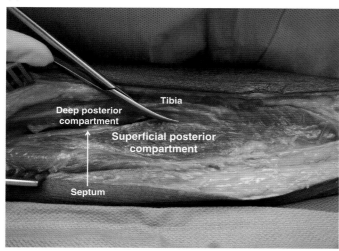

Fig. 38.14(a). Left leg fasciotomy, medial incision. The superficial compartment is decompressed with a fascial incision, made about two finger breadths posterior to the tibia. The deep posterior compartment is decompressed through a fascial incision just behind the edge of the tibia.

(b)

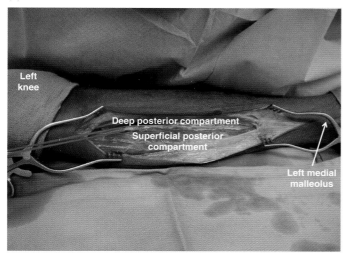

Fig. 38.14(b). Identification of the posterior tibial neurovascular bundle (red vessel loop) ensures that the deep compartment has been properly identified.

Foot fasciotomy

The most common cause of foot compartment syndrome is crush injury.

Incisions

- The compartments of the foot are usually decompressed through three incisions: one medial incision and two dorsal incisions over the interosseous compartments.

Procedure

- The medial incision extends from a point below the medial malleolus to the metatarsophalangeal joint. This incision risks injury to the neurovascular bundle and some surgeons avoid it in favor of only two dorsal incisions.
- The two dorsal incisions are placed over the second and fourth metatarsal shafts. Maintain a wide skin bridge to avoid necrosis. Skin flaps are raised to identify each of the interosseous compartments.

(a)

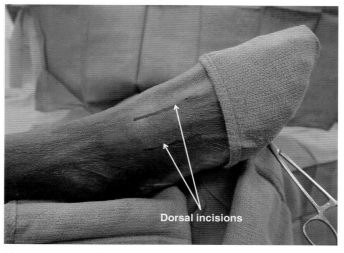

Fig. 38.15(a). Foot fasciotomy. The two dorsal incisions are placed over the second and fourth metatarsal shafts.

(b)

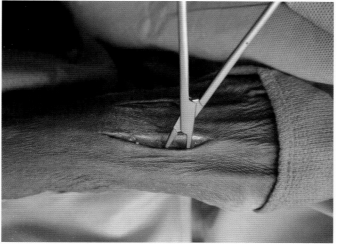

Fig. 38.15(b). The interosseous compartments are identified and opened.

333

(a)

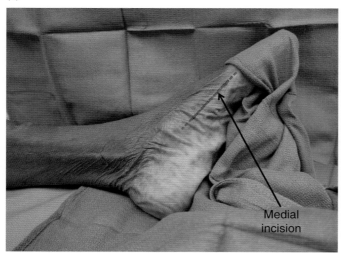

Medial
incision

(b)

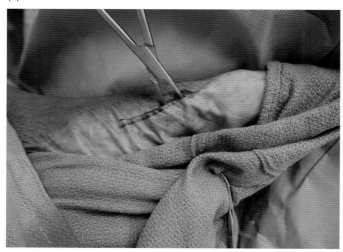

Fig. 38.16(a),(b). Foot fasciotomy: medial incision.

(a)

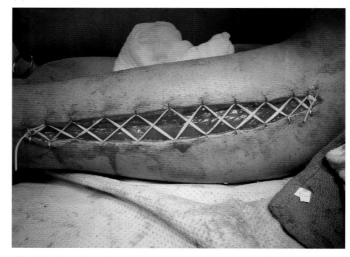

Fig. 38.17(a). Vessel-loop shoelace wound closure of the fasciotomy wound.

(b)

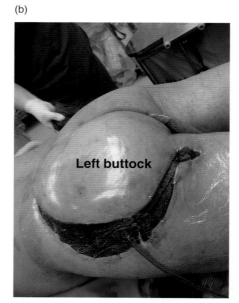

Left buttock

Fig. 38.17(b). Negative pressure therapy of a left buttock fasciotomy.

Fasciotomy wound management

- Negative pressure therapy dressing (VAC) is a useful modality to manage the fasciotomy sites. It prevents wound retraction, removes excessive soft tissue edema and facilitates delayed primary skin closure. However, its application in the presence of incomplete hemostasis may result in severe bleeding. It is advisable that this dressing is used after the second look operation, when hemostasis is complete.
- Vessel-loop shoelace wound closure is a useful technique to achieve delayed primary skin closure.

- Split-thickness skin graft may be necessary for wound closure, if delayed primary closure is not possible.

Tips and pitfalls

- Delayed diagnosis is the most common problem in the management of the compartment syndrome. A high index of suspicion, serial clinical examinations, compartment pressure measurements, and serial CK levels remain the cornerstone of early diagnosis and timely fasciotomy.

- The CK levels may be normal in delayed recognition of the compartment syndrome and completely dead muscle.
- In suspected compartment syndrome, the pressures should be measured in all compartments. The pressures may be normal in one compartment and abnormal in the adjacent one.
- Poor knowledge of the anatomy of the extremity muscle compartments is the most common cause of incomplete fasciotomy or iatrogenic damage to the neurovascular bundle.
- The superficial peroneal nerve is the most commonly injured nerve.

- The deep posterior compartment of the lower leg is the most commonly missed or incompletely released compartment. The easiest location to identify the deep posterior compartment is distal in the calf.
- Short skin incisions may result in an inadequate fasciotomy and progression of the ischemic neuromuscular damage or renal failure.
- Open fractures do not preclude compartment syndrome in the affected compartments.

39 Orthopedic damage control

Eric Pagenkopf, Daniel J. Grabo, and Peter Hammer

General principles

- The treatment goals of damage control surgery in orthopedics (DCO) include the following.
  - Improving vascular flow and subsequent tissue perfusion by reducing and realigning long bone fractures.
  - Treatment of open fractures and associated soft tissue wounds.
  - Stabilizing long bone fractures.
  - Giving priority to other more severe, life-threatening associated injuries.
- Through these goals, patients will have reduced pain, decreased blood loss, and a lower systemic inflammatory response.

Special equipment

- Damage control surgery in orthopedics is centered around the placement of external fixators on both reduced and stabilized fractures. Placement of this hardware requires a set of specialized tools, generally available in any facility that treats patients with orthopedic injuries.
- Instrument trays are manufactured by several different companies but all will share similar components.
  - *Pins*: placed into the cortex of the bone as the anchor point for the external fixator.
  - *Pin clamps*: secured around two pins, providing the bridge between the pins and the connecting rods. Each pin clamp can be affixed with two posts (straight, 30 degree, 90 degree) and can be rotated into 12 different positions, thus giving maximal flexibility to the structure of the external fixator.
  - *Pin-to-rod coupler*: can connect a pin to a connecting rod when a pin clamp is not used.
  - *Rod-to-rod coupler*: can connect a connecting rod to a post or another connecting rod.
  - *Drill*: can be either pneumatic-driven or battery powered.

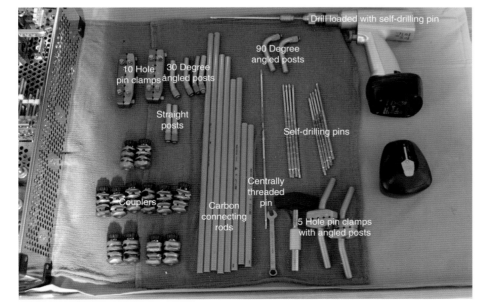

Fig. 39.1. A representative sample of equipment found in a standard external fixator set.

Atlas of Surgical Techniques in Trauma, ed. Demetrios Demetriades, Kenji Inaba, and George Velmahos. Published by Cambridge University Press. © Cambridge University Press 2015.

o For pin selection, the choice is between a blunt and a self-drilling pin. Blunt pins require pre-drilling of holes in the cortex. Self-drilling pins can be mounted directly on to the drill and drilled into place.

o Another screw that may be necessary is a centrally threaded pin. This long pin has a self-drilling tip, but the threads are located in the middle of the pin, not at the end. This pin is placed across the calcaneus when an ankle-bridging external fixator must be placed.

(a)

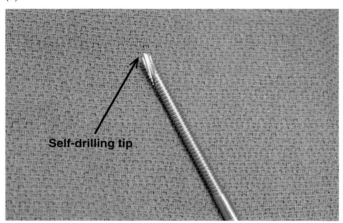

Fig. 39.2(a). A self-drilling pin. Pre-drilling the bone prior to placement is not required.

(b)

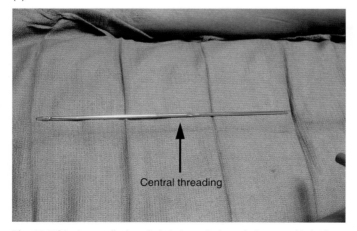

Fig. 39.2(b). A centrally threaded pin is used when placing an ankle-bridging external fixator. The pin is placed through the calcaneus with the central threads engaging the cortex on both sides.

Positioning of patient

Placement of external fixators on the lower extremities requires the patient to be in the supine position with the legs in a neutral position.

Management of specific fractures

Mid shaft tibia fracture

- After the decision has been made to stabilize a tibial fracture with an external fixator, the locations of the anchoring pins must be decided. Two pins should be placed on each side of a fracture site. One pin is inadequate to provide stability.

  o When choosing a location, the pin closest to the fracture site must be greater than 2 cm away. Pin placement too close to the fracture could prevent adequate stabilization.

  o Care must be taken to avoid placing a pin in the metaphysis or intra-articular area.

  o If the fracture is very proximal or distal and there isn't adequate tibial shaft to place pins, an articular-spanning fixator must be placed (see below). The safest area to place pins into the tibia is anywhere between the anterior tibial ridge and 60° medially.

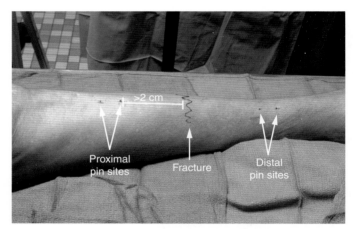

Fig. 39.3. Pin site placement in relation to the fracture. Safe placement is along the anterior aspect of the tibia, with pins placed > 2 cm from fracture. Avoid the metaphysis.

- Make a 4 mm incision over the intended pin sites with a scalpel and carry down through the periosteum. With the self-drilling pin loaded on the drill, place the tip of the pin directly on the cortex. Apply partial power to the drill until the pin adequately engages. Then increase power on the drill. After the tip of the pin passes through the first layer of cortex and into the medulla, there will be decreased resistance. As the tip engages to the far cortex, the resistance will increase again. Be sure to allow for several more revolutions of the pin to be sure that there is secure bicortical purchase. Without bicortical purchase, the pins can become loose and the external fixator can fail to adequately hold reduction.

- Repeat the above process with the second pin. When judging how far to place the second pin from the first, use a 5- or 10-hole pin clamp as your guide. One should place the pins as far apart as possible, but still be able to fit them into one clamp. The second pin should be placed parallel to the first.

(a)

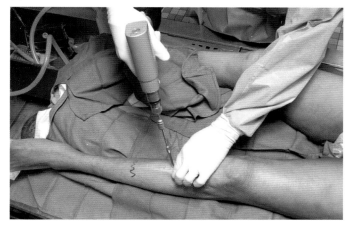

Fig. 39.4(a). Drilling the pin into the tibia. It is important that the pin has a bicortical purchase for maximum stability.

(b)

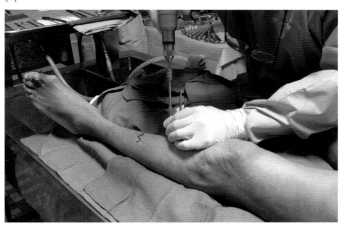

Fig. 39.4(b). Placement of the second pin. The pin should be placed parallel to the first, with the largest distance between the two pins allowed by the pin clamp.

(c)

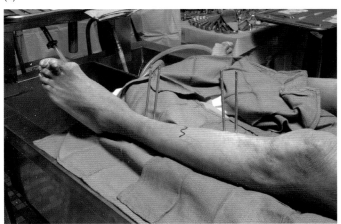

Fig. 39.4(c). Repeat the previous step distal to the fracture site.

- Repeat the above process with the distal pins.
- Pin clamps must now be secured around the pins. The clamp should be placed roughly 1.5 – 2 cm from the skin, or two finger breadths.
- Tighten all fasteners with a full hand torque while applying a counter-torque to prevent damage to the fixator hardware.

(a)

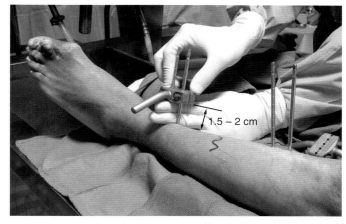

Fig. 39.5(a). Pin clamp placement. The 5-hole pin clamps used here have 30 degree angled posts. Pin clamps allow for placement of different angled posts, pointing in any direction. The clamp should be placed approximately 1.5 – 2 cm from the skin/soft tissue. Two finger breadths is a good way to judge adequate placement.

(b)

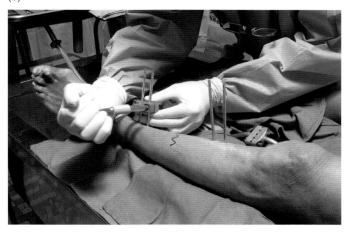

Fig. 39.5(b). Tighten all bolts with full torque while applying counter-torque to prevent damage to the fixator hardware.

- Attach rod-to-rod couplers to the posts, one on each side of the clamp. The optimal location is mid post.

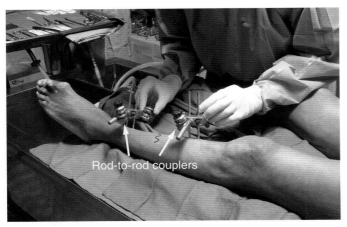

Fig. 39.6. Applying the couplers to the angled posts. They should be placed near mid post to provide better stability.

- At least two connecting rods should be placed parallel to the long bone, preferably one medial and one lateral. When placing the connecting rods, a second person should pull the limb out to length and reduce the fracture. With the fracture reduced, the rod-to-rod couplers should be tightened, thus securing the limb in place.

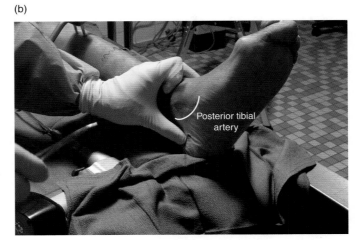

Fig. 39.7. Final hardware apparatus after insertion of the connecting rods and tightening of all fasteners.

Distal tibia and fibula fracture/ankle instability

- In the event that a tibial fracture is too distal to allow for pin placement above the metaphysis, an ankle-bridging

external fixator must be placed. The proximal pins are placed in the tibia as described above. For the distal pin, a calcaneal pin must be placed. An incision is made over the medial aspect of the center of the calcaneus.

- Using a centrally threaded pin, drill the pin medial to lateral. Care must be taken to avoid the posterior tibial artery. This should be inserted until the threads have a bicortical purchase in both sides of the calcaneus.

(a)

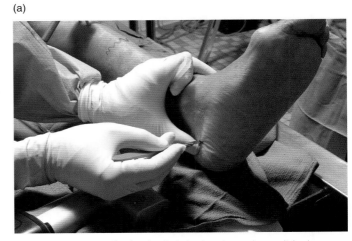

Fig. 39.8(a). Incision for the distal pin is placed over the medial calcaneus.

(b)

Fig. 39.8(b). Take care to avoid injury to the posterior tibial artery. Semicircle representing tibial artery needs to be moved clockwise to run along posterior portion of medical malleolus from superior to inferior.

(a)

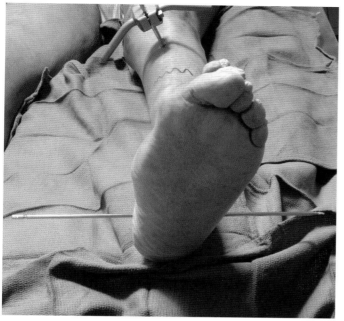

Fig. 39.9(a). The centrally threaded pin in place, with the threads engaged in the cortex on both sides of the calcaneus.

(b)

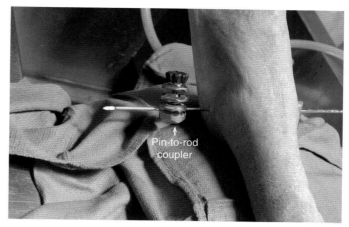

Fig. 39.9(b). For the single pin, a pin-to-rod coupler is used.

- Since a single pin is used, a pin-to-rod coupler must be used. One should be placed on each side of the foot.
- The connecting rods should be placed in the same fashion as for a mid shaft tibia fracture.
- If there is concern that the patient could develop skin breakdown over the ankle, a posterior semi-circular connecting rod could be placed.

Mid-shaft femur fractures

- When stabilizing a mid shaft femur fracture, the same principles apply as to a tibial fracture. Pins should be placed no closer to the fracture than 2 cm. The safest approach to the femur is laterally.

(a)

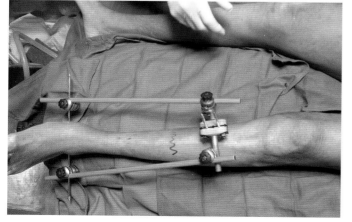

Fig. 39.10(a). The distal fixation hardware in place with bilateral connecting rods.

(b)

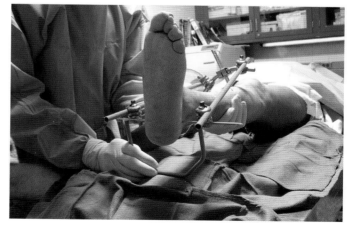

Fig. 39.10(b). A semi-circular rod can be placed posteriorly to elevate the ankle off the bed, thus preventing a potential pressure sore.

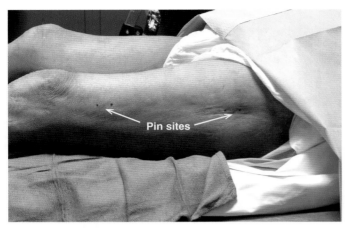

Fig. 39.11. Pin site selection for a mid shaft femur fracture. Safe placement is from the lateral approach.

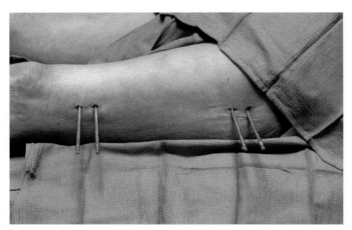

Fig. 39.12. Fixation pins in place in the femur.

- Pin clamp selection is the same as for the tibia. Be sure that they are two finger breadths away from the skin.
- Angled or straight posts can be used.

(a)

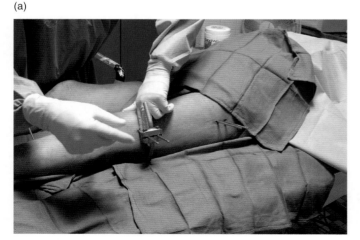

Fig. 39.13(a). Pin clamp with angled posts being placed two finger breadths from the skin.

(b)

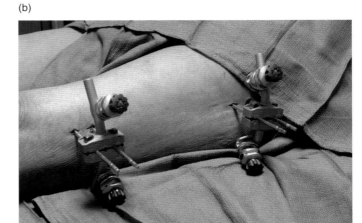

Fig. 39.13(b). Both pin clamps in place with attached post-to-rod couplers.

(c)

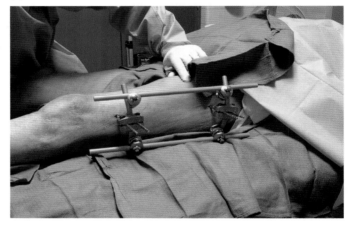

Fig. 39.13(c). The final femur external fixation hardware with connecting rods in place.

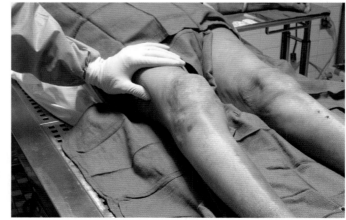

Fig. 39.14. Proximal and distal pin sites for treatment of distal femur/proximal tibia fractures. For the proximal pins, the lateral approach is safest.

(a)

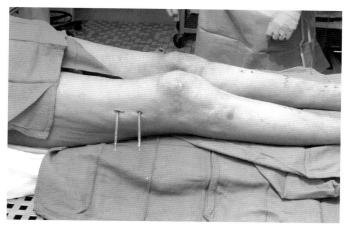

Fig. 39.15(a). Proximal pins in place.

(b)

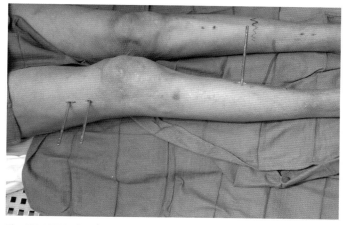

Fig. 39.15(b). Distal pin placement into the tibia. As with a tibia fracture, the safe pin approach is along the anterior surface.

(c)

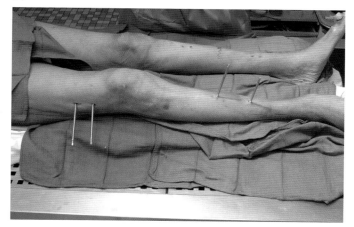

Fig. 39.15(c). Distal pins are in place. Since the length of the external fixator is significantly longer when bridging the knee, placing the distal pins further apart will provide an increase in stability.

- As with the tibia, the femur should be pulled to length before completely tightening the fasteners on the connecting rods.

Distal femur/proximal tibia

- For fractures involving the distal femur or proximal tibia that preclude safe pin placement outside of the knee joint, a knee-spanning fixator may be required. Pin site selection criteria on the femur are the same as for a mid shaft femur fracture. Since the entire weight of the lower leg will be resting on the knee-spanning apparatus, further spaced pin placement in the tibia may be necessary.

(a)

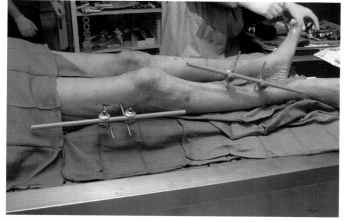

Fig. 39.16(a). Pin-to-rod couplers in place. Because the pins were placed far apart to increase stability, pin clamps will likely not be long enough to use. Couplers are necessary for connecting hardware.

(b)

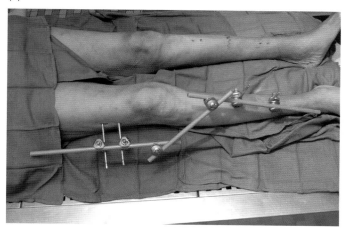

Fig. 39.16(b). The knee-spanning external fixator in place. Only one spanning rod is present in the picture. If the surgeon feels that there isn't enough stability, a second spanning bar could be placed.

"Floating knee"

- A special case could arise where there is both a distal femur fracture and proximal tibia fracture. A knee-spanning external fixator would provide stability to the lower leg, but the bony structures of the knee joint would still be unstable. This would be an instance where a long-leg splint would need to be placed in addition to the knee-spanning external fixator.

Pin care

- External fixator pin sites can be a focus of infection. The pin sites should be cleaned daily with chlorhexidine gluconate and dressed with iodine-soaked gauze.

Tips and pitfalls

- Not every patient who suffers a long bone fracture will require a damage control intervention. Knowing when to apply the principles of early definitive fixation vs. DCO requires clinical knowledge and skill in managing these types of fractures. Communication between all members of the team is critical to achieving optimal outcomes in these multisystem injuries.
- As with any reduction of a comminuted fracture, after application of external fixation hardware, a postreduction neurovascular check must be performed and documented in the record.
- Pin placement in relation to the fracture site is very important. Pins placed too close to the site will not provide adequate stability to reduce and stabilize long bone fractures. When placing the two pins, try to place the pins far apart but still able to fit into the pin clamp.
- When placing an ankle bridging external fixator, attention must be paid to anatomy to avoid neurovascular structures, such as the posterior tibial artery.
- All screws and bolts must be tightened to full torque to prevent equipment slippage and loss of fracture reduction. Counter-torque must be held on the hardware to prevent damage during tightening.

Index

Figures and illustrations are indicated in bold typeface

abdominal aorta
  anatomy of, **240**, 240–241
  complications, 256
  instruments, 242
  patient positioning, 242
  surgical principles, 242
  surgical technique, 242–256,
    **243, 245, 248, 250, 252, 253,
    254, 255**
abdominal injuries
  aorta, 240–256
  DC in, 172–179
  duodenum, 189–197
  gastrointestinal tract, 180–188
  general principles, 165–171
  iliac, 257–261
  inferior vena cava, 262–272
  liver, 198–208
  pancreas, 219–227
  spleen, 209–218
  urological, 228–239
above-knee amputation (AKA),
  315, 315, **317, 318**
ABThera technique, 175–179,
  177
acute epidural hematomas
  (EDH)
  surgical principles, 35–38, **36**
  surgical technique, **41**, 41–45,
    44
adductor canal, **303**, 303
air embolism
  arrhythmias, **26**
  in cardiac injuries, 115
  lung injuries, **149**
  neck trauma, 52
  thoracic vessels, 135, 139
airway management
  cricothyrotomy, 6
  neck trauma, 52
amputations (lower extremity)
  anatomy of, 314
  complications, 319, 321
  instruments, **315**
  patient positioning, 315
  postoperative care, 322
  surgical principles, 314

surgical technique, **315**, 315,
  317, 318, 320, 322
amputations (upper extremity)
  anatomy of, **294**, 294
  complications, 302
  instruments, **295**, 295, **296**
  surgical principles, 294–295
  surgical technique, 295–301,
    296, 297, 300, 301
anastomosis
  esophageal, 152, 161
  intestinal, 171, **185**
  popliteal artery, 312–313
  ureter, 235–236
angioembolization (vertebral
  artery), 93
aorta
  abdominal, 240–256
  cross-clamping, 27
  thoracotomy cross-clamping,
    26
artery
  brachial, 281–287
  carotid, 53–68, 135–136
  celiac, 251
  femoral, 303–306
  mesenteric, 252–253, 256
  renal, 253–255
  subclavian, 72–81
axillary artery, 83–87
axillary vessels
  complications, 86–87
  instruments, 84
  patient positioning, 84, 86
  surgical anatomy, **83**
  surgical principles, 84
  surgical technique, 84, 84–86,
    86

Barker's vacuum technique, 174,
  179
below-knee amputation,
  319–322, **320, 322**
billary tract injuries, 207
bladder
  anatomy of, 229
  complications, 239

postoperative care, 239
  surgical principles, 238
  surgical technique, **238**
bleeding. *See also* hemorrhage
  abdominal injuries, **169**,
    169–171, **170**, 173, 179
  and EDH/SDH, 36
  and laryngotracheal injuries,
    100
  cardiac repair, **120**, 120–122,
    122
  kidney, **229**, 229–231, **231**
  liver, **203**, 203–207, **205**
  operating room supply, **3**
  spleen, 212
blunt trauma
  abdominal, 184, 204, 262
  and EDH/SDH, 35
  arterial, 66, 135, 137, 254, 308
  cardiac rupture, 115
  lung, 142
  parenchymal damage, 205
  retroperitoneal hematoma,
    242, 264
  spleen, 211
Bogota bag technique, 174
brachial artery
  anatomy of, **281**, 281
  complications, 287
  instruments, 282
  patient positioning, 282
  surgical principles, 282
  surgical technique, **283**,
    283–286, **285, 286**
Burr holes, **41**, 41–43, **42**

cardiac arrest. *See also* heart
  failure
  air embolism, **26**
  pharmacological treatment of,
    23
cardiac defibrillation
  (thoracotomy), 24
cardiac injuries
  anatomy of, **115**, 115
  instruments, **116**
  patient positioning, 116

surgical principles, 115
  surgical technique, **116**,
    116–123, **117, 118, 120, 122,
    123**
  thoracic vessels, 126–139
cardiac massage, **22, 24**
carotid artery
  anatomy of, **53**, 53, **54**
  complications, 68
  instruments, 56
  patient positioning, 56
  surgical principles, 55–56
  surgical technique, 56–68, **57,
    60, 65, 66, 135**, 135–136
catheter
  EVD, 30, 34
  ICP, 29–34
celiac artery, **251**
cerebral spinal fluid (CSF),
  32–33
cervical esophagus
  anatomy of, **101**
  complications, 101–105
  instruments, 101
  patient positioning, 101
  surgical principles, 101
  surgical technique, **102**, 102,
    103, 104
chest trauma
  cardiac injuries, 115–125
  DC in, 172
  general operation principles,
    107–114
clamshell incision
  general chest operation, 108,
    113, 114
  lung injuries, 143
  thoracic vessel, **130**
clavicular incision
  general neck trauma, **52**
  subclavian vessels, 72–77, **73,
    75**
  supra, **80**
  with median sternotomy, 78
collar incision
  general neck trauma, **51**, 51
  trachea and larynx, **96**, 96

colon
  anatomy of, 185
  complications, 187
  surgical principles, 185–187,
    186
common bile duct injuries
    (CBD), 207
compartment pressure
    measurement technique,
    324, 324–325
compartment syndrome
  and axillary vessels, 87
  upper extremity fasciotomy,
    293
complications
  abdominal DC, 179
  cardiac injuries, 118, 120, 125
  gastrointestinal tract, 183
  general neck trauma, 52
  thoracostomy tube, 17
craniectomy incision, 39–40, **40**
cricothyrotomy
  anatomy of, **5**, 5
  difficulties with, 11
  instruments, **6**, 6
  patient positioning, **7**
  surgical principles, 6
  surgical technique, 7–11, **8**, **9**,
    10

damage control (DC)
  abdominal, 172–179, **173**, **174**,
    175, **177**
  extremities, 172
  orthopedic, 337–344
  pelvic, **275**, 275–280, **278**, **279**
  surgical principles, 172
  vascular trauma, 172
DC, *See* damage control
diaphram
  anatomy of, 162
  complications, 164
  instruments, 162
  surgical principles, **162**
  surgical technique, 162–164,
    163, **164**
distal femur fracture, 342, **343**
distal tibia fracture, **340**
duodenum
  anatomy of, **189–190**
  complications, 197
  instruments, 191
  patient positioning, 191
  surgical principles, **190–191**
  surgical technique, **191**,
    191–197, **194**, **196**

EDH. *See* acute epidural
    hematoma
epicardial pacing, **24**, 24–27
epidural intracranial pressure
    monitoring (ICP), 30, 34
esophagus
  anatomy of, 150–152, **151**
  anesthesia, 152

cervical, 101–105
complications, 161
instruments, 152
patient positioning, 152–153,
  153
surgical principles, 152, **181**, **183**
surgical technique, **153**, 153,
  154, **156**, **158**
EVD. *See* external ventricular
    drain
external ventricular drain (EVD),
    30, 34

fasciotomies (lower extremity)
  anatomy of, 323
  complications, 334–335
  instruments, 324
  surgical principles, 323
  surgical technique, **324**,
    324–325, **325**, **327**, 327, **328**,
    331
fasciotomies (upper extremity)
  anatomy of, 288
  complications, 293
  instruments, 289
  patient positioning, 289
  surgical principles, 288
  surgical technique, **289**, **291**,
    292
femoral artery
  anatomy of, **303**, 303
  complications, 306
  patient positioning, 304
  surgical principles, 304
  surgical technique, 304–306,
    305
femoral triangle, 303
femur fracture, 341–343, **342**
fibula fracture, **340**
floating knee, 344
foot fasciotomy, 333
forearm fasciotomies, **290**, **292**
fractures
  femur, **340**, 340, **342**, 342
  management of, **338**, 338–344,
    339, **342**
  pelvic, 187–188, 273–274
  rib, 107, 114, 153
  skull, 36–37
  spinal, 88
  tibia, **338**, 338–340, **339**, **340**

gallbladder injuries, 207
general abdominal operation
  anatomy of, **165**, 165
  complications, 171
  instruments, 167
  patient positioning, **166**
  surgical principles, 165–166
  surgical technique, **167**,
    167–171, **169**, **170**
general chest operation
  anatomy of, **107**, 107
  complications, 114
  patient positioning, **108**, 108

surgical principles, 107
surgical technique, **108**,
  108–113, **110**, **111**, **113**, **114**
general gastrointestinal operation
  instruments, 180
  patient positioning, 180
  surgical technique, 180
gluteal compartment fasciotomy,
  325–326
guillotine amputation (below
  knee), 322
gunshot wounds
  cardiac injuries, 115
  liver, 204
  mediastinal artery, 135
  to neck, 48

hand fasciotomies, **290**, **292**
head trauma procedures
  hemotomas, 35–45
  intracranial pressure
    monitoring, 29–34
heart failure, 149, *See also* cardiac
    arrest
hematomas
  abdominal aorta, 242
  abdominal injuries, **169**,
    169–171, **170**
  duodenum, 196
  retroperitoneal, 264
hematomas (cranial)
  anatomy of, **35**, 35
  instruments, 39
  patient positioning, 39
  problems, 41, 43
  surgical principles, 35–38, **36**
  surgical technique, **40**, **41**, **44**,
    45
hemorrhage. *See also* bleeding
  IVC, **266**, 266–270, **267**, **269**
  pelvic, 273–280
hilar occlusion, 26
hilar twist, 26

ICP. *See* intracranial pressure
    monitoring
iliac injuries
  anatomy of, **257**, 257
  complications, 261
  instruments, 258
  patient positioning, 258
  surgical principles, 257–258
  surgical technique, **258**,
    258–261, **261**
incision
  abdominal aorta, 242
  above-elbow amputation,
    295–296, **296**, **297**
  axillary vessels, **84**
  below-elbow amputation, **299**
  brachial artery, **283**, 283
  cardiac injuries, **116**, 116–123,
    117, **118**, **122**, **123**
  carotid artery, 56
  duodenum, 191

esophageal, **153**, 153, **154**
femoral artery, 304–305, **305**
foot fasciotomy, 333
general abdominal operation,
  167, 167–169, **169**
general chest operation, **108**,
  108–113, **110**, **111**, **113**, **114**
gluteal compartment
  fasciotomy, 325, 325–326
iliac injuries, 258
IVC, 263
kidney, 229
liver, **201**, 201, **202**
lower leg fasciotomy, **329**, 329,
  330, **331**
lung injuries, 143
neck trauma, **50**, 50, **51**, **52**
pancreatic, 220
popliteal artery, **309**, 309–310
spleen, 212
subclavian vessels, 72–81, **73**,
  75, **78**, **81**
thigh fasciotomy, 326, **328**
thoracic vessels, **129–130**
thoracotomy, **19**, 19–21, **21**, 27
trachea and larynx, **96**, 96, **98**
upper extremity, 289–291, **290**
vertebral artery, **89**, 89, **91**, **92**
indications
  DC, 172
  enteric contamination, 258
  for EDH/SDH surgery, 34, 38
  pelvic, 274
  thoracotomy, 18
  upper extremity operation, 282
inferior mesenteric artery, 256
inferior vena cava (IVC)
  anatomy of, **262**
  complications, 272
  instruments, 263
  patient positioning, 263
  surgical principles, 262–263
  surgical technique, **263**, 263,
    264, **265**, **266**, **267**, **269**, **271**
innominate artery, 135, **135–136**
intestines
  small, 183–185, **184**, **185**
  spillage control, 174
intracranial pressure monitoring
    (ICP)
  anatomy of, **29**
  and SDH/EDH, 45
  instruments, 30
  patient positioning, 31
  problems, 34
  surgical principles, 29
  surgical technique, **31**, 31, **32**
  types of, 30
intraparenchymal intracranial
    pressure monitoring (ICP),
    30, 33
intraventricular intracranial
    pressure monitoring (ICP),
    30, **31**, **32**
IVC. *See* inferior vena cava

kidney
    anatomy of, **228**, 228
    complications, 234
    patient positioning, 229
    postoperative care, 234
    surgical principles, 229
    surgical technique, **229**, 229–233, **231**, **234**

laparoscopy (diaphragm), 162–164, **163**
laparotomy
    abdominal, **167**, 167–169, **169**, 242
    duodenum, 191
    gastrointestinal tract, 180
    iliac injuries, 258
    IVC, 263
    kidney, 229
    liver, **201**, **202**
    pancreatic, 220
larynx
    anatomy of, **94**, 94
    complications, **100**
    instruments, 95
    patient positioning, **95**
    surgical principles, 95
    surgical technique, **97**, **99**
Lazy S incision, 290–291, **291**
left thoracotomy incision (cardiac injuries), 118
liver
    anatomy of, **198**, 198–199, **199**
    complications, 208
    instruments, 200
    patient positioning, 200
    surgical principles, 200
    surgical technique, **201**, 201, **202**, **203**, **204**, **205**, **206**
lower extremity injuries
    amputations, 314–322
    fasciotomies, 323–335
    femoral artery, 303–306
lower leg fasciotomy, **329**, 329, **330**, **331**
lung injuries
    anatomy of, **140**, 140
    anesthesia, 143
    complications, **149**
    diaphragm, 162–164
    instruments, 143
    patient positioning, 143
    surgical principles, 142–143
    surgical technique, **143**, 143–149, **144**, **146**, **148**
    thoracic esophagus, 150–161

median sternotomy incision
    cardiac injuries, **116**, **117**, **123**, 123
    general chest operation, **108**, 108–110, **110**, 114
    liver, 202

lung injuries, 143
    thoracic vessel, **129**
mediastinal artery injuries, 135–139, **136**, **137**
mediastinal vein injuries, 135
mesenteric artery (inferior and superior), **252**, 252–253, **253**, 256
mesh
    abdominal, 173
    facial defects, 179
    liver, 205
    spleen, 213

neck trauma
    axillary vessels, 83–87
    carotid artery, 53–68
    cervical esophagus, 101–105
    general operation principles, 47–52
    instruments, 50
    patient positioning, **49**
    subclavian vessels, 69–82
    surgical anatomy, 47–48
    surgical principles, **48**, 48–49
    surgical technique, **50**, 50, **51**, 52
    trachea and larynx, 94–100
    vertebral artery, 88–93
negative pressure therapies (NPT)
    abdominal, **174**, 174, **175**, 177
    lower extremity fasciotomy, 334
    upper extremity fasciotomy, 293
nephrectomy, 232–233, **234**

open cricothyrotomy, **9**, 9–10, **10**
operating room
    blood supply for, **3**
    composition of, 1, **2**
    equipment, 2
    set-up, **2**
    temperature of, 2
orthopedic damage control (DCO)
    complications, 344
    instruments, **337**, 337–338, **338**
    patient positioning, 338
    surgical principles, 337
    surgical technique, **338**, 338–344, **339**, **342**

pancreas
    anatomy of, 219, **220**
    complications, 227
    instruments, 220
    patient positioning, 220
    surgical principles, 220
    surgical technique, 220–227, **221**, **223**, **224**, **226**

pediatrics
    anastomosis, 171
    cricothyrotomy, 6, 11
    EDH, 38
    thoracostomy, 13
pelvis
    anatomy of, **273**, 273
    blood control, 274
    complications, 280
    instruments, 275
    patient positioning, 275
    surgical principles, 274
    surgical technique, **275**, 275, **278**, **279**
percutaneous cricothyrotomy, 7–8, **8**
pericardiotomy incision (cardiac), **118**, 118–120
pitfalls. See complications
pneumonectomy, **147**, 148
pneumonorrhaphy, **143**
popliteal artery
    anatomy of, **307**
    instruments, 308
    patient positioning, **308**
    surgical principles, 308
    surgical technique, **309**, 309–313, **311**, **312**, **312**
posterolateral thoracotomy
    esophageal, **153**, 154
    general chest operation, 108, 113–114, **114**
    thoracic vessel, 130
postoperative care
    bladder, 239
    kidney, 234
    lower extremity amputations, 322
    lower extremity fasciotomy, **334**, 334
    orthopedics, 344
    ureter, 237
problems. See complications
proximal tibia fracture, 342, **343**
pyloric injuries, 183

rectum
    anatomy of, 187
    complications, 187–188, **188**
    surgical principles, 187
renal artery, 253–255, **254**, **255**
resection
    colon, 187
    liver, 205–207, **206**
    lung, **145**, **146**
    pancreatic, **226**, 226
    small intestine, 185
resuscitative procedures
    cricothyrotomy, 5–11
    thoracostomy tube, 12–17
    thoracotomy, 18–27
retrohepatic inferior vena cava, 270–272, **271**

SDH. See subdural hematomas
sepsis, 161, 179, 234
small intestine
    anatomy of, 183–184
    complications, 185
    surgical principles, **184**, **185**
spleen
    anatomy of, 209–211, **210**
    complications, 218
    instruments, 212
    patient positioning, 212
    surgical principles, 211
    surgical technique, **212**, 212, **213**, **215**, **216**
splenectomy
    partial, **215**, 215, **216**
    total, **213**, 213–215
splenorrhaphy, **215**, 215–216
stabbing wounds
    cardiac injuries, 115
    mediastinal artery, 135
    to neck, 48
sternocleidomastoid incision
    general neck trauma, 50, **51**
    trachea and larynx, 97–99, **98**
    vertebral artery, **91**, 91–92, 92
stomach
    anatomy of, 180–181
    surgical principles, **181**
subarachnoid bolt, 30, **33**
subclavian vessels
    anatomy of, **69**, 69, **70**, **72**
    complications, 82
    instruments, 72
    patient positioning, 72
    surgical principles, 72
    surgical technique, 72–81, **73**, **75**, **78**, **81**, 137
subdural hematomas (SDH)
    surgical principles, 35–38, **36**
    surgical technique, **41**, 41–45, **44**
superior mesenteric artery, **252**, 252–253, **253**
supraceliac aortic control, **243**, 243, **245**, 248
supraclavicular incision
    subclavian vessels, **80**, 80
    vertebral artery, **89**, 91
supramesocolic aorta, 248–251, **249**

temperature (operating room), 2
thigh fasciotomy, **327**, 327, **328**
thoracic vessels
    anatomy of, **126**, 126–128, **128**
    complications, 139
    instruments, 129
    patient positioning, 129
    surgical principles, 129

thoracic vessels (cont.)
  surgical technique, **129**, 129, **130**, **131**, **133**, **136**, 137
thoracostomy tube
  autotransfusion in, 17
  difficulties with, 17
  insertion site, **12**
  patient positioning, 12
  removal, 17
  surgical principles, 12
  surgical technique, 12–17, **14**, 15
thoracotomy
  anatomy of, 18
  instruments, **19**
  patient positioning, 19
  posterolateral, 108, 113–114, **114**, 130, **153**, **154**
  problems, 27

surgical principles, 18
surgical technique, **19**, 19–27, **21**, **24**
thoracotomy incision
  abdominal injuries, 242
  general chest operation, 108, 110–112, **111**, 114
  lung injuries, 143
tibia fracture, **338**, 338–340, **339**, **340**
trachea
  anatomy of, **94**
  complications, **100**, 105
  instruments, 95
  patient positioning, **95**
  surgical principles, 95
  surgical technique, **96**, 96, **98**
tracheostomy
  and cricothyrotomy, 6

laryngotracheal, 99
tractotomy
  liver, 204
  lung, **144**
trap door incision (subclavian vessels), **81**, 94–100

ultrasound, 82
upper arm fasciotomy, **289**
upper extremities
  amputations, 294–302
  brachial artery injury, 281–287
  fasciotomies, 288–293
ureter
  anatomy of, 228
  complications, 236
  postoperative care, 237
  surgical principles, 234–235

surgical technique, **235**, 235, **236**, **238**
urological trauma, 228–239

vacuum-assisted closure technique (VAC), **176**
vascular trauma
  abdominal aorta, **240**, 240
  damage control, 172
  DC in, 172
  popliteal artery, 308
  retroperitoneum, **165**, 165
vertebral artery
  complications, 93
  instruments, 89
  patient positioning, 89
  surgical anatomy, **88**, 88
  surgical principles, 88
  surgical technique, **89**, 89, **91**, **92**